CRITICAL CARE
NURSING CARE PLANS

Sheree Comer

Contributor:

Barbara Sagel R.N., M.S., C.C.R.N.

SKIDMORE-ROTH PUBLICATIONS

Skidmore-Roth

Developmental Editor: Molly Sullivan, B.A.
Copy Editor: Kathryn Head, B.A.
Cover Design: Barbara Barr, Visual Impact
Typesetting: Barbara Barr, Visual Impact

ISBN 1-56930-035-6

Notice: The author(s) and the publisher of this volume have taken care to make certain all information is correct and compatible with the standards generally accepted at the time of publication.

Skidmore-Roth Publishing
400 Inverness Drive South
Suite 260
Englewood, Colorado 80112

TABLE OF CONTENTS

CARDIOVASCULAR SYSTEM

Congestive Heart Failure

Myocardial Infarction (MI)

Pericarditis

Infective Endocarditis (IE)

Hypertension

Thrombophlebitis

Intra-Aortic Balloon Pump (IABP)

Pacemakers

Cardiac Surgery

Aortic Aneurysm

Congestive Heart Failure

Heart failure is the inability of the heart to supply blood flow to meet physiologic demands, without utilizing compensatory changes. There may be failure involving one or both sides of the heart, and over time, causes the development of pulmonary and systemic congestion and complications. Congestive heart failure, or CHF, is a common complication after myocardial infarction and can be attributed to one-third of the deaths of patients with MIs. Usually following MI, the heart failure is left-sided since most infarctions involve damage to the left ventricle.

Heart failure can also be classified as acute or chronic. In chronic heart failure, the body experiences a gradual development as the heart becomes unable to pump a sufficient amount of blood to meet the body's demands. Chronic heart failure can become acute without any overt cause.

Often, the patient will have no early symptoms of left-sided heart failure. Symptoms of decreased cardiac output will develop once the heart fails to pump enough blood into the systemic circulation. The pressure in the left ventricle increases, which in turn causes retrograde increases of pressure in the left atrium because of the increased difficulty for blood to enter the atrium from the pulmonary veins. Blood backs up in the lung vasculature, and when the pulmonary capillary pressure is exceeded by the oncotic pressure of the proteins in the plasma fluid (usually > 30 mmHg), the fluid leaks into the interstitial spaces. When this fluid moves into the alveoli, shortness of breath, coughing, and crackles (rales) occur, and the patient progresses into overt pulmonary edema, with the classic sign of coughing up copious amounts of pink frothy sputum.

Right-sided heart failure is usually caused by left-sided heart failure, but can also be caused by pulmonary emboli, pulmonary hypertension, COPD, and the presence of right ventricular infarctions.

The lungs can accept a certain amount of fluid build-up, but eventually, if no intervention is taken, the pressure in the lungs increases to the point whereby the right ventricle cannot eject its blood into the lungs. The right ventricle fails and then the blood in the right atrium cannot drain completely, and thus cannot accept the total amount of blood from the vena cavae. Venous pooling occurs with the impairment of venous blood flow, and eventually the organs become congested with venous blood.

Treatment of heart failure involves attempts to improve contractility of the ventricle by use of positive inotropic drugs, decrease of afterload by the use of nitrates and vasodilators, and in some instances, by use of the IABP, and decrease of preload by the use of diuretics, IV nitroglycerin, and fluid/sodium restrictions.

MEDICAL CARE

Oxygen: to increase available oxygen supply

Morphine: used to induce vasodilation, decrease venous return to the heart, reduce pain and anxiety, and decrease myocardial oxygen consumption

Cardiac glycosides: digitalis (Digoxin, Lanoxin) PO or IV to increase the force and strength of ventricular contractions and to decrease rate of contractions in order to increase cardiac output

Diuretics: furosemide (Lasix) PO or IV, chlorothiazide (Diuril) PO, bumetanide (Bumex) PO or IV to promote excess fluid removal, to decrease edema and pulmonary venous pressure by preventing sodium and water reabsorption

Vasodilators: hydralazine (Apresoline) PO or IV, isosorbide dinitrate (Isordil) SL or PO, prazosin (Minipress) PO, minoxidil (Loniten) PO, diazoxide (Hyperstat) IV, sodium nitroprusside (Nipride) IV, nitroglycerine (Nitrostat, Tridil) PO, SL, IV to relax vascular smooth muscle, decrease preload and afterload, decrease oxygen demand, decrease systemic vascular resistance, and increase venous capacitance

Renin-angiotensin system inhibitors: captopril (Capoten) PO used to inhibit angiotensin converting enzyme to reduce the production of angiotensin II to enable the decrease in vasoconstriction and to reduce afterload

Inotropic agents: dopamine, dobutamine (Dobutrex) IV, amrinone (Inocor) IV used to increase myocardial contractility, without increasing the heart rate, to produce peripheral vasodilation and decrease preload and afterload

Electrolytes: mainly potassium to replace that which is lost during diuretic therapy

Laboratory: electrolyte levels to monitor for imbalances; renal profiles to monitor for kidney function problems; digoxin levels to monitor for toxicity; platelet count to monitor for thrombocytopenia from amrinone

Chest x-ray: shows any enlargement of the heart and pulmonary vein, presence of pulmonary edema or pleural effusion

Electrocardiography: used to monitor for dysrhythmias which may occur as a result of the heart failure or as a result of digitalis toxicity

Echocardiography: used to study structural abnormalities and blood flow through the heart

Intra-aortic balloon pump: decreases the workload on the heart, decreases myocardial oxygen demand, increases coronary perfusion, decreases afterload, decreases preload, improves cardiac output and tissue perfusion

NURSING CARE PLANS

Fluid volume excess

Related to: increased sodium and water retention, decreased organ perfusion, compromised regulatory mechanisms, decreased cardiac output, increased ADH production

Defining characteristics: edema, weight gain, intake greater than output, increased blood pressure, increased heart rate, shortness of breath, dyspnea, orthopnea, crackles (rales), S_3 gallop, oliguria, jugular vein distention, pleural effusion, specific gravity changes, altered electrolyte levels

Outcome Criteria

Blood pressure will be maintained within normal limits and edema will be absent or minimal in all body parts.

Fluid volume will be stabilized with balanced intake and output.

INTERVENTIONS	RATIONALES
Monitor vital signs and hemodynamic readings if available.	Fluid volume excess will cause increases in blood pressure, and CVP and pulmonary artery pressures, and these changes will be reflected from the development of pulmonary congestion and heart failure.
Auscultate lungs for presence of crackles (rales), or other adventitious breath sounds. Observe for presence of cough, increased dyspnea, tachypnea, orthopnea or paroxysmal nocturnal dyspnea.	May indicate pulmonary edema from cardiac decompensation and pulmonary congestion. Pulmonary edema symptoms reflect left-sided heart failure. Right-sided heart failure may have slower onset, but symptoms of dyspnea, orthopnea, and cough are more difficult to reverse.

INTERVENTIONS	RATIONALES
Observe for jugular vein distention and dependent edema. Note presence of generalized body edema (anasarca).	May indicate impending congestive failure and fluid excess. Peripheral edema begins in feet and ankles, or other dependent areas and ascends as failure progresses. Pitting will usually occur only after 10 or more pounds of excess fluid is retained. Anasarca will be seen only with right heart failure or bi-ventricular failure.
Investigate abrupt complaints of dyspnea, air hunger, feeling of impending doom or suffocation.	Excessive fluid build-up can promote other complications such as pulmonary edema or pulmonary embolus and intervention must be immediate.
Determine fluid balance by measuring intake and output, and observing for decreases in output and concentrated urine.	Renal perfusion is impaired with excessive fluid volume, which causes decreased cardiac output leading to sodium and water retention and oliguria.
Weigh daily and notify MD of greater than 2 lb/day increase.	Abrupt changes in weight usually indicate excess fluid.
Provide patient with fluid intake of 2 L/day, unless fluid restriction is warranted.	Fluids may need to be restricted due to cardiac decompensation. Fluids maintain hydration of tissues.
Administer diuretics as ordered (furosemide, hydralazine, spirolactone with hydrochlorothiazide).	Drugs may be necessary to correct fluid overload depending on emergent nature of problem. Diuretics increase urine flow rate and may inhibit reabsorption of sodium and chloride in the renal tubules.
Monitor electrolyte for imbalances. Note increasing lethargy, hypotension, or muscle cramping.	Hypokalemia can occur with the administration of diuretics. Signs of potassium and sodium deficits may occur due to fluid shifts with diuretic therapy.

INTERVENTIONS	RATIONALES
Place and maintain patient in semi-Fowler's position.	Diuresis may be enhanced by recumbent position due to increased glomerular filtration and decreased production of ADH.
Auscultate bowel sounds and observe for abdominal distention, anorexia, nausea, or constipation. Provide small, easily-digestible meals.	CHF progression can impair gastric motility and intestinal function. Small, frequent meals may enhance digestion and prevent abdominal discomfort.
Measure abdominal girth if warranted.	Progressive right-sided heart failure can cause fluid to shift into the peritoneal space and cause ascites.
Palpate abdomen for liver enlargement; note any right upper quadrant tenderness or pain.	Progressive heart failure can lead to venous congestion, abdominal distention, liver engorgement, and pain. Liver function may be impaired and can impede drug metabolism.
Assist with dialysis or hemofiltration as warranted.	Mechanically removing excess fluid may be performed to rapidly reduce circulating volume in cases refractory to other medical therapeutics.

Instruction, Information, Demonstration

INTERVENTIONS	RATIONALES
Instruct patient regarding dietary restrictions of sodium.	Fluid retention is increased with intake of sodium.
Instruct patient to observe for weight changes and report these to MD.	Weight gain may be first overt sign of fluid excess and should be monitored to prevent complications.
Consult with dietitian.	May be required to ensure adequacy of caloric intake with fluid and sodium restriction requirements.

INTERVENTIONS	RATIONALES
Instruct patient in medications prescribed after discharge, with dose, effect, side effects, contraindications.	Promotes knowledge and compliance with treatment regimen.
Monitor chest x-rays.	Reveal changes in pulmonary status regarding improvement or deterioration.

Discharge or Maintenance Evaluation

- Patient will have no edema or fluid excess.

- Fluid balance will be maintained and blood pressure will be within normal limits of baseline.

- Lung fields will be clear, without adventitious breath sounds, and weight will be stable.

- Patient will be able to accurately verbalize understanding of dietary restrictions and medications.

Decreased cardiac output

Related to: damaged myocardium, decreased contractility, dysrhythmias, conduction defects, alteration in preload, alteration in afterload, vasoconstriction, myocardial ischemia, ventricular hypertrophy, accumulation of blood in lungs or in systemic venous system

Defining characteristics: dependent edema, elevated blood pressure, elevated mean arterial pressure greater than 120 mmHg, elevated systemic vascular resistance greater than 1400 dyne-seconds/cm^5, cardiac output less than 4 L/min or cardiac index less than 2.5 L/min/m^2, tachycardia, cold, pale extremities, absent or decreased peripheral pulses, EKG changes, hypotension, S$_3$ or S$_4$ gallops, decreased urinary output, diaphoresis, orthopnea, dyspnea, crackles (rales), frothy blood-tinged sputum, jugular vein distention, edema, chest pain, confusion, restlessness

Outcome Criteria

Vital signs and hemodynamic parameters will be within normal limits for patient, with no dysrhythmias noted.

Patient will be eupneic with no adventitious breath sounds or abnormal heart tones.

INTERVENTIONS	RATIONALES
Determine level of cardiac function and existing cardiac and other conditions.	Additional disease states and complications may place an additional workload on an already compromised heart.
Auscultate apical pulses and monitor heart rate and rhythm. Monitor BP in both arms.	Decreased contractility will be compensated by tachycardia, especially concurrently with heart failure. Blood volume will be lowered if blood pressure is increased resulting in increased afterload. Pulse decreases may be noted in association with toxic levels of digoxin, and peripheral pulses may be hard to accurately determine if perfusion is decreased. Hypotension may occur as a result of ventricular dysfunction and poor perfusion of the myocardium.
Measure cardiac output and cardiac index, and calculate hemodynamic pressures every 4 hours and prn.	Provides measurement of cardiac function and calculated measurements of preload and afterload to facilitate titration of vasoactive drugs and manipulation of hemodynamic pressures.
Monitor EKG for dysrhythmias and treat as indicated.	Conduction abnormalities may occur due to ischemic myocardium affecting the pumping efficiency of the heart.
Observe for development of new S$_3$ or S$_4$ gallops.	S$_3$ gallops are usually associated with congestive heart failure but can be found with mitral regurgitation and left

INTERVENTIONS	RATIONALES
	ventricular overload after MI. S$_4$ gallops can be associated with myocardial ischemia, ventricular rigidity, pulmonary hypertension, or systemic hypertension, which can decrease cardiac output.
Auscultate for presence of murmurs and/or rubs.	Indicates disturbances of normal blood flow within the heart related to incompetent valves, septal defects, or papillary muscle/chordae tendonae complications post-MI. Presence of a rub with an MI is associated with pericarditis and/or pericardial effusion.
Observe lower extremities for edema, distended neck veins, cold hands and feet, mottling, oliguria.	Reduced venous return to the heart can result in low cardiac output; oliguria results from decreased venous return due to fluid retention.
Position in semi-Fowler's position.	Promotes easier breathing and prevents pooling of blood in the pulmonary vasculature.
Administer cardiac glycosides, nitrates, vasodilators, diuretics, and antihypertensives as ordered.	Used in the treatment of vasoconstriction and to reduce heart rate and contractility, reduces blood pressure by relaxation of venous and arterial smooth muscle which then in turn increases cardiac output and decreases the workload on the heart.
Titrate vasoactive drugs as ordered per MD parameters.	Maintains blood pressure and heart rate at levels to optimize cardiac output function.
Weigh every day.	Weight gain may indicate fluid retention and possible impending congestive failure.
Arrange activities so as to not over-tax patient.	Avoids over-fatiguing patient and decreasing cardiac output further. Balancing rest with activity minimizes energy expenditure and myocardial oxygen demands by maintaining cardiac output.

INTERVENTIONS	RATIONALES
Avoid Valsalva-type maneuvers with straining, coughing or moving.	Increasing intra-abdominal pressure results in an abrupt decrease in cardiac output by preventing blood from being pumped into the thoracic cavity and thus, less blood being pumped into the heart which then decreases the heart rate. When the pressure is released, there is a sudden overload of blood which then increases preload.
Provide small, easy to digest, meals and restrict caffeine.	Large meals increase the workload on the heart. Caffeine directly stimulates the heart and increases heart rate.
Have emergency equipment and medications available at all times.	Coronary occlusion, lethal dysrhythmias, infarct extensions or intractable pain may precipitate cardiac arrest that requires life support and resuscitation.

Information, Instruction, Demonstration

INTERVENTIONS	RATIONALES
Instruct on medications, dose, effects, side effects, contraindications, and avoidance of over-the-counter drugs without MD approval.	Promotes knowledge and compliance with regimen. Prevents any adverse drug interactions.
Instruct in activity limitations. Demonstrate exercises to be done.	Promotes compliance. Reduces decrease in cardiac output by lessening the workload placed on the heart.
Instruct to report chest pain.	May indicate complications of decreased cardiac output.
Instruct patient/family regarding placement of pulmonary artery catheter, and post-procedure care.	Alleviates fear and promotes knowledge. Pulmonary artery catheter necessary for direct measurement of cardiac output and for obtaining values for other hemodynamic measurements.

INTERVENTIONS	RATIONALES
Assist with insertion and maintainance of pacemaker when needed.	Cardiac pacing may be necessary during the acute phase of MI or may be necessary as a permanent measure if the MI severely damages the conduction system.

Discharge or Maintenance Evaluation

- Patient will have no chest pain or shortness of breath.

- Vital signs and hemodynamic parameters will be within normal limits for age and disease condition.

- Minimal activity will be tolerated without fatigue or dyspnea.

- Urinary output will be adequate.

- Cardiac output will be adequate to ensure adequate perfusion of all body systems.

Impaired gas exchange

Related to: ventilation/perfusion imbalance caused from excess fluid in alveoli and reduction of air exchange area in lung fields, fluid collection shifts into the interstitial space

Defining characteristics: confusion, restlessness, irritability, hypoxia, hypercapnea, dyspnea, orthopnea, abnormal ABGs, abnormal oxygen saturation

Outcome Criteria

Patient will have adequate oxygenation with respiratory status within limits of normal based on age and other conditions, and ABGs will be within normal limits.

INTERVENTIONS	RATIONALES
Monitor respiratory status for rate, regularity, depth, ease of effort at rest or with exertion, inspiratory/expiratory ratio.	Changes in respiratory pattern or patency of airway may result in gas exchange imbalances.
Observe for presence of cyanosis and mottling; monitor oximetry for oxygen saturation; monitor ABGs for ventilation/perfusion problems.	Cyanosis results from decreases in oxygenated hemoglobin in the blood and this reduction leads to hypoxia. Reading of 90% on pulse oximeter correlates with pO_2 of 60.
Monitor for mental status changes, deterioration in level of consciousness, restlessness, irritability, easy fatigueability.	Hypoxia affects all body systems and mental status changes can result from decreased oxygen to brain tissues.
Position in semi- or high-Fowler's position.	Promotes breathing and lung expansion to enhance gas distribution.
Administer oxygen via nasal cannula at 2-3 L/min, or other delivery systems.	Maintains adequate oxygenation without depression of respiratory drive. CO_2 may be retained with higher flow rates when used in patients with COPD.
Assist with placement of ETT and placement on mechanical ventilation.	Mechanical ventilation may be required if respiratory failure is progressive and adequate oxygen levels cannot be maintained by other delivery systems.

Instruction, Information, Demonstration

INTERVENTIONS	RATIONALES
Instruct in breathing exercises as warranted.	Assists to restore function to diaphragm, decreases work of breathing, and improves gas exchange.
Assess for nausea and vomiting.	May indicate effects of hypoxia on gastrointestinal system.
Avoid activities that promotes dyspnea or fatigue. Allow for periods of rest between activities.	Activity increases oxygen consumption and demand, and can impair breathing pattern.

INTERVENTIONS	RATIONALES
Instruct in safety concerns with oxygen use.	Promotes safety with oxygen and provides knowledge.
Instruct patient/family in need for placement on mechanical ventilation, what to expect, what benefits are to be received, what potential problems may be encountered.	Promotes knowledge and decreases anxiety and fear of the unknown.

Discharge or Maintenance Evaluation

- Patient will exhibit no ventilation/perfusion imbalances.

- Patient will be eupneic with no adventitious breath sounds.

- ABGs will be within acceptable ranges for patient with adequate oxygenation of all tissues.

- Patient will be able to verbalize/demonstrate the correct use of oxygen.

Risk for impaired skin integrity

Related to: bed rest, decreased tissue perfusion, edema, immobility, decreased peripheral perfusion, shearing forces or pressure, secretions, excretions, altered sensation, skeletal prominence, poor skin turgor, altered metabolic rate

Defining characteristics: disruption of skin surface, pressure areas, reddened areas, blanched areas, mottling, warmth, firmness to area of skin, irritated tissues, excoriation of skin, maceration of skin, lacerations of skin, pruritis, dermatitis

Outcome Criteria

Patient will have and maintain skin integrity.

INTERVENTIONS	RATIONALES
Monitor mobility status and patient's ability to move self.	Immobility is the primary cause of skin breakdown.
Inspect all skin surfaces, especially bony prominences, for skin breakdown, altered circulation to areas, or presence of edema.	Skin is at risk because of decreased tissue perfusion, immobility, decreased peripheral perfusion, and possible nutritional alterations.
Provide skin care to blanched or reddened areas.	Stimulates blood flow and decreases tissue hypoxia. Excess dryness or moistness of skin can promote breakdown.
Provide eggcrate mattress, alternating pressure mattress, sheepskin, elbow protectors, heel protectors, etc.	These items can reduce pressure on skin and may improve circulation.
Reposition frequently, at least every 2 hours. Assist with ROM exercises. Maintain body alignment. Raise head of bed no higher than 30 degrees.	Improves circulation by reduction of time pressure is on any one area. Proper body alignment prevents contractures. Elevations higher than this may promote pressure and friction from sliding down, and shearing force may result in breakdown of skin.
Avoid subcutaneous or IM injections when possible.	Edema and tissue hypoxia impede circulation which can cause decreased absorption of medication and can predispose patient to tissue breakdown and development of abscess/infection.

Instruction, Information, Demonstration

INTERVENTIONS	RATIONALES
Instruct on safety precautions in bed—avoiding bumping against rails, falls, etc.	May cause breaks in skin integrity.
Instruct on hazards of immobility; avoid lying or sitting in one position for prolonged time.	Bedrest promotes pressure to skin and tissues.
Instruct on the use of lotions and oil to apply to skin.	Prevents skin dryness and chance of tissue breakdown.

Discharge or Maintenance Evaluation

- Patient will have intact skin, free of redness, irritation, rashes, or bruising.

- Patient will be able to verbally relate measures to reduce chance of tissue injury.

Anxiety
[See MI]

Related to: change in health status, fear of death, threat to body image, threat to role functioning, pain

Defining characteristics: restlessness, insomnia, anorexia, increased respirations, increased heart rate, increased blood pressure, difficulty concentrating, dry mouth, poor eye contact, decreased energy, irritability, crying, feelings of helplessness

Knowledge deficit
[See MI]

Related to: lack of understanding, lack of understanding of medical condition, lack of recall

Defining characteristics: questions regarding problems, inadequate follow-up on instructions given, misconceptions, lack of improvement of previous regimen, development of preventable complications

LEFT-SIDED HEART FAILURE

Burden placed on cardiovascular system by any of the following: hypertension, myocardial infarction, valvular heart disease, dysrhythmias, tachy/bradycardia, cardiomyopathy, cardiac tamponade, constrictive pericarditis, aortic stenosis, mitral insufficiency, or anemia ↓

Decreased cardiac output → - → Sympathetic nervous system stimulated
Fatigue, weakness

    Heart rate increases
    Arteriolar vasoconstriction
    Myocardial contractility increases
            Venous tone increases
            Venous and ventricular filling
            pressures increase

↓

Decreased effective arterial blood volume

↓

Renal compensatory changes occur
    Renal blood flow decreases
    GFR decreases
    Cortical blood flow decreases
    Renin and angiotensin increase
    Aldosterone increases
    ADH increases

↓

Sodium reabsorption and free water clearance decreases
Effective blood volume increases

↓

Accumulation of blood in lungs

↓

LV cannot pump blood from lungs into systemic circulation

↓

LV pressures and LV volume increase

↓

LA pressures and volume increase

↓

Fluid backs up into pulmonary vasculature = pulmonary congestion
    Paroxysmal nocturnal dyspnea, orthopnea

↓

Pulmonary hypertension, PA diastolic and PCWP pressure increases

↓

Fluid leaks into interstitial and alveoli

↓

Pulmonary edema
    Cough
    Frothy, blood-tinged sputum
    Rales (crackles)

↓

Decreased oxygen in blood
Impaired gas exchange and hypoxia
        Tachypnea   Restlessness
        Cyanosis   Pulmonary effusion
        Confusion   Pulsus alternans

RIGHT-SIDED HEART FAILURE

Burden placed on the cardiovascular system by any of the following: left-sided heart failure, pulmonary hypertension, COPD, cor pulmonale, pulmonary embolus, anemia, thyrotoxicosis, pulmonary stenosis, or mitral stenosis.

Accumulation of blood in systemic venous system
Lung pressure increases
Pressure in pulmonary vasculature increases

Increased right atrial and ventricular pressures
Increased peripheral venous pressure

Right heart cannot pump blood into pulmonary system
Right-sided heart failure
Bounding pulses
Dysrhythmias
S_3 or S_4 gallop

Venous return decreases
Organs become congested with blood
Peripheral dependent edema occurs

Congestion of portal circulation
Hepatomegaly, hepatojugular reflux
JVD, weight gain
Anorexia
Ascites, abdominal pain, anorexia, nausea
Fatigue, cyanosis

Advanced heart failure

Air hunger, gasping
Tachycardia
Crackles, frothy blood-tinged sputum
Skin cool and moist
Cyanotic lips, nailbeds
Confusion, stupor
Enlarged RA and RV
Tricuspid murmur

Myocardial Infarction (MI)

Myocardial infarction (MI) is a critical emergency that requires timely management to save heart muscle and limit damage that may evolve over several hours. Blood flow is abruptly decreased or stopped through the coronary arteries and results in ischemia and necrosis to the myocardium if not treated. Many people die prior to receiving medical care due to the denial that anything may be wrong and postponement of seeking medical care. Cardiac dysrhythmias, mainly ventricular fibrillation, is usually the cause of death in these individuals. An MI is diagnosed based on type of chest pain, electrocardiographic changes, and increase of cardiac enzymes, such as CK, SGOT, and LDH. Precordial pain is similar to but usually more intense and prolonged than anginal pain, and in the instance of MI, the chest pain is usually constant and not relieved with nitroglycerin or rest.

Atherosclerosis of the arteries is usually the most common finding in patients. Atherosclerosis and arteriosclerosis are used interchangeably when discussing the fatty plaques that adhere to the inner layer of the arteries. The continuous build-up of these plaques, as well as the potential for hemorrhage at the intimal layer may result in alterations of the blood flow through the coronary arteries and abnormalities in platelet aggregation may contribute to changes in coronary perfusion. Infarction may occur without coronary artery disease or occlusion, and if the patient has developed an adequate collateral circulation, coronary occlusion may occur without infarction.

MI is usually a disease involving the left ventricle but the damage may extend to other areas, such as the atria or right ventricle. A right ventricular myocardial infarction usually has high right ventricular filling pressures and often has severe tricuspid regurgitation. Transmural infarcts involve the entire thickness of the myocardium and are characterized by Q waves on the electrocardiogram. Nontransmural infarcts are characterized by S-T segment and T wave changes. Subendocardial infarcts usually involve the inner portion of the myocardium where wall tension is highest and the blood flow is most vulnerable to circulatory problems. Occlusion of the right coronary artery will result in an inferior infarction that may also include posterior portions of the heart. Occlusion of the left main artery, known as "the widow maker," usually results in death due to the extensive damage. Occlusion of the left anterior descending artery results in an anterior infarction and may include some inferior parts of the heart, and occlusion of the circumflex artery results in a lateral infarction.

Precipitating factors that preclude MIs include heredity, age, gender, presence of hypertension, presence of diabetes mellitus, cigarette smoking, hyperlipidemia, obesity, sedentary lifestyles, and stress.

The main goals in treating myocardial infarction are to increase blood flow to the coronary arteries and thus decrease infarction size, increase oxygen supply and decrease oxygen demand to prevent myocardial death or injury, and control or correct dysrhythmias.

MEDICAL CARE

Oxygen: to increase available oxygen supply

Analgesics: morphine is the drug of choice, given in incremental doses IV every 5 minutes as needed; IM injections are avoided because they can raise the enzyme levels and do not act as quickly

Thrombolytic agents: Streptokinase, Urokinase, or Tissue Plasminogen Activator (tPa) given either intracoronary or intravenously to activate the body's own fibrinolytic system to dissolve the clot and resume coronary blood perfusion

Cardiac glycosides: digitalis to increase force and strength of ventricular contractions and to decrease the conduction and rate of contractions in order to increase cardiac output; usually not used in the acute phase

Diuretics: furosemide (Lasix) to promote excess fluid removal, to decrease edema and pulmonary venous pressure by preventing sodium and water reabsorption

Vasodilators: hydralazine (Apresoline), nifedipine (Procardia, Adalat), nitroglycerin (Nitropaste, Nitrodur, Nitrostat, Tridil, Nitroglycerine), prazosin (Minipres), captopril (Capoten)—used to relax venous and/or arterial smooth muscle to decrease preload, decrease afterload, and decrease oxygen demand

Beta-adrenergic blockers: used to decrease blood pressure, decrease elevated plasma renins, and with non-selective blockers, may do so without related reflex tachycardias; used to treat ventricular dysrhythmias and for the prophylaxis of angina

Aspirin: used to decrease platelet aggregation and helps with vasodilation of peripheral vessels

Thrombolytics: used in the treatment of acute MI; acts by activating mechanisms for conversion of plasminogen to plasmin which is able to dissolve the clot; commonly used are streptokinase, urokinase, alteplase, or anistreplase

Heparin: used with thrombolytic protocols, and in the treatment of MI; prevents conversion of fibrinogen to fibrin and prothrombin to thrombin by its action on antithrombin III

Laboratory: leukocyte count, sed rate and blood glucose may be elevated; creatinine phosphokinase (CK, CPK) will normally increase within 4-6 hours, peak between 12-24 hours, and last 2-3 days but should not be used as sole indicator due to possibility of elevation with other problems such as surgery or trauma; lactate dehydrogenase (LDH) will normally increase within 8-12 hours, peak between 2-4 days, and last 10-14 days but should not be used as sole indicator due to possibility of elevation with other problems such as liver failure; serum glutamic oxaloacetic transaminase (SGOT) is occasionally used as an infarct indicator; isoenzymes of CPK are very specific with CPK-MB most specific for MI, and levels will not rise with transient chest pain or in surgical procedures; a definitive level for CPK-MB is greater than or equal to 4% of the total CPK; LDH isoenzymes, specifically LDH1 is more specific for MI; if the total LDH is elevated and LDH1 is most predominant, MI is confirmed; both CPK-MB and LDH1 will return to normal 72-96 hours after elevation

Chest x-ray: shows any enlargement of the heart and pulmonary vein, presence of pulmonary edema or pleural effusion

Electrocardiography: shows indicative changes associated with sites of acute infarcts using Q waves, S-T segment elevation, and T wave inversion. Also reveals changes with atrial and ventricular enlargement, rhythm and conduction abnormalities, ischemia, electrolyte abnormalities, drug toxicity, and presence of dysrhythmias

Echocardiography: used to study structural abnormalities and blood flow through the heart; M-mode echocardiography measures structures with a single ultrasonic beam that provides a narrow view of the heart; two-dimensional (2D) echocardiography shows a two-dimensional and wider look at the heart that is more useful in diag-nosing right ventricular infarcts; documents increased right ventricular size, performance and segmental wall motion abnormalities, and blood flow through the heart

Nuclear cardiologic testing: MUGA (multiple gated acquisition study) provides information that approximates ejection fractions and the analysis of the ventricular wall motion; 99mTc (Technetium-99 pyrophosphate scan) shows infarcted areas as increased levels of radioactivity, or "hot spots" that appear 12-36 hours after infarct and remain for 4-7 days; PET (positron emission tomography) allows measurement of myocardial blood flow, fatty acid and glucose metabolism, and blood volume; thallium scans can determine size and location of damage as a "cold spot"

Magnetic resonance imaging (MRI): provides a three-dimensional view that can detect changes in tissues before structural damage is done and is safe for pregnant women and children

Cardiac catheterization: used to assess pathophysiology of the patient's cardiovascular disorder, to provide left ventricular function information, to allow for measurement of heart pressures and cardiac output, to evaluate stenotic lesions, and to measure blood gas content

Intra-aortic balloon pump (IABP): decreases the workload on the heart, decreases myocardial oxygen demand, increases coronary perfusion, decreases afterload, decreases preload, and helps to limit infarct size if quickly initiated, improves cardiac output and tissue perfusion; used in cardiogenic shock, for support post cardiac surgery, intractable chest pain, and in cardiac catheterizations or other cardiovascular procedures of high-risk patients

Ventricular assist device (VAD): used on either or both ventricles to provide total support to the heart and circulation in order to allow recovery to the heart; usually indicated in patients who are awaiting cardiac transplantation or in those patients with cardiogenic shock and ventricular failure; may be used in conjunction with IABP

Pacemakers: either temporary or permanent, used in anticipation of lethal dysrhythmias and/or conduction problems

Surgery: coronary artery bypass grafting to reroute the coronary blood flow around the diseased vessel to enable coronary perfusion

NURSING CARE PLANS

Alteration in comfort

Related to: chest pain due to decreased blood flow to myocardium, myocardial ischemia or infarct, post-procedure discomfort, chest wall pain post-surgery, pericarditis

Defining characteristics: chest pain with or without radiation, facial grimacing, clutching of hands or chest, restlessness, diaphoresis, changes in pulse and blood pressure, dyspnea, dizziness

Outcome Criteria

Chest pain will be relieved or controlled to patient's satisfaction.

INTERVENTIONS	RATIONALES
Evaluate chest pain as to type, location, severity, relief, change with activity or rest, other symptoms concurrently noted, such as pallor, diaphoresis, radiation of pain, nausea, vomiting, shortness of breath, and vital sign changes.	Variations may occur with patients regarding specific complaints and behavior. Most MI patients look acutely ill and can only focus on their pain. Respirations may be increased as a result of anxiety and pain. Heart rate

INTERVENTIONS	RATIONALES
	may increase due to increased catecholamines, stress, and pain, which can also increase blood pressure.
Obtain description of intensity using 0-10 scale, with 0 being no pain and 10 being the worst pain experienced.	Pain is a subjective experience and personal to that patient. Intensity scales are useful to gauge improvement or deterioration as perceived by the patient.
Obtain history (when possible) of previous cardiac pain and familial history of cardiac problems.	This provides information that may help to differentiate current pain from previous problems, as well as identify new problems and complications.
Administer oxygen by nasal cannula or mask as indicated.	Supplemental oxygen can increase the available oxygen and can relieve pain associated with myocardial ischemia.
Administer analgesic as ordered, such as morphine sulfate, meperidine (Demerol), or Dilaudid IV.	Morphine is the drug of choice to control MI pain, but other analgesics may be used to reduce pain and reduce the workload on the heart. IM injections should be avoided because they can alter cardiac enzymes and are not absorbed well in tissue that is non- or under-perfused.
Administer beta-blockers as ordered (such as atenolol, pindolol, and propranolol).	These drugs block sympathetic stimulation, reduce heart rate and systolic blood pressure, and thus lowers the myocardial oxygen demand. Beta-blockers should not be given in severely impaired contractility states due to the negative inotropic properties.

INTERVENTIONS	RATIONALES
Administer calcium-channel blockers as ordered (such as verapamil, diltiazem, or nifedipine).	These drugs can increase coronary blood flow and collateral circulation, reduce preload and myocardial oxygen demands, which can decrease pain due to ischemia.
Maintain bedrest during pain, with position of comfort; nurse to stay with patient during pain.	Reduces oxygen consumption, and demand; alleviates fear and provides caring atmosphere.
Maintain relaxing environment to promote calmness.	Reduces competing stimuli and reduces anxiety.

Information, Instruction, Demonstration

INTERVENTIONS	RATIONALES
Instruct to notify nurse immediately of any chest pain.	Delay in notification can delay pain relief and may require increased amounts of medication in order to finally achieve relief. Pain can cause further damage to an already-injured myocardium, and may signal extension of MI, spasm, or other complication.
Instruct in relaxation techniques, deep breathing, guided imagery, visualization, etc.	Helps to decrease pain and anxiety and provides distraction from pain.
Instruct in nitroglycerin SL administration after hospitalization; 1 q5 minutes up to 3 times, and if pain is unrelieved, patient should seek emergency medical care.	Knowledge facilitates cooperation and compliance with medical regimen. Pain unrelieved with NTG may be indicative of MI.
Instruct in activity alterations and limitations.	Decreases myocardial oxygen demand and workload on the heart.
Instruct in medication effects, side effects, contraindications, and symptoms to report.	Promotes knowledge and compliance with therapeutic regimen. Alleviates fear of unknown.

Discharge or Maintenance Evaluation

- Patient will report pain being absent or controlled with medication administration.

- Medication will be administered prior to pain becoming severe.

- Patient will be able to recall effects, side effects, and contraindications of medications accurately.

- Activity will be modified in such a way as to prevent onset of chest pain.

Altered tissue perfusion: cardiopulmonary, cerebral, peripheral

Related to: tissue ischemia, reduction or interruption of blood flow, vasoconstriction, hypovolemia, shunting, depressed ventricular function, dysrhythmias, conduction defects

Defining characteristics: abnormal hemodynamic readings, dysrhythmias, decreased peripheral pulses, cyanosis, decreased blood pressure, shortness of breath, dyspnea, cold and clammy skin, decreased mental alertness, changes in mental status, oliguria, anuria, sluggish capillary refill, abnormal electrolyte and digoxin levels, hypoxia, ABG changes, chest pain, ventilation perfusion imbalances, changes in peripheral resistance, impaired oxygenation of myocardium, EKG changes (S-T segment, T wave, U wave), LV enlargement, palpitations

Outcome Criteria

Blood flow and perfusion to vital organs will be preserved and circulatory function will be maximized.

Patient will be free of dysrhythmias.

Hemodynamic parameters will be within normal limits.

INTERVENTIONS	RATIONALES
Monitor vital signs. Obtain hemodynamic values, noting deviations from baseline values.	Provides information about the hemodynamics of the patient and facilitates early intervention for problems.
Monitor EKG for disturbances in conduction and for dysrhythmias and treat as indicated.	Decreased cardiac perfusion may instigate conduction abnormalities. Ventricular fibrillation is the most common dysrhythmia following MI. Reperfusion dysrhythmias may occur after the administration of thrombolytic therapy.
Administer oxygen by nasal cannula as ordered, with rate dependent on disease process and condition.	Provides oxygen necessary for tissues and organ perfusion.
Auscultate lungs for crackles (rales), rhonchi, or wheezes.	May indicate fluid overload that will further decrease tissue perfusion.
Auscultate heart sounds for S_3 or S_4 gallop, new murmurs, presence of jugular vein distention, or hepatojugular reflex.	May indicate impending or present heart failure.
Monitor oxygen status with ABGs, S_vO_2 monitoring, or with pulse oximetry.	Provides information about the oxygenation status of the patient. Continuous monitoring of saturation levels provide an instant analysis of how activity affects oxygenation and perfusion for the patient.
Monitor for changes in respiratory status, increased work of breathing, dyspnea, etc.	Decreased cardiac perfusion may result in pump failure and precipitate respiratory distress and failure.
Determine the presence and character of peripheral pulses, capillary refill time, skin color and temperature.	May indicate decreased perfusion resulting from impaired coronary blood flow.

INTERVENTIONS	RATIONALES
Discourage any non-essential activity.	Ambulation, exercise, transfers, and Valsalva-type maneuvers can increase blood pressure and decrease tissue perfusion.
Assist patient with planned, graduated levels of activity.	Allows for balance between rest and activity to decrease myocardial workload and oxygen demand. Gradual increases help to increase patient tolerance to activity without pain.
Titrate vasoactive drugs as ordered.	Maintain blood pressure and heart rate at parameters set by MD for optimal perfusion with minimal workload on heart.
Administer thrombolytic drugs as ordered.	Drugs lyse the clot that may be occluding the coronary artery and promote restoration of oxygen and blood flow to increase perfusion.
Auscultate for bowel sounds and monitor for complaints of nausea, vomiting, anorexia, abdominal distention, abdominal pain, or constipation.	Decreased perfusion to mesentery may result in loss or change in peristalsis, resulting in GI use of analgesics, and change in surroundings may contribute to changes in GI status.
Monitor urine output for adequate amounts, character of urine, presence of sediment, and specific gravity.	Decreased perfusion to renal arteries may result in oliguria. Dehydration secondary to nausea and vomiting may affect renal perfusion.
Monitor labwork such as renal or liver profiles.	May indicate organ dysfunction and decreased perfusion.

Information, Instruction, Demonstration

INTERVENTIONS	RATIONALES
Instruct on medications, dosage, effects, side effects, and contraindications.	Promotes compliance with regimen and knowledge base.
Instruct to refrain from smoking.	Smoking causes vasoconstriction with can decrease perfusion.
Instruct in dietary requirements, menu planning, sodium restrictions, foods to avoid.	Reduction of high-cholesterol and sodium foods will help to control atherosclerosis, hyperlipidemia, fluid retention, and the effects on coronary blood flow.

Discharge or Maintenance Evaluation

- Lung fields will be clear and free of adventitious breath sounds.

- Extremities will be warm and pink, with easily palpable pulses.

- Vital signs and hemodynamic parameters will be within normal limits for patient.

- Oxygenation will be optimal as evidenced by pulse oximetry greater than 90%, S_vO_2 greater than 75%, or normal ABGs.

- Patient will be free of chest pain and shortness of breath.

- Patient will be able to verbalize information accurately regarding medications, diet and activity limitations.

Decreased cardiac output

Related to: damaged myocardium, decreased contractility, dysrhythmias, conduction defects, alteration in preload, alteration in afterload, vasoconstriction, myocardial ischemia, ventricular hypertrophy

Defining characteristics: elevated blood pressure, elevated mean arterial pressure greater than 120 mmHg, elevated systemic vascular resistance greater than 1400 dyne-seconds/cm^5, cardiac output less than 4 L/min or cardiac index less than 2.7 L/min/m^2, tachycardia, cold, pale extremities, absent or decreased peripheral pulses, EKG changes, hypotension, S_3 or S_4 gallops, decreased urinary output, diaphoresis, orthopnea, dyspnea, crackles (rales), jugular vein distention, edema, chest pain

Outcome Criteria

Vital signs and hemodynamic parameters will be within normal limits for patient, with no dysrhythmias noted.

INTERVENTIONS	RATIONALES
Auscultate apical pulses and monitor heart rate and rhythm. Monitor BP in both arms.	Decreased contractility will be compensated by tachycardia, especially concurrently with heart failure. Blood volume will be lowered if blood pressure is increased resulting in increased afterload. Pulse decreases may be noted in association with toxic levels of digoxin. Hypotension may occur as a result of ventricular dysfunction and poor perfusion of the myocardium.
Monitor EKG for dysrhythmias. and treat as indicated.	Conduction abnormalities may occur due to ischemic myocardium affecting the pumping efficiency of the heart.
Determine level of cardiac function and existing cardiac and other conditions.	Additional disease states and complications may place an additional workload on an already compromised heart.
Measure CO and perform other hemodynamic calculations.	Provides direct measurement of cardiac output function, and calculated measurement of preload and afterload.

INTERVENTIONS	RATIONALES
Monitor for development of new S_3 or S_4 gallops.	S_3 gallops are usually associated with congestive heart failure but can be found with mitral regurgitation and left ventricular overload after MI. S_4 gallops can be associated with myocardial ischemia, ventricular rigidity, pulmonary hypertension, or systemic hypertension, which can decrease cardiac output.
Auscultate for presence of murmurs and/or rubs.	Indicates disturbances of normal blood flow within the heart related to incompetent valves, septal defects, or papillary muscle/chordae tendonae rupture post-MI. Presence of a rub with an MI may be associated with pericarditis and/or pericardial effusions.
Observe lower extremities for edema, distended neck veins, cold hands and feet, mottling, oliguria. Notify MD if urine output is < 30 cc/hr.	Reduced venous return to the heart can result in low cardiac output; oliguria results from decreased venous return due to fluid retention.
Position in semi-Fowler's position.	Promotes easier breathing by allowing for chest expansion and prevents pooling of blood in the pulmonary vasculature.
Administer cardiac glycosides, nitrates, vasodilators, diuretics, and antihypertensives as ordered.	Used in the treatment of vasoconstriction and to reduce heart rate and contractility, reduces blood pressure by relaxation of venous and arterial smooth muscle which then in turn increases cardiac output and decreases the workload on the heart.
Titrate vasoactive drugs as ordered per MD parameters.	Maintains blood pressure and heart rate at levels to optimize cardiac output function.
Weigh every day.	Weight gain may indicate fluid retention and possible impending congestive failure.

INTERVENTIONS	RATIONALES
Arrange activities so as to not overwhelm patient.	Avoids fatiguing patient and decreasing cardiac output further. Balancing rest with activity minimizes energy expenditure and myocardial oxygen demands by maintaining adequate cardiac output.
Avoid Valsalva-type maneuvers with straining, coughing or moving.	Increasing intra-abdominal pressure results in an abrupt decrease in cardiac output by preventing blood from being pumped into the thoracic cavity and thus, less blood being pumped into the heart which then decreases the heart rate. When the pressure is released, there is a sudden overload of blood which then increases preload and the workload on the heart.
Provide small, easy to digest, meals and restrict caffeine.	Large meals increase the workload on the heart by diverting blood flow to that area. Caffeine directly stimulates the heart and increases heart rate.
Have emergency equipment and medications available at all times.	Coronary occlusion, lethal dysrhythmias, infarction extensions or intractable pain may precipitate cardiac arrest that requires life support and resuscitation.

Information, Instruction, Demonstration

INTERVENTIONS	RATIONALES
Instruct on medications, dose, effects, side effects, contra-indications, and avoidance of over-the-counter drugs without MD approval.	Promotes knowledge and compliance with regimen. Prevents any adverse drug interactions.
Instruct in activity limitations. Demonstrate exercises to be done.	Promotes compliance. Reduces potential for decrease in car-

INTERVENTIONS	RATIONALES
	diac output by lessening the workload placed on the heart.
Instruct to report chest pain immediately.	May indicate complications of decreased cardiac output.
Instruct patient/family regarding placement of pulmonary artery catheter, and post-procedure care.	Alleviates fear and promotes knowledge. Pulmonary artery catheter necessary for direct measurement of cardiac output and for obtaining values for other hemodynamic measurements.
Assist with insertion and maintenance of pacemaker when needed.	Cardiac pacing may be necessary during the acute phase of MI or may be necessary as a permanent measure if the MI severely damages the conduction system.

Discharge or Maintenance Evaluation

- Patient will have no chest pain or shortness of breath.

- Vital signs and hemodynamic parameters will be within normal limits for age and disease condition.

- Minimal activity will be tolerated without fatigue or dyspnea.

- Urinary output will be adequate.

- Cardiac output will be adequate to ensure adequate perfusion of all body systems.

Risk for fluid volume excess

Related to: increased sodium and water retention, decreased organ perfusion

Defining characteristics: edema, weight gain, intake greater than output, increased blood pressure, increased heart rate, shortness of breath, dyspnea, orthopnea, crackles (rales), oliguria, jugular vein distention, pleural effusion, specific gravity changes, altered electrolyte levels

Outcome Criteria

Blood pressure will be maintained within normal limits and edema will be absent or minimal in all body parts.

INTERVENTIONS	RATIONALES
Auscultate lungs for presence of crackles (rales).	May indicate pulmonary edema from cardiac decompensation.
Observe for jugular vein distention and dependent edema.	May indicate impending congestive failure and fluid excess.
Determine fluid balance by measuring intake and output, and observing for decreases in output and concentrated urine.	Renal perfusion is impaired with decreased cardiac output, which leads to sodium and water retention and oliguria.
Weigh daily and notify MD of greater than 2 lb/day increase.	Abrupt changes in weight usually indicate excess fluid.
Provide patient with fluid intake of 2 L/day, unless fluid restriction is warranted.	Fluids provide hydration of tissues. Fluids may need to be restricted due to cardiac decompensation.
Administer diuretics as ordered (furosemide, hydralazine, spirolactone, hydrochlorothiazide).	Drugs may be necessary to correct fluid overload depending on emergent nature of problem.
Monitor electrolyte for imbalances.	Hypokalemia can occur with the administration of diuretics.

Instruction, Information, Demonstration

INTERVENTIONS	RATIONALES
Instruct patient regarding dietary restrictions of sodium.	Fluid retention is increased with intake of sodium.
Instruct patient to observe for weight changes and report these to MD.	Weight gain may be first overt sign of fluid excess and should be monitored to prevent complications.

INTERVENTIONS	RATIONALES
Instruct patient in medications prescribed after discharge, with dose, effect, side effects, contraindications.	Promotes knowledge and compliance with treatment regimen.

Discharge or Maintenance Evaluation

- Patient will have no edema or fluid excess.

- Fluid balance will be maintained and blood pressure will be within normal limits of baseline.

- Lung fields will be clear, without adventitious breath sounds, and weight will be stable.

- Patient will be able to verbalize understanding of dietary restrictions and medications.

Anxiety

Related to: change in health status, fear of death, threat to body image, threat to role functioning, pain

Defining characteristics: restlessness, insomnia, anorexia, increased respirations, increased heart rate, increased blood pressure, difficulty concentrating, dry mouth, poor eye contact, decreased energy, irritability, crying, feelings of helplessness

Outcome Criteria

Patient will be able to use coping mechanisms effectively, will appear less anxious, and be able to verbalize feelings.

INTERVENTIONS	RATIONALES
Identify patient's perception of illness or situation. Encourage expressions of anger, grief, sadness, fear, and loss.	Patient may be afraid of dying and be anxious about his immediate problem as related to his lifestyle and the problems that have been left unattended.
Explain all procedures to patient in concise and reassuring manner. Repeat information	Knowledge reduces fear of the unknown. Establishes feelings of trust and concern. Informa-

INTERVENTIONS	RATIONALES
as needed based on patient's ability to comprehend.	tion may need to be repeated or reinforced due to competing stimuli.
Encourage the patient to discuss his fears and feelings. Provide an atmosphere of acceptance without judgment. Accept his use of denial, but do not reinforce false beliefs. Avoid confrontations and upsets.	Assists the patient in verbalizing concerns and provides the opportunity to deal with matters of import to the patient. Accepting the patient's feelings may decrease his anxiety which can facilitate a therapeutic environment for instruction. Denial can be useful to decrease anxiety but can postpone dealing with the reality of the problem. Confrontations can lead to anger and exacerbate the use of denial and decrease cooperation.
Provide opportunities for the family to visit and assist with care if possible. Orient to routines.	Familiar people can decrease anxiety of the patient, as well as provide a more conducive atmosphere for learning and recovery. Predictability can decrease anxiety. Supportive family members can comfort the patient and relieve worries.
Provide private time for patient and family member(s) to verbalize feelings.	Allows time for expression of concerns and feelings, and relieves tension by establishing a more normal routine.
Provide opportunities for patient to control his environment and activities as much as feasible based on condition.	Allows the patient to have some control over his situation and facilitates compliance with care of which patient is not in control.
Provide opportunity for patient to rest without interruption as much as possible.	Facilitates coping mechanism by conserving energy, and by providing required rest.
Administer antianxiety drugs as ordered (diazepam, flurazepam, lorazepam).	Promotes rest and reduces anxiety.

Information, Instruction, Demonstration

INTERVENTIONS	RATIONALES
Instruct patient and family as to all procedures, tests, medications, and care in a factual consistent manner. Reinforce as needed.	Accurate information reduces anxiety, facilitates the relationship between patient and nurse, and allows the patient and family to deal with the problem in a realistic manner. Repetition, when needed, helps in the retention of information when the attention span is diminished.
Instruct patient in relaxation techniques. Provide for diversionary activities.	Reduces anxiety and stress.
Instruct about post-discharge care, activities, limitations, symptoms to report, problems that might be encountered, and goals.	Reduces anxiety and promotes increased independence and self-confidence; decreases fear of abandonment that can occur with discharge from hospital; assists patient and family to identify realistic goals and decreases the chances of discouragement with limitations during recuperation.

Discharge or Maintenance Evaluation

- Patient is able to recognize feelings and identify mechanisms to cope and identify causes.

- Patient has significant reduction in fear and anxiety and appears less tense, with normal vital signs.

- Patient/family can appropriately utilize problem-solving skills.

- Patient can verbalize concerns easily and has increased energy.

- Patient can make appropriate decisions based on factual information regarding his condition and is able to discuss future plans.

Knowledge deficit

Related to: lack of understanding, lack of understanding of medical condition, lack of recall

Defining characteristics: verbalized questions regarding problems, inadequate follow-up on instructions given, misconceptions, lack of improvement of previous regimen, development of preventable complications

Outcome Criteria

Patient will be able to verbalize and demonstrate understanding of information given regarding condition, medications, and treatment regimen.

Information, Instruction, Demonstration

INTERVENTIONS	RATIONALES
Determine patient's baseline of knowledge regarding disease process, normal physiology, and function of the heart.	Provides information regarding patient's understanding of condition as well as a baseline from which to base teaching.
Monitor patient's readiness to learn and determine best methods to use for teaching. Attempt to incorporate family members in learning process. Reinstruct/reinforce information as needed.	Promotes optimal learning environment when patient shows willingness to learn. Family members may assist with helping the patient to make informed choices regarding his treatment. Anxiety or large volumes of instruction may impede comprehension and limit learning.
Provide time for individual interaction with patient.	Promotes relationship between patient and nurse, and establishes trust.
Instruct patient on procedures that may be performed.	Provides knowledge and promotes the ability to make informed choices.
Instruct patient on medications, dose, effects, side effects, contraindications, and signs/symptoms to report to MD.	Provides information to the patient to manage medication regimen and ensure compliance.

INTERVENTIONS	RATIONALES
Instruct in dietary needs and restrictions, such as limiting caffeine and sodium or increasing potassium, etc.	Patient may need to increase dietary potassium if placed on diuretics; caffeine should be limited due to the direct stimulant effect on the heart; sodium should be limited due to the potential for fluid retention.
Provide printed materials when possible for patient/family to review.	Provides references for patient and family to refer to once discharged, and can enhance the understanding of verbally-given instructions.
Demonstrate and instruct on technique for checking pulse rate and regularity. Instruct in situations where immediate action must be taken.	Self-monitoring promotes self-independence and can provide timely intervention for abnormalities or complications. Heart rates that exceed set parameters may require further medical alteration in medications or regimen.
Have patient demonstrate all skills that will be necessary for post-discharge.	Provides information that patient has gained a full understanding of instruction and is able to demonstrate correct information.
Instruct/demonstrate exercises to be performed, avoiding over-taxing activities, signs/symptoms that may require the cessation of any activity, and to report symptoms that may require medical attention.	Exercise programs are helpful in improving cardiac function.

Discharge or Maintenance Evaluation

• Patient will be able to verbalize understanding of condition, treatment regimen, and signs/symptoms to report.

• Patient will be able to correctly perform all tasks prior to discharge.

• Patient will be able to verbalize understanding of cardiac disease, risk factors, dietary restrictions, and lifestyle adaptations.

MYOCARDIAL INFARCTION (MI)

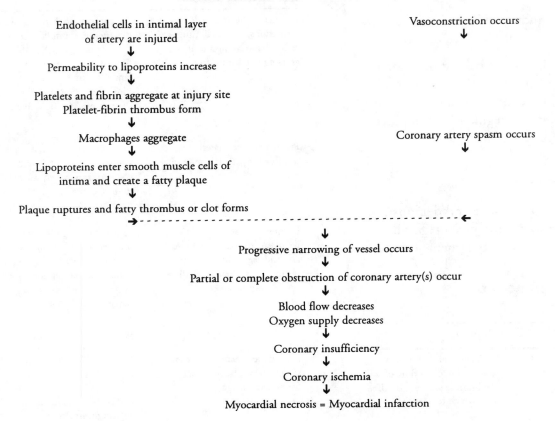

Endothelial cells in intimal layer
of artery are injured
↓
Permeability to lipoproteins increase
↓
Platelets and fibrin aggregate at injury site
Platelet-fibrin thrombus form
↓
Macrophages aggregate
↓
Lipoproteins enter smooth muscle cells of
intima and create a fatty plaque
↓
Plaque ruptures and fatty thrombus or clot forms
- ←

Vasoconstriction occurs
↓

Coronary artery spasm occurs
↓

Progressive narrowing of vessel occurs
↓
Partial or complete obstruction of coronary artery(s) occur
↓
Blood flow decreases
Oxygen supply decreases
↓
Coronary insufficiency
↓
Coronary ischemia
↓
Myocardial necrosis = Myocardial infarction

COMPLICATIONS RESULTING FROM MI THAT MAY LEAD TO DEATH IF NOT TREATED:

Congestive heart failure

Dysrhythmias

Conduction problems

Cardiogenic shock

Systemic embolus

Pulmonary embolus

Papillary muscle rupture

Dressler's syndrome

Ventricular rupture

Ventricular septal defects

Pericarditis

Pericarditis is an inflammation of the pericardium that can occur due to a variety of circumstances. The inflammation is usually a manifestation of another disease process, but may be drug induced, from agents such as procainamide, hydralazine, phenytoin, penicillin, phenylbutazone, minoxidil, or daunorubicin. Other causes for pericarditis include idiopathic causes, viral, bacterial, fungal, protozoal, uremia, MI, tuberculosis, neoplasms, trauma, surgical procedures, autoimmune disorders (lupus, rheumatoid arthritis, scleroderma), inflammatory disorders (amyloidosis), dissecting aortic aneurysms, or radiation treatments to the thorax.

Pericarditis may be classified as acute or chronic, as well as constrictive or restrictive. Constrictive pericarditis occurs when fibrin material is deposited on the pericardium and adhesions form between the epicardium and pericardium. Restrictive pericarditis results when effusion into the pericardial sac occurs. Both types cause interference with the heart's ability to fill properly, which causes increases in systemic and pulmonary venous pressures. Eventually systemic blood pressure and cardiac output decrease.

The visceral pericardium is a serous membrane that is separated from a fibrous sac, or parietal pericardium, by a small (less than 50 cc) amount of fluid. If the fluid increases to the point where the heart function is compromised, pleural effusion occurs and cardiac tamponade becomes a critical concern. The pericardium is important because it holds the heart in a fixed position to minimize friction between it and other structures. Other functions include prevention of exercise- or hypervolemic-induced dilatation of the cardiac chambers and assistance with atrial filling during systole.

The main symptoms of pericarditis include sharp, retrosternal and/or left precordial pain that worsens while in a supine position, and a pericardial friction rub best auscultated at the lower left sternal border. The pain may be exacerbated by coughing, swallowing, breathing, or twisting. Other symptoms may be seen depending on the severity of the pericarditis and the rapidity in which the fluid accumulates. Volumes of 100 cc that accumulates quickly may produce a more life-threatening complication, cardiac tamponade, than a larger accumulation of fluid that is generated over a long period of time.

MEDICAL CARE

Oxygen: to increase available oxygen supply

Analgesics: morphine or meperidine used to alleviate pain

Steroids: large doses of corticosteroids, such as prednisone, are given to reduce inflammation and control the symptoms of pericarditis

NSAIDs: aspirin or indomethacin are used to reduce fever and inflammation

IV fluids: given to help restore left ventricular filling volume and to offset any compressive effects of intrapericardial pressure increases

Inotropic drugs: isoproterenol or dobutamine IV given for their positive inotropic effects as well as peripheral vasodilating properties

Laboratory: white blood cell count may be elevated, sed rate may be elevated from non-specific inflammatory response; CKMB may be mildly elevated; blood cultures done to identify organism responsible for infective process and to ascertain appropriate drug for eradication; renal profile done to evaluate for uremic pericarditis and worsening renal status

Electrocardiography: used to monitor for S-T elevation, T wave changes associated with pericarditis, and to monitor for dysrhythmias

Echocardiography: used to establish presence of pericardial fluid and an estimate of volume, any vegetation on valves, and to observe for right atrium and right ventricular dilatation

Chest x-ray: used to show cardiomegaly and to assess lung fields

Pericardiocentesis: used to relieve fluid build-up and pressure in emergency situations where the patient is deteriorating or is in shock

Surgery: open surgical drainage is usually the treatment of choice for cardiac tamponade

NURSING CARE PLANS

Alteration in comfort
[See MI]

Related to: chest pain due to pericardial inflammation

Defining characteristics: chest pain with or without radiation, facial grimacing, clutching of hands or chest, restlessness, diaphoresis, changes in pulse and blood pressure, dyspnea

Altered tissue perfusion: cardiopulmonary, renal, peripheral, cerebral

Related to: tissue ischemia, reduction or interruption of blood flow, vasoconstriction, hypovolemia, shunting, depressed ventricular function, dysrhythmias, conduction defects

Defining characteristics: abnormal hemodynamic readings, dysrhythmias, decreased peripheral pulses, cyanosis, decreased blood pressure, shortness of breath, dyspnea, cold and clammy skin, decreased mental alertness and changes in mental status, oliguria, anuria, sluggish capillary refill, abnormal electrolyte and digoxin levels, hypoxia, ABG changes, chest pain, ventilation perfusion

imbalances, changes in peripheral resistance, impaired oxygenation of myocardium, EKG changes (S-T segment, T wave, U wave), LV enlargement, palpitations, abnormal renal function studies

Outcome Criteria

Blood flow and perfusion to vital organs will be preserved and circulatory function will be maximized.

Patient will be free of dysrhythmias.

Hemodynamic parameters will be within normal limits.

INTERVENTIONS	RATIONALES
Obtain vital signs. Obtain hemodynamic values, noting deviations from baseline values.	Provides information about the hemodynamics of the patient.
Determine the presence and character of peripheral pulses, capillary refill time, skin color and temperature.	May indicate decreased perfusion resulting from impaired coronary blood flow.
Discourage any non-essential activity.	Ambulation, exercise, transfers, and Valsalva-type maneuvers can increase blood pressure and decrease tissue perfusion.
Monitor EKG for disturbances in conduction and for dysrhythmias and treat as indicated.	Decreased cardiac perfusion may instigate conduction abnormalities. Dysrhythmias may occur due to compromised function of ventricles due to pressure exerted on them by excess fluid.
Titrate vasoactive drugs as ordered.	Maintain blood pressure and heart rate at parameters set by MD for optimal perfusion with minimal workload on heart.
Administer oxygen by nasal cannula as ordered, with rate dependent on disease process and condition.	Provides oxygen necessary for tissues and organ perfusion.

INTERVENTIONS	RATIONALES
Auscultate lungs for crackles (rales), rhonchi, or wheezes.	Suggestive of fluid overload that will further decrease tissue perfusion.
Auscultate heart sounds for S_3 or S_4 gallop, new murmurs, presence of jugular vein distention, or hepatojugular reflex.	Suggestive of impending or present heart failure.
Monitor oxygen status with ABGs, S_vO_2 monitoring, or with pulse oximetry.	Provides information about the oxygenation status of the patient. Continuous monitoring of saturation levels provide an instant analysis of how activity can affect oxygenation and perfusion.
Assist patient with planned, graduated levels of activity.	Allows for balance between rest and activity to decrease myocardial workload and oxygen demand. Gradual increases help to increase patient tolerance to activity without pain occurring.

Information, Instruction, Demonstration

INTERVENTIONS	RATIONALES
Instruct on medications, dosage, effects, side effects, and contraindications.	Promotes compliance with regimen and knowledge base.
Instruct to refrain from smoking.	Smoking causes vasoconstriction with can decrease perfusion.
Instruct in dietary requirements, menu planning, sodium restrictions, foods to avoid.	Reduction of high-cholesterol and sodium foods will help to control atherosclerosis, hyperlipidemia, fluid retention, and the effects on coronary blood flow.

Discharge or Maintenance Evaluation

- Lung fields will be clear and free of adventitious breath sounds.

- Extremities will be warm, pink, with easily palpable pulses of equal character.

- Vital signs and hemodynamic parameters will be within normal limits for patient.

- Oxygenation will be optimal as evidenced by pulse oximetry greater than 90%, S_vO_2 greater than 75%, or normal ABGs.

- Patient will be free of chest pain and shortness of breath.

- Patient will be able to verbalize information correctly regarding medications, diet and activity limitations.

Decreased cardiac output
[See MI]

Related to: fluid in pericardial sac from pericardial effusion, potential for cardiac tamponade because of effusion, damaged myocardium, decreased contractility, dysrhythmias, conduction defects, alteration in preload, alteration in afterload, vasoconstriction, myocardial ischemia, ventricular hypertrophy

Defining characteristics: decreased blood pressure, tachycardia, pulsus paradoxus greater than 10 mmHg, distended neck veins, increased central venous pressure, dysrhythmias, decreased QRS voltage or electrical alternans, diminished heart sounds, dyspnea, friction rub, cardiac output less than 4 L/min, cardiac index less than 2.5 L/min/m^2

Anxiety
[See MI]

Related to: change in health status, fear of death, threat to body image, threat to role functioning, pain

Defining characteristics: restlessness, insomnia, anorexia, increased respirations, increased heart rate, increased blood pressure, difficulty concentrating, dry mouth, poor eye contact, decreased energy, irritability, crying, feelings of helplessness

Knowledge deficit
[See MI]

Related to: lack of understanding, lack of understanding of medical condition, lack of recall

Defining characteristics: questions regarding problems, inadequate follow-up on instructions given, misconceptions, lack of improvement of previous regimen, development of preventable complications

PERICARDITIS

Inflammation

↓

Infiltration of neutrophils

↓

Increased pericardial vascularity

↓

Increased deposits of fibrin

↓

Fibrinous adhesions form between pericardium and epicarium

↓

Fluid accumulates in pericardial sac

↓

Pericardial effusion

↓

Heart function restricted

↓

Cardiac output decreased

↓

Pressures in heart equalize

↓

Cardiogenic shock occurs

↓

Death

Infective Endocarditis (IE)

Bacterial endocarditis is now referred to as infective endocarditis due to the presence of other organisms besides bacteria being the causative agent. It is an infection of the cardiac valves and inner lining of the heart that is characterized as a systemic illness. Endocarditis may be misdiagnosed as other infections in the early stages if signs and symptoms of cardiac involvement are not present. Common complaints range from fever with temperature less than 102 degrees, chills, arthralgia, lethargy, and anorexia. Acute endocarditis may result in death within a matter of hours if not treated. Antimicrobial therapy can decrease mortality to 15%, but heart failure secondary to valvular scarring and damage can occur after the infection is resolved.

Almost any organism can cause endocarditis but the most common ones noted have been Streptococcus viridans, Staphylococcus aureus, Enterococci, Staphylococcus epidermidis, Streptococcus pneumoniae, Pseudomonas aeruginosa, Candida albicans, and Aspergillus fumigatus.

Endocarditis may be subdivided into the acute and subacute classes, depending on the virulence of the organism involved and the length of duration. Acute infective endocarditis (AIE) has less than one month duration whereas subacute infective endocarditis (SIE) is usually greater than one month in duration. SIE usually involves congenitally-deformed or damaged heart valves, and AIE usually involves normal heart valves. Trauma in many forms can occur to the epithelial layer of the valves/endocardium causing injury and deposits of platelets and fibrin to adhere to this surface. This is known as nonbacterial thrombotic endocarditis

(NBTE). After this stage, the heart is then set up for vegetation to colonize from bacteria from other areas of the body during transient episodes of bacteremia. As these organisms grow, more platelets and fibrin adhere and eventually valves are destroyed, vegetation breaks off and embolizes to other areas of the body, and a systemic immune response occurs.

Patients who are at risk for endocarditis include those with rheumatic heart disease, open-heart surgery, congenital heart defects, prosthetic valve replacements, dental procedures, gynecological surgery or procedures, genitourinary surgery or procedures, invasive tests or lines, infected peripheral or central venous lines, IUDs, AV shunts or fistulas, skin abnormalities in preexisting cardiac disease, immunosuppressive therapy, and IV drug use.

Patients who have had prosthetic valves placed and who develop endocarditis are divided into early (occurring less than two months postoperatively) and late (occurring greater than two months postoperatively) classes, and develop chills, fever, leukocytosis, and/or a new murmur. Mortality is higher in early prosthetic valve endocarditis and is a serious problem.

MEDICAL CARE

Antibiotics: penicillin is the treatment of choice for Streptococcus viridans, with cephalothin or vancomycin being alternate choices; penicillin plus gentamicin is the treatment of choice for Steptococcus faecalis; synthetic penicillins, such as oxacillin or nafcillin, cephalothin and/or gentamicin are used in Staphylococcus epidermidis

Laboratory: a series of blood cultures is done to isolate the causative organism and sensitivity to antimicrobial agents; CBC is used to assess for anemia that may occur in up to 70% of patients, to monitor leukocyte levels, and to assess platelet counts; sedimentation rates may increase; immune titers show antigen-antibody response

Electrocardiography: shows alterations in conduction, dysrhythmias, ischemia

Echocardiography: used to establish diagnosis, to determine underlying cardiac disease, to estimate myocardial contractility, and demonstrate early mitral valve closure and aortic insufficiency

Nuclear cardiologic testing: Technetium-99 scans and gallium-67 imaging used to evaluate the extent of the infective process and to evaluate potential as a surgical candidate

Surgery: valve replacement is necessary if patient develops intractable congestive heart failure with hemodynamic compromise, persistent bacteremia despite antimicrobial treatment, prosthetic valve endocarditis, major systemic emboli, gram negative or fungal infection; drainage of abscesses or empyema; repair of peripheral or cerebral mycotic aneurysms

Prophylaxis: prophylactic antibiotic therapy must be prescribed prior to dental procedures, urethral or gynecological procedures, or surgery

NURSING CARE PLANS

Risk for altered tissue perfusion: cardiopulmonary, cerebral, renal, gastrointestinal, and peripheral

Related to: valvular vegetation emboli, platelet-fibrin emboli, and immunologic responses causing allergic vasculitis; embolu

Defining characteristics: petechiae, arthritis, arthralgia, myalgias, decreased peripheral pulses, Janeway's lesions, Roth's spots, Osler's nodes, lower back pain, splinter hemorrhages to subungual

areas, hematuria, oliguria, anuria, chest pain, shortness of breath, dyspnea, confusion, weakness, convulsions, coma, hemiplegia, aphasia, hemiparesis, cardiac tamponade, pericardial friction rub, murmur, dysrhythmias, conduction defects, cold clammy skin, cyanosis, mental status changes, hypotension, tachycardia, decreased urinary output, increased BUN

Outcome Criteria

Patient will achieve and maintain adequate tissue perfusion to all body systems.

INTERVENTIONS	RATIONALES
Determine mental status and level of consciousness. Observe for hemiparesis, paralysis, aphasia, convulsions, visual field defects, or coma, and notify MD.	Symptoms may indicate embolization to cerebrum which may require emergency treatment.
Monitor EKG for conduction abnormalities, especially prolonged PR interval, new left bundle branch block, new right bundle branch block with or without left anterior hemiblock. Treat as indicated per protocol.	Due to the close proximity of aortic valve cusps to the conduction system, bacterial invasion and proliferation may extend the infection process into the myocardium and cause dysrhythmias. Extension of the infection from the mitral valve to the Bundle of His and AV node may result in junctional tachycardia, Mobitz I, second degree or third degree AV blocks.
Observe for sudden shortness of breath, tachypnea, pleurisy-type pain, pallor or cyanosis.	Arterial emboli may affect the heart and other vital organs. Venous congestion may result in thrombus formation in deep veins and cause embolization to lungs, or embolization of vegetation thrombi may result in pulmonary embolus.
Evaluate chest pain, tachycardia, decreased blood pressure. Auscultate heart sounds for new	Arterial emboli may affect the heart and cause myocardial infarction. New murmurs may

INTERVENTIONS	RATIONALES
or changed murmurs, pericardial friction rubs, or abnormal lung sounds (crackles, rales).	occur as a result of valve scarring and distortion, valve aneurysm, septal rupture, papillary muscle rupture, or myocardial abscess rupture. Rupture into the pericardial sac can cause cardiac tamponade, in which heart tones will be muffled. Pericardial friction rubs may indicate pericarditis. Abnormal lung sounds may indicate impending congestive heart failure.
Observe extremities for swelling, erythema, tenderness, pain, positive Homans' sign, positive Pratt's sign. Observe for decreased peripheral pulses, pallor, coldness, cyanosis.	Bedrest promotes venous stasis which can increase the risk of thromboembolus formation. Actual vegetation emboli can migrate and occlude peripheral arteries, leading to tissue ischemia and necrosis.
Monitor for complaints of abdominal pain to left upper abdomen with radiation to left shoulder, abdominal rigidity, tenderness, nausea, or vomiting.	May indicate embolization to spleen. Vegetative emboli may occlude mesenteric artery and cause bowel infarction. Splenomegaly may be caused by antigen stimulation and allergic vasculitis.
Observe urine for hematuria, oliguria, anuria, complaints of flank or back pain.	Allergic vasculitis from endocarditis can result in focal, acute, or chronic glomerulonephritis and progress to renal insufficiency, renal failure, and uremia.
Observe for petechiae on mucous membranes, conjunctiva, neck, wrists, and ankles. Observe for splinter hemorrhages in subungual areas, Osler's nodes to distal fingers and toes, sides of fingers, palms or thighs, and for Janeway's lesions to the palms, soles of feet, arms and legs.	Petechiae is one of the classic symptoms of endocarditis as a result of allergic vasculitis. Petechiae are usually 1-2 mm in diameter, flat, red with white or gray centers, non-tender, and groups fade within a few days. Petechiae may be noted in other diagnoses and they should be ruled out. Hemorrhages to the subungual areas may be seen in early infective endocarditis but may be seen in trauma, with hemo- or peritoneal dialysis, or in mitral stenosis. Osler's nodes are nodules that range from

INTERVENTIONS	RATIONALES
	1-10 mm in diameter, red with white centers, overtly tender, and are usually a late sign of endocarditis, typically found in subacute endocarditis infections. Janeway's lesions are non-tender reddened or pink macular lesions, 1-5 mm in diameter, and usually change to tan and fade within 2 weeks. These are usually an early sign of endocarditis.
Evaluate complaints of arthritis, arthralgia, and severe lower back pain. Medicate as needed.	Occur in endocarditis due to localized immune responses or in decreased perfusion.
Monitor blood culture and sensitivity reports.	Usually 3-6 blood cultures are done in a series to assess for sustained bacteremia because bacteria are continually released into the system in endocarditis. The series prevents the possibility of false readings. Cultures determine the specific organism responsible for the bacteremia, and sensitivity results enable the choice of antimicrobials to be suited to the specific infection.
Administer antimicrobials as ordered.	Antibiotics should not be started until culture series is completed in subacute IE, but with acute IE, empiric antibiotics are given until cultures are available. In some instances, early negative results may indicate only that the culture could not be grown due to low levels of bacteria or an unusual organism being present. Obtaining cultures after antibiotics have been started do not give accurate information.

Instruction, Information, Demonstration

INTERVENTIONS	RATIONALES
Instruct patient in signs/ symptoms to report to MD.	Promotes knowledge and compliance with regimen.

Discharge or Maintenance Evaluation

- Patient will have adequate tissue perfusion to all body systems.

- Patient will be mentally lucid, with no confusion or neurological deficits.

- Patient will have adequate urinary output with no hematuria, and renal function studies will be within normal limits.

- Patient will be able to recall accurately the information instructed.

Decreased cardiac output [See MI]

Related to: complications with infected heart valves, potential for cardiac tamponade because of effusion, damaged myocardium, decreased contractility, dysrhythmias, conduction defects, alteration in preload, alteration in afterload, vasoconstriction, myocardial ischemia, ventricular hypertrophy

Defining characteristics: decreased blood pressure, tachycardia, pulsus paradoxus greater than 10 mmHg, distended neck veins, increased central venous pressure, dysrhythmias, decreased QRS voltage or electrical alternans, diminished heart sounds, dyspnea, friction rub, cardiac output less than 5 L/min, cardiac index less than 2.5 L/min/m^2, change in mental status, change or new cardiac murmur, arterial emboli, decreased urine output, cyanosis, cold clammy skin

Hyperthermia

Related to: bacteremia, allergic vasculitis, arterial occlusion/infarction, abscess

Defining characteristics: body temperature greater than normal range, flushed warm skin, chills, increased heart rate, increased respiratory rate

Outcome Criteria

Patient will maintain body temperature within normal limits and be free of infection.

INTERVENTIONS	RATIONALES
Monitor temperature every 2-4 hours and prn. Observe for chills and diaphoresis.	Endocarditis usually results in temperatures less than 102 degrees; temperatures greater than this indicate an acute infective process. Chills frequently precede a temperature spike.
Monitor environment temperature and limit or add blankets as warranted. Change linens as needed.	Room temperature may be altered to assist with maintenance of normal body temperature.
Monitor I&O; provide adequate fluids.	Diaphoresis and increased metabolic rate from temperature elevations increase fluid loss and may cause dehydration.
Give tepid sponge baths prn.	May assist in lowering temperature by means of evaporation. Using cooler water or alcohol may cause chilling and thus increase body temperature.
Place on cooling blanket as warranted.	Cooling blankets are usually only used for severe fever greater than 104 degrees when risk of brain damage or seizures is imminent.
Administer antipyretic medications as warranted.	Reduces fever by action on the hypothalamus. Low grade temperatures may be beneficial to the body's immune system and ability to retard the growth of organisms.

Information, Instruction, Demonstration

INTERVENTIONS	RATIONALES
Instruct on procedures for decreasing temperature.	Provides knowledge and reduces fear and enhances compliance.
Instruct to take temperature frequently and to notify MD for elevations immediately.	Temperature elevations indicate infection and prompt notification will allow for prompt treatment.
Instruct on medications, effects, side effects, contraindications, symptoms to report.	Promotes knowledge and compliance.

Discharge or Maintenance Evaluation

• Patient will be normothermic with no overt signs/symptoms of infection.

Risk for infection

Related to: inhibition of antibodies due to immunological system action, inflammatory processes due to vegetation growth, predisposition to bacteremia, septic emboli, myocardial abscess, occlusion of arteries leading to necrosis of body systems, invasive procedures and lines, dental procedures, nosocomial infections, lack of recognition of infection, lack of prophylactic treatment, suprainfection

Defining characteristics: elevated temperature, elevated WBC count, positive blood cultures, reddened, draining IV sites

Outcome Criteria

Patient will be free of infection, afebrile, with no over symptoms of infection or infective process noted.

INTERVENTIONS	RATIONALES
Monitor temperature trends.	Decreases in body temperature below 96 degrees may indicate advanced shock states and is a critical indicator of decreased tissue perfusion and lack of the body's ability to muster enough defense to raise the temperature. Temperatures greater than 101 degrees are due to the effect of endotoxins on the hypothalamus and of pyrogen-released endorphins.
Monitor for signs/symptoms of deterioration of patient and failure to improve within a timely manner.	May indicate ineffective antibiotic therapy or abundance of resistant organisms.
Observe mouth for patches of white plaque and perineal areas for vaginal drainage or itching, and notify MD.	Thrush or yeast infections may occur as a secondary infection when normal flora is killed by massive antibiotic therapy.
Inspect wounds, IV sites, catheter sites, invasive devices and lines, changes in drainage or body fluids.	May indicate local secondary infection or inflammation.
Maintain aseptic or sterile technique as warranted.	Reduces the risk of opportunistic infection and chances of cross-contamination.
Obtain urine, blood, sputum, wound, and invasive line/catheter specimens for culture and sensitivity and Gram stain as warranted.	Assists with identification of source of infection, causative organism, and antibiotic of choice to enable prompt and effective treatment.
Reposition patient every 2 hours; encourage coughing and deep breathing.	Frequent changes in position and breathing exercises enhance pulmonary toilet and may help to prevent pneumonia.

INTERVENTIONS	RATIONALES
Administer antibiotics as ordered.	Antibiotics may be started prior to receiving final culture reports based on the likelihood of the infective organism. Specific antibiotics are determined by the culture information.

Information, Instruction, Demonstration

INTERVENTIONS	RATIONALES
Instruct patient to cover mouth and nose during coughing/sneezing. Instruct in handwashing and disposal of contaminated materials.	Prevents spread of infection from airborne organisms. Good handwashing reduces spread of infection. Infection control procedures limit contamination and spread of infective materials.
Instruct patient in good dental hygiene to use soft toothbrush; to avoid water pik and toothpicks; to obtain regular dental exams.	Avoids trauma to gums which may promote reinfection. Water pik and toothpicks may cause bleeding and promote infection.
Instruct patient to take temperature every day for 1 month post discharge.	Temperature elevations may indicate infection/reinfection.
Prepare patient for surgery as warranted.	Surgery may be required to remove necrotic tissue or limbs and to remove purulent material in order to enhance healing. Surgery may be required to replace damaged heart valves due to vegetative infection.
Instruct patient in obtaining prophylactic antibiotic therapy prior to procedures.	Prophylaxis will be required for any invasive procedure due to likelihood of reinfection.

Discharge or Maintenance Evaluation

- Patient will have normal temperature and vital signs.

- Patient will exhibit no overt symptoms or signs of infection.

- Patient will be able to recall instructions accurately.

- Patient will seek prophylactic antibiotic therapy prior to any procedure and will have no evidence of reinfection.

Anxiety
[See MI]

Related to: change in health status, fear of death, threat to body image, threat to role functioning, pain

Defining characteristics: restlessness, insomnia, anorexia, increased respirations, increased heart rate, increased blood pressure, difficulty concentrating, dry mouth, poor eye contact, decreased energy, irritability, crying, feelings of helplessness

Knowledge deficit
[See MI]

Related to: lack of understanding, lack of understanding of medical condition, lack of recall

Defining characteristics: questions regarding problems, inadequate follow-up on instructions given, misconceptions, lack of improvement of previous regimen, development of preventable complications

INFECTIVE ENDOCARDITIS

Trauma to valves predispose epithelial surface to injury
(valvular insufficiency, ventricular septal defects, artificial valves, and indwelling catheters and lines)

↓

Platelets and fibrin deposit

↓

Microscopic platelet-fibrin thrombi
(known as NBTE—nonbacterial thrombotic endocarditis)

↓

Bacteria lodge on endocardium/valves

↓

Bacteria increase
Platelets, fibrin, RBCs, and PMN leukocytes deposited

↓

Vegetations formed

↓

Vegetations embolize	Valvular tissue deformed	Inflammation adjacent to vegetation
↓	↓	↓
Arteries occlude	Valves incompetent	Immunologic antibodies inhibit PMNs
	↓	Humoral immunity system stimulated
	CHF	Cellular immunity system decreased
	↓	↓
	Ruptured perforated cusps	Hypergammaglobulinemia
	↓	↓
	Myocardial abscess	Cryoglobulins increase
	↓	Hypersensitivity reaction
	Rupture to pericardial sac	↓
	↓	Allergic vasculitis
	Pericarditis	↓
	↓	Petechiae
	Tamponade	Arthritis
		Myalgias
		Janeway's lesions
		Roth's spots
		Osler's nodes

Cerebral	Cardiac	Pulmonary	GI	GU	Peripheral
TIA	Myocardial ischemia	Pulmonary embolus	Bowel infarction	Renal infarction	Claudication to extremities
CVA	Myocardial infarction	Dyspnea	Mesentery infarct	Glomerulonephritis	Arterial insufficiency
Mycotic cerebral Anysm.	CHF		Splenic infarction	Renal insufficiency	Pain
Confusion	Pericarditis		Radiating pain	Renal failure	Pulselessness
Weakness	Cardiac tamponade		Fever	Flank pain	Cyanosis
Mental changes	Chest pain		Abdominal pain	Hematuria	Pallor
Hemiparesis	Radiating pain			Oliguria	Mottling
Hemiplegia	Nausea, vomiting			Azotemia	
Aphasia	Sweating, diaphoresis			Albuminuria	
Convulsions	Dyspnea				
Coma					

Hypertension

Essential hypertension, which is an elevated blood pressure of unknown origin, and secondary hypertension, which is an elevated blood pressure resulting from a known cause, will cause inflammation and necrosis in the arterioles which then result in decreased blood flow to vital body organs, and places stress on the heart and vessels. Uncontrolled hypertension is associated with permanent damage to body systems. Blood pressure is considered to be hypertension if the systolic pressure is greater than 140 mmHg or the diastolic pressure is greater than 90 mmHg, and is classified based on the severity from a high normal to malignant hypertension. Hypertensive crisis is defined as a sustained increase in diastolic blood pressure above 120 mmHg, which is high enough to cause irreversible damage to organs and tissue death.

Hypertension may result from several origins—adrenal origin (as in pheochromocytoma, Cushing's disease, brain tumor, etc.), renal origin (as in pyelonephritis), cardiovascular origin (as in atherosclerosis or coarctation of the aorta, etc.), or unknown origin which accounts for the majority of all known hypertension.

Untreated, hypertension will result in death due to cerebrovascular accident, congestive heart failure, intracerebral hemorrhage, kidney failure, or dissecting aneurysms.

Systolic blood pressure is the pressure that the heart pumps against to force blood from the left side of the heart to the aorta and to major arteries. Diastolic blood pressure is the pressure required to permit filling of the ventricles before the next systole cycle. The pulse pressure, which is the value of the difference between the systolic and diastolic pressures, may be used to indicate perfusion prob-lems. The mean arterial pressure, or MAP (or MABP) is the average pressure attempting to push the blood through the circulatory system and should be greater than 60 mmHg in order to adequately perfuse organs.

Elevated blood pressure may occur as a result of emotional stress with as much as 40 mmHg increase, and may also result from ventilatory insufficiency, post-seizures, electroconvulsive therapy, intracerebral injury, CNS disorders due to the massive stimulation of catecholamines, coronary artery bypass surgery, myocardial infarction, heart failure, renal insufficiency, eclampsia/toxemia, endocrine disorders, and some drugs.

Risk factors include: ages between 30 and 70 years of age, race (black), use of birth control pills, obesity, familial history, smoking, stress, diabetes mellitus, and sedentary lifestyle.

Treatment is aimed at lowering blood pressure by use of antihypertensive medications, diuretics to increase urinary output, and by eliminating factors that promote the elevation of blood pressure. A "stepped care" regimen is used most often, with step one involving the use of thiazide diuretics and calcium ion antagonists; step two involves the supplemental use of beta-adrenergic blockers; step three includes vasodilators; and step four involves guanethidine.

MEDICAL CARE

Diuretics: chlorothiazide (Diuril), spironolactone (Aldactone), chlorthalidone (Hygroton), hydrochlorothiazide (Esidrix, HydroDiuril), triamterene (Dyrenium), metolazone (Zaroxolyn, Diulo), ethacrynic acid (Edecrin), furosemide (Lasix) to promote diuresis and block reabsorption of sodium and water in the kidney

Calcium ion antagonists: verapamil (Calan), diltiazem (Cardizem), nifedipine (Procardia), nitrendipine to produce vasodilation on vascular smooth muscle

Adrenergic inhibitors: reserpine, methyldopa (Aldomet), propranolol (Inderal), prazosin hydrochloride (Minipress) used to impair synthesis of norepinephrine, suppression of sympathetic outflow by central alpha-adrenergic stimulation, or blocking of preganglionic to postganglionic autonomic transmission

Vasodilators: hydralazine (Apresoline), minoxidil (Loniten), nadolol (Corgard) to relax smooth muscle of arterioles and reduce peripheral vascular resistance and thus, blood pressure

ACE inhibitors: captopril (Capoten) used to lower total peripheral resistance by inhibiting angiotensin-converting enzyme

Electrolytes: potassium chloride (KCl, K Dur, K tabs) to replace potassium lost through diuresis

Chest x-ray: shows any enlargement of the heart and pulmonary vein, presence of pulmonary edema or pleural effusion

Electrocardiography: used to monitor for changes in rate and rhythm, conduction abnormalities, left ventricular hypertrophy, ischemia, electrolyte abnormalities, drug toxicity, and presence of dysrhythmias

Laboratory: cholesterol levels and lipid profile used to determine cholesterol and triglyceride levels and their pertinence to atherosclerosis; electrolyte profiles used to monitor for hypokalemia and hypernatremia which may be prevalent due to diuretic therapy; CBC used to identify potential renal failure and polycythemia; glucose levels used to identify potential causes of hypertension; BUN and creatinine levels used to identify renal dysfunction; urinalysis used to identify proteinuria for possible indication of renal disease and hema-

turia for possible indication of nephrosclerosis; thyroid profile used to identify hyperthyroidism which may lead to vasoconstriction and hypertension; aldosterone level used to identify primary aldosteronism; urine VMA to identify elevation of catecholamine metabolites which may indicate pheochromocytoma

Radiographic testing: IVP may be used to identify presence of kidney disease; renal arteriogram may be used to show renal artery stenosis or other causes of hypertension

NURSING CARE PLANS

Risk for decreased cardiac output

Related to: vasoconstriction, increased preload, increased afterload, ventricular hypertrophy, ischemia

Defining characteristics: elevated blood pressure, decreased cardiac output, decreased stroke volume, increased peripheral vascular resistance, increased systemic vascular resistance

Outcome Criteria

Patient will have no elevation in blood pressure above normal limits and will have adequate cardiac output, and will maintain blood pressure within acceptable limits.

INTERVENTIONS	RATIONALES
Monitor blood pressure every 1-2 hours, or every 5 minutes during active titration of vasoactive drugs. Measure pressure in both arms using appropriate size of cuff. When possible, obtain pressures lying, sitting, and standing.	Changes in blood pressure may indicate changes in patient status requiring prompt attention. Comparing pressures in both sides provides information as to amount of vascular involvement. Blood pressure may vary depending on body position and postural hypotension may result in syncope.

INTERVENTIONS	RATIONALES
Monitor EKG for dysrhythmias, conduction defects, and for heart rate and rhythm changes. Treat as indicated.	Decreases in cardiac output may result in changes in cardiac perfusion causing dysrhythmias.
Observe skin for color, temperature, capillary refill time, and diaphoresis.	Peripheral vasoconstriction may result in pale, cool, clammy skin, with prolonged capillary refill time due to cardiac dysfunction and decreased cardiac output.
Auscultate lungs for adventitious breath sounds.	Crackles (rales) or wheezing may indicate pulmonary congestion due to cardiac failure as a result of increased blood pressure.
Ausculate heart tones.	Hypertensive patients often have S_4 gallops due to atrial hypertrophy. Ventricular hypertrophy may result in S_3 gallops.
Administer thiazide, loop, or potassium-sparing diuretics as ordered.	Thiazides are used to reduce blood pressure in patients with normal renal function and these limit fluid retention. Loop diuretics inhibits reabsorption of sodium and chloride and are used in patients who have renal dysfunction. Potassium-sparing diuretics are used in conjunction with thiazides to decrease the amount of potassium lost.
Administer sympathetic inhibitors as ordered.	These drugs reduce blood pressure by decreasing peripheral resistance, reducing cardiac output, inhibiting sympathetic activity, and suppressing the release of renin which is a potent vasoconstrictor.
Administer vasodilators as ordered.	May be used in severe hypertension to increase coronary blood flow and decrease afterload to improve cardiac output.
Administer antiadrenergic drugs as ordered.	Prevents blood vessels from constricting and increasing blood pressure.

Information, Instruction, Demonstration

INTERVENTIONS	RATIONALES
Instruct on fluid and diet requirements and restrictions of sodium.	Restrictions can assist with decrease in fluid retention and hypertension, thereby improving cardiac output.
Instruct on medications, effects, side effects, contraindications, signs to report.	Promotes knowledge and compliance with drug regimen.
Prepare patient for surgery if warranted.	Pheochromocytoma may require surgical intervention for removal of the tumor in order to correct hypertension.

Discharge or Maintenance Evaluation

- Patient will be normotensive, with adequate cardiac output and index.

- Medications will be taken as ordered with no side effects.

- Patient will have stable heart rate, rhythm, and heart tones, with no adventitious breath sounds.

- Patient will be able to verbalize instructions accurately.

Risk for altered tissue perfusion: cardiopulmonary, cerebral, renal, gastrointestinal, and peripheral

Related to: increased catecholamine stimulation, increased blood pressure, decreased cardiac output, decreased baroreceptor sensitivity, changes in cerebrospinal fluid pressure, angiotensin and aldosterone stimulation, sodium intake, environmental factors, genetic factors, strain on arterial wall, atherosclerosis

Defining characteristics: increased blood pressure, retinopathy, retinal hemorrhage, headache, epistaxis, tachycardia, rales, S_3 or S_4 gallops, restlessness, bruits to femoral, carotids, abdominal aorta, blurred vision, chest pain, shortness of breath, optic disc papilledema, seizures, coma, nystagmus, mental changes

Outcome Criteria

Patient will achieve and maintain adequate tissue perfusion to all body systems.

INTERVENTIONS	RATIONALES
Monitor for sudden onset of chest pain.	May indicate dissecting aortic aneurysm.
Monitor EKG for changes in rate, rhythm, dysrhythmias, and conduction defects. Treat as indicated.	Decreased perfusion may result in dysrhythmias due to decrease in oxygen.
Monitor hemodynamic parameters closely and titrate vasoactive drugs as warranted.	Provides immediate information regarding efficacy of medication and status of hypertension.
Observe for shift of point of maximal impulse (PMI) to left.	Shift occurs in cardiac enlargement.
Auscultate over peripheral arteries for bruits.	Atherosclerosis may cause bruits by obstructing blood flow.
Observe extremities for swelling, erythema, tenderness, pain, positive Homans' sign, positive Pratt's sign. Observe for decreased peripheral pulses, pallor, coldness, cyanosis.	Bedrest promotes venous stasis which can increase the risk of thromboembolus formation. Actual vegetation emboli can migrate and occlude peripheral arteries, leading to tissue ischemia and necrosis.

Instruction, Information, Demonstration

INTERVENTIONS	RATIONALES
Instruct patient in signs/ symptoms to report to MD, such as headache upon rising, increased blood pressure, chest pain, shortness of breath, increased heart rate, weight gain of > 2 lb/day or 5 lb/wk, edema, visual changes, nosebleeds, dizziness, syncope, muscle cramps, nausea/vomiting, impotence or decreased libido.	Promotes knowledge and compliance with treatment. Promotes prompt detection and facilitates prompt intervention.

Discharge or Maintenance Evaluation

- Patient will have adequate tissue perfusion to all body systems.

- Patient will be mentally lucid, with no confusion or neurological deficits.

- Patient will have adequate urinary output with no hematuria, and renal function studies will be within normal limits.

- Patient will be able to recall accurately the information instructed.

Anxiety
[See MI]

Related to: change in health status, fear of death, threat to body image, threat to role functioning, pain

Defining characteristics: restlessness, insomnia, anorexia, increased respirations, increased heart rate, increased blood pressure, difficulty concentrating, dry mouth, poor eye contact, decreased energy, irritability, crying, feelings of helplessness

Knowledge deficit

Related to: lack of understanding, lack of understanding of medical condition, lack of recall

Defining characteristics: questions regarding problems, inadequate follow-up on instructions given, misconceptions, lack of improvement of previous regimen, development of preventable complications

Outcome Criteria

Patient will be able to verbalize and demonstrate understanding of information given regarding condition, medications, and treatment regimen.

Information, Instruction, Demonstration

INTERVENTIONS	RATIONALES
Determine patient's baseline of knowledge regarding disease process, normal physiology, and function of the heart.	Provides information regarding patient's understanding of condition as well as a baseline from which to base teaching.
Monitor patient's readiness to learn and determine best methods to use for learning. Attempt to incorporate family/significant other in learning process. Reinstruct/reinforce information as needed.	Promotes optimal learning environment when patient shows willingness to learn. Family members may assist with helping the patient to make informed choices regarding his treatment. Anxiety or large volumes of instruction may impede comprehension and limit learning.
Provide time for individual interaction with patient.	Promotes relationship between patient and nurse, and establishes trust.
Instruct patient on procedures that may be performed.	Provides knowledge and promotes the ability to make informed choices.

INTERVENTIONS	RATIONALES
Instruct patient in medications, dose, effects, side effects, contraindications, and signs/symptoms to report to MD.	Promotes understanding that side effects are common and may subside over time, and facilitates compliance.
Instruct in dietary needs and restrictions, such as limiting caffeine and sodium, or increasing potassium and calcium.	Patient may need to increase dietary potassium if placed on diuretics; caffeine should be limited due to the direct stimulant effect on the heart; sodium should be limited due to the potential for fluid retention. Additional calcium has been shown to lower blood pressure. Excessive intake of fat and cholesterol are additional risk factors in hypertension. Low fat diets can decrease BP through prostaglandin balance.
Instruct on hypertension, effects on the blood vessels, heart, brain, and kidneys. Instruct on normal values for BP.	Promotes understanding of the disease process and enhances compliance with treatment.
Instruct on maintaining medication regimen to keep blood pressure well controlled, and in keeping medical appointments.	Assist patient to understand need for life-long compliance to reduce incidence of CVA, MI, cardiac and renal dysfunction. Lack of compliance is the major reason for failure of antihypertensive therapy.
Instruct on ways to modify risk factors, such as smoking, obesity, high fat diets, stressful lifestyle, etc.	Risk factors contribute to disease and complications associated with hypertension, as well as exacerbate symptoms. Nicotine increases catecholamine release and increases heart rate, blood pressure, and myocardial oxygen demand.
Instruct in self-monitoring for blood pressure; technique to be used post discharge.	Provides reinforcement and the ability to monitor response to medical regimen.
Instruct to take diuretics in am.	Decreases incidence of nocturia.

INTERVENTIONS	RATIONALES
Instruct to weigh daily at same time on same scale.	Monitors effectiveness of diuretics and for fluid retention.
Instruct on leg exercises and position changes.	Decreases venous pooling that can be potentiated by vasodilators and prolonged time in one position.
Instruct to avoid hot baths, saunas, hot tubs, and alcohol intake.	These promote vasodilation and when combined with diuretics, may increase chance of orthostatic hypotension and syncope.
Instruct to avoid over-the-counter medications unless prescribed by MD.	Some drugs contain sympathetic stimulants that can increase blood pressure or may cause drug interactions.
Instruct to rise slowly, allowing time between position changes.	Assist body to equilobrate and adjust in order to decrease the risk of syncope.
Provide printed materials when possible for patient/family to review.	Provides references for patient and family to refer to once discharged, and can enhance the understanding of verbally-given instructions.
Demonstrate and instruct on technique for checking pulse rate and regularity. Instruct in situations where immediate action must be taken.	Self-monitoring promotes self-independence and can provide timely intervention for abnormalities or complications. Heart rates that exceed set parameters may require further medical alteration in medications or regimen.
Have patient demonstrate all skills that will be necessary for post-discharge.	Provides information that patient has gained a full understanding of instruction and is able to demonstrate correct information.

Discharge or Maintenance Evaluation

- Patient will be able to verbalize understanding of condition, treatment regimen, and signs/symptoms to report.

- Patient will be able to correctly perform all tasks prior to discharge.

- Patient will be able to verbalize understanding of cardiac disease, risk factors, dietary restrictions, and lifestyle adaptations.

HYPERTENSION

Genetic Factors   Environmental Factors
Family history   Sodium intake, alcohol, stress, obesity

Strain on arterial wall
↓
Loss of elasticity
↓
Increased collagen and calcification of arterial media
↓
Atherosclerosis in intima
Narrowing of blood vessel lumen
↓
Stiffness of aortic and peripheral arteriae
↓
Constriction of arterioles

Cardiovascular   Neurologic   Renal
↓   ↓   ↓
Increased TPR, PVR, CO   Decreased baroreceptor sensitivity   Sympathetic stimulation
↓

Impaired myocardial oxygen   ↓
Increased workload on heart   Chronic hypertension   Angiotension/aldosterone release
Increased myocardial oxygen consumption   ↓   Decreased renal blood flow
                              Changes in CSF pressures   Decreased renal oxygenation
↓   Decrease in cerebral perfusion   ↓
Dyspnea on exertion   Decrease in cerebral oxygen supply   Ischemia of renal tissues
Ventricular hypertrophy   ↓   Renin/aldosterone secretion
Chest pain   Memory impairment   Increased blood pressure
↓   Dull headache in a.m.   ↓
Cardiac decompensation   Vertigo, tremors   Nocturia
Coronary artery disease   ↓   Sodium/water retention
Myocardial infarction   Cerebral edema   Increased blood volume
Cardiac failure   ↓   Decreased GFR
                              Retinal hemorrhage, blurred vision   ↓
                              TIAs, epistaxis   Azotemia
                              Cerebral hemorrhage   Renal failure
                              Cerebral aneurysm
                              Cerebral thrombosis, CVA

Thrombophlebitis

Thrombophlebitis occurs when a clot forms in a vein secondary to inflammation or when the vein is partially occluded from some disease process. As a general rule, two out of the following three factors occur prior to the formation of a thrombus—blood stasis, injury to the vessel, and altered blood coagulation.

Deep vein thrombosis, or DVT, pertains to clots that are formed in the deep veins and may result in complications such as pulmonary embolus and postphlebotic syndrome, or chronic venous insufficiency. This can be a residual effect of thrombophlebitis in which the veins are partially occluded or valves in the vessels have been damaged. This chronic insufficiency may cause increased venous pressure and fluid accumulation in the interstitial tissues, which results in chronic edema, tissue fibrosis, and induration.

DVT may be asymptomatic, but usually produces side effects such as fever, pain, edema, cyanosis or pallor to the involved extremity, and malaise.

Superficial vein thrombophlebitis causes may include trauma, infection, chemical irritations, frequent IVs, and recreational drug abuse.

The goals in treatment of thrombophlebitis are to control thrombotic development, relieve pain, improve blood flow, and prevent complications.

MEDICAL CARE

Venography: used to visualize the vascular system and locate any impairment in blood flow

Plethysmography: a non-invasive measurement of changes in calf volume that corresponds to changing blood volume as a result of impairment in blood flow

^{125}I **Fibrinogen uptake test:** a radioactive scan performed after radioactive fibrinogen is injected, which concentrates in the area of clot formation; not sensitive to thrombi high on the iliofemoral region or with inactive thrombi

Anticoagulants: heparin, coumadin, warfarin to prolong clotting time to prevent further clot formation

NURSING CARE PLANS

Alteration in tissue perfusion: peripheral

Related to: impaired blood flow, venous stasis, venous obstruction

Defining characteristics: pain, tissue edema, decreased peripheral pulses, prolonged capillary refill time, pallor, cyanosis, erythema, paresthesia

Outcome Criteria

Patient will have improved peripheral perfusion, with palpable and equal pulses, normal skin color, temperature, and sensation, and have no evidence of edema.

INTERVENTIONS	RATIONALES
Observe lower extremities for edema, color, and temperature. Measure calf circumference every shift. Monitor for capillary refill time.	Findings may help to differentiate between superficial thrombophlebitis and deep vein thrombosis. Measurements can facilitate early recognition of edema and changes. Edema, redness, and warmth are indicative of superficial phlebitis whereas DVT usually is exhibited by cool pale skin. DVT may prolong capillary refill time.
Observe extremity for prominence of veins, knots, bumps, or stretched skin.	Superficial veins may become distended because of backflow through veins. Evidence of thrombophlebitis to superficial veins may be visible or easily palpable.

INTERVENTIONS	RATIONALES
Maintain bedrest.	Activity limitation may minimize the potential for dislodgment of the clot.
Elevate legs while in bed or sitting in chair.	Reduces swelling and increases venous return. Some experts believe that elevation may actually enhance the release of thrombi.
Observe for positive Homan's sign (pain in calf upon dorsiflexion of foot).	Homan's sign may or may not be present consistently and should not be used as a sole indicator of thrombophlebitis.
Perform active or passive ROM exercises while at bedrest.	Promote increased venous blood return and decrease venous stasis.
Apply TED hose after acute phase is over. Remove for at least 1 hour every shift.	Assists to minimize postphlebotic syndrome and increases blood flow to deep veins. Removal allows time for compression of veins to be relaxed.
Apply warm moist soaks as ordered.	Promotes vasodilation and may improve venous return and decrease in edema.
Administer anticoagulants as ordered.	Heparin is used initially because of its action on thrombin formation and the removal of the intrinsic pathway to prevent further clot formation. Coumadin is usually used for long-term therapy.
Monitor laboratory studies for PT, PTT, APTT, and CBC.	Monitors efficacy of anticoagulant therapy and potential for clot formation due to hemoconcentration/dehydration.

Information, Instruction, Demonstration

INTERVENTIONS	RATIONALES
Instruct on avoidance of rubbing or massaging extremity involved.	May promote risk of dislodging clot and causing embolization.
Avoid crossing legs, prolonged positions with legs dangling, or knees bent.	Positions tend to restrict circulation and increases venous stasis, and increases edema.
Instruct in deep breathing exercises.	Promotes emptying of large veins by increasing negative pressure in the thorax.
Instruct on maintaining fluid intake of at least 2 L/day.	Dehydration promotes increased viscosity of blood, and increases venous stasis.
Prepare patient for surgery if warranted.	Surgical intervention may be required if circulation is severely compromised. Recurrent episodes of thrombi may require a vena caval umbrella to filter out thrombi going to lungs.
Instruct on lying in a slightly reversed trendelenburg position.	Promotes blood flow to dependent extremities; preferable to have extremities full of blood as opposed to empty.

Discharge or Maintenance Evaluation

- Patient will have palpable pulses of equal strength to all extremities.

- Skin will be within normal limits of coloration, temperature, and sensation.

- Patient will be able to recall all instructions accurately.

- Patient will have no complications from anticoagulation therapy.

Risk for impaired skin integrity

Related to: edema, venous stasis, bedrest, surgery, pressure, altered circulation and blood flow, altered metabolic states

Defining characteristics: skin surface disruptions, incisions, ulcerations, wounds that do not heal

Outcome Criteria

Patient will have no evidence of impairment to skin tissues.

Patient will have surgical wound approximated and well-healed with no evidence of infection.

INTERVENTIONS	RATIONALES
Monitor extremities for presence of ulcers, wounds, symptoms of decreased circulation.	Provides prompt assessment and treatment for impaired tissues.
If surgery is required, change dressing using aseptic or sterile technique as warranted. Leave wound open to air as soon as is feasible, or apply light dressing.	Prevents drainage accumulations from excoriating skin, provides assessment to monitor for changes in wound appearance and deterioration/improvement, and prevents wound from contamination. Allowing air to reach wound facilitates drying and promotes the healing process. Sutures may be abrasive to skin or get caught on garments and irritation may be reduced with a light gauze dressing.
Cleanse wound as ordered with each dressing change.	Various agents can be used to remove exudate or necrotic material from wound to promote healing. Any packing of the wound should be done using sterile technique to reduce the risk of contamination.
Monitor wound for skin integrity to incision and surrounding tissues, noting increases and changes in characteristics of drainage.	Prompt recognition of problems with healing may prevent exacerbation of wound. Increased drainage or malodorous drainage may indicate infection and delayed wound healing.

INTERVENTIONS	RATIONALES
Monitor any drainage tubes for amounts and character of drainage. Use ostomy bags over tubes when drainage is massive.	Provides indication of decreasing or increasing wound drainage and assessment of healing process. Collection of drainage in bags facilitates more accurate measurement of fluid loss and prevents excoriation of skin from copious drainage.
Use skin prep, moisture barrier, or benzoin to skin prior to tape application. Use hypoallergenic tape or Montgomery straps to secure dressings.	Provides protection to skin and reduces potential for skin trauma. Reduces potential for skin/wound disruption when frequent dressing changes are required.

Information, Instruction, Demonstration

INTERVENTIONS	RATIONALES
Instruct to avoid scratching, hitting or bumping legs, or other injurious activities.	Injuries may damage tissues that may deteriorate into ulcer formation.
Instruct on signs/symptoms of infection to wound/skin and to report to nurse/MD.	Provides prompt notification to enhance prompt treatment.
Instruct on cleansing incision area post discharge.	Reduces skin surface contaminants and prevents infection.

Discharge or Maintenance Evaluation

- Patient will have approximated, healed surgical wound with no drainage, erythema, or edema to site.

- Patient will be able to recall instructions accurately.

- Patient will be compliant with avoiding injurious activities, and will seek medical help when injury occurs.

Alteration in comfort
[See MI]

Related to: inflammation, impaired blood flow, intermittent claudication, venous stasis, lactic acid in tissues, surgical procedures, fever

Defining characteristics: complaints of pain, tenderness to touch, aching, burning, restlessness, facial grimacing, guarding of extremity

Knowledge deficit

Related to: lack of understanding, lack of understanding of medical condition, lack of recall

Defining characteristics: questions regarding problems, inadequate follow-up on instructions given, misconceptions, lack of improvement of previous regimen, development of preventable complications

Outcome Criteria

Patient will be able to verbalize and demonstrate understanding of information given regarding condition, medications, and treatment regimen.

Information, Instruction, Demonstration

INTERVENTIONS	RATIONALES
Determine patient's baseline of knowledge regarding disease process, normal physiology, and function.	Provides information regarding patient's understanding of condition as well as a baseline from which to base teaching.
Monitor patient's readiness to learn and determine best methods to use for learning. Attempt to incorporate family/significant other in learning process. Reinstruct/reinforce information as needed.	Promotes optimal learning environment when patient shows willingness to learn. Family members may assist with helping the patient to make informed choices regarding his treatment. Anxiety or large volumes of instruction may impede comprehension and limit learning.
Provide time for individual interaction with patient.	Promotes relationship between patient and nurse, and establishes trust.
Instruct patient on procedures that may be performed.	Provides knowledge and promotes the ability to make informed choices.
Instruct on signs/symptoms of possible complications, such as pulmonary emboli, venous insufficiency, and venous stasis ulcers.	Provides knowledge and assists patient to understand health care needs.
Instruct on care to lower extremities and to notify MD for development of any lesion.	Chronic venous stasis may occur and promotes risk of infection and/or ulcer formation.
Instruct patient in medications, dose, effects, side effects, contraindications, and signs/symptoms to report to MD.	Promotes understanding that side effects are common and may subside over time, and facilitates compliance.
Instruct on leg exercises and position changes. Assist with setting up activity program post-discharge.	Decreases venous pooling that can be potentiated by vasodilators and prolonged time in one position. Exercise may assist in developing collateral circulation and enhances venous return.
Instruct to rise slowly, allowing time between position changes.	Assist body to equilobrate and adjust in order to decrease the risk of syncope.
Instruct to balance rest with activity.	Rest decreases oxygen demands of compromised tissue and decreases potential for embolization of thrombus. Balancing rest with graduated activity prevents exhaustion and impairment of tissue perfusion.
Instruct on proper application of TED stockings.	Improper application may cause a tourniquet-like effect and impede circulation.
Avoid valsalva-type maneuvers. Provide increased fiber to diet and administer stool softeners as warranted.	Increases venous pressure in the leg which increases potential for thrombophlebitis.

INTERVENTIONS	RATIONALES
Instruct on anticoagulation therapy—dosage, effects, side effects, when to administer, other medications to avoid.	Promotes compliance with medical regimen and decreases potential for improper dosage and adverse drug interactions. Aspirin and salicylates decrease prothrombin activity, vitamin K increases prothrombin activity, antibiotics may interfere with vitamin K synthesis, and barbiturates can potentiate anticoagulant effect.
Instruct on importance of keeping MD appointments for follow-up laboratory studies.	Promotes compliance with treatment and decreases potential for non-therapeutic levels of anticoagulation therapy.
Provide printed materials when possible for patient/family to review.	Provides references for patient and family to refer to once discharged, and can enhance the understanding of verbally-given instructions.
Have patient demonstrate all skills that will be necessary for post-discharge.	Provides information that patient has gained a full understanding of instruction and is able to demonstrate correct information.

Discharge or Maintenance Evaluation

- Patient will be able to verbalize understanding of condition, treatment regimen, and signs/symptoms to report.

- Patient will be able to correctly perform all tasks prior to discharge.

- Patient will be able to verbalize understanding of safety precautions, correct dosage and administration of all medications, and activity limitations.

THROMBOPHLEBITIS

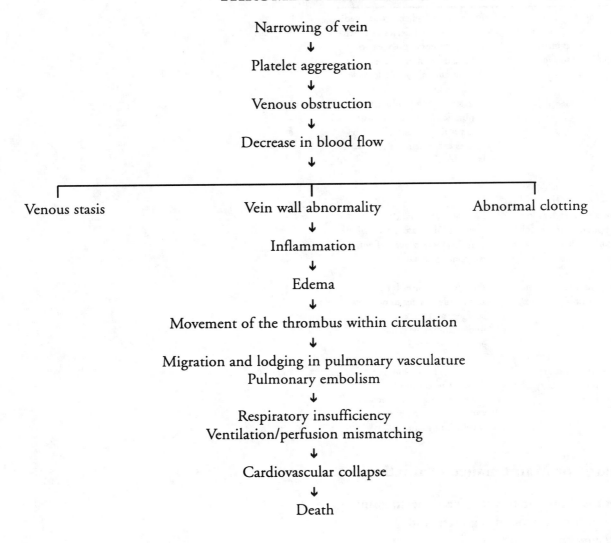

Narrowing of vein
↓
Platelet aggregation
↓
Venous obstruction
↓
Decrease in blood flow
↓

Venous stasis   Vein wall abnormality   Abnormal clotting
↓
Inflammation
↓
Edema
↓
Movement of the thrombus within circulation
↓
Migration and lodging in pulmonary vasculature
Pulmonary embolism
↓
Respiratory insufficiency
Ventilation/perfusion mismatching
↓
Cardiovascular collapse
↓
Death

Intra-Aortic Balloon Pump (IABP)

The intra-aortic balloon pump (IABP) is an advanced procedure that is used in the management of cardiovascular problems that are refractory to routine medical therapeutics. An intra-aortic balloon catheter (IAB) is inserted into the descending aorta, most commonly by way of the femoral artery. The IAB is then attached to the IABP which inflates and deflates the balloon in synchronization with the cardiac cycle. The balloon inflates during diastole when the aortic valve closes and increases the aortic pressure when the blood distally to the balloon is forced back towards the aortic valve. The coronary arteries are supplied with additional blood to improve coronary blood flow and perfusion and to decrease preload. Deflation occurs prior to the onset of systole and decreases the aortic pressure and ventricular resistance and makes it easier for the ventricle to contract and expel its normal volume of blood, thus decreasing afterload. This counterpulsation and displacement of blood decreases myocardial oxygen demand by decreasing myocardial workload and increases coronary perfusion and cardiac output.

Indications for use of IAB counterpulsation include cardiogenic shock, valvular disease, intractable chest pain resistant to medical treatment, prophylactic support during coronary angiography or anesthesia induction, papillary muscle rupture, ventricular septal defects, complications of acute myocardial infarctions, weaning from the cardiopulmonary bypass, septic shock, and as a bridge to cardiac transplantation. Counterpulsation is contraindicated in patients with severe aortic insufficiency, dissecting aneurysms, peripheral vascular disease, organic brain syndrome, irreversible brain damage, absent femoral pulses, trauma that has resulted in internal bleeding, active bleeding ulcers, blood dyscrasias, or previous aortofemoral or aortoiliac bypass grafts.

Because the potential for complications is high, this procedure should be utilized only by personnel well-versed and competent in all aspects of the IABP function and troubleshooting complications.

Two of the major complications associated with the use of the IABP are compromise of the left circulation and difficulty with weaning the patient from the IABP.

MEDICAL CARE

Oxygen: to increase available oxygen supply

Nitrates: (nitroglycerin, isosorbide dinitrate, Nitro-bid, Nitrostat) used to relax vascular smooth muscle to produce vasodilation, decrease preload, decrease afterload, decrease venous return, decrease peripheral vascular resistance, decrease oxygen demand

Beta-blockers: (propranolol, metoprolol, nadolol, atenolol, timolol, pindolol) used to reduce myocardial oxygen demand by blocking catecholamine and sympathetic induced increases in heart rate, contractility and blood pressure; slows AV node conduction; decreases sodium and water retention by reduction of renin secretion; decreases platelet aggregation and may reduce vasospasm

Calcium-channel blockers: (verapamil, nifedipine, diltiazem) used for decreasing myocardial oxygen demand and to enhance relaxation in hypertrophic cardiomyopathies, reduces blood pressure and afterload, and help prevent coronary spasm from decreased oxygen supply

Sympathomimetic drugs: (dopamine, Intropin) used for treatment of hypotension in normovolemic states and in the treatment of severe heart failure and cardiogenic shock

Placement of IAB: necessary for counterpulsation to begin

Cardiac catheterization: used to define lesions and evaluate their severity, to provide information on ventricular function, and to allow for measurement of heart pressures and cardiac output

Labwork: PT, PTT, and platelets are obtained to monitor anticoagulation status; general chemistry profiles and renal profiles are monitored every day for chemical imbalances and impending hepatic or renal problems; cardiac isoenzymes are used to monitor for heart damage; CBC and differentials are done every day to monitor for infection and changes in hematologic status; cultures of blood, urine and sputum are done for temperature elevations greater than 102 degrees to assess for infection/suspected organisms

Arterial blood gases: used to assess oxygenation status

Chest x-ray: used daily to monitor placement of IAB and watch for migration, to assess enlargement of the heart and/or pulmonary vessels, and to assess pulmonary fluid status and atelectasis

Electrocardiography: reveals changes with atrial and ventricular enlargement, rhythm and conduction abnormalities, ischemia, electrolyte abnormalities, drug toxicity, and presence of dysrhythmias

Pacemakers: either temporary or permanent, used in anticipation of lethal dysrhythmias and/or conduction problems

NURSING CARE PLANS

Altered tissue perfusion: cardiopulmonary, cerebral, gastrointestinal, renal, peripheral

Related to: cardiac failure, tissue ischemia, vasoconstriction, hypovolemia, shunting, depressed ventricular function, dysrhythmias, conduction defects, hypoxia, reduction or interruption of blood flow

Defining characteristics: visual disturbances, paresthesias, mental changes, change in level of consciousness, confusion, restlessness, pulse and blood pressure changes, changes in cardiac output, changes in peripheral resistance, impaired oxygenation of myocardium, chest pain, cardiac dysrhythmias, changes in EKG (S-T segment, T wave, U wave), LV enlargement, dyspnea, shortness of breath, tachypnea, palpitations, nausea, vomiting, slow digestion, oliguria, anuria, electrolyte imbalance, cold, clammy skin, decreased peripheral pulses, mottling, cyanosis, diaphoresis

Outcome Criteria

Blood flow and perfusion to vital organs will be preserved and circulatory function will be maximized.

Patient will be free of dysrhythmias and hemodynamic parameters will be within normal limits.

INTERVENTIONS	RATIONALES
Monitor vital signs every 15 to 30 minutes until stable, then every hour. Notify MD of deviations from parameters.	IABP timing is based on heart rate, and when rate changes > 10 beats/minute, adjustments in timing are necessary to ensure optimal counterpulsation. Dysrhythmias hamper optimal oxygenation and function of the IABP.

INTERVENTIONS	RATIONALES
Monitor mean arterial blood pressure every hour.	Assesses volume status to help monitor for efficacy of counter-pulsation. MABP can be calculated by adding 1/3 (systolic BP-diastolic BP) + diastolic BP. MABP is a function of cardiac output and systemic vascular resistance. Levels < 60 have little, if any, perfusion to brain.
Obtain pulmonary artery pressures every hour.	Provides information as to fluid status and heart pressures. PA systolic pressures represent RV pressures with normals ranging from 20-30 mmHg. PA diastolic pressures reflects the LVEDP and is an indirect measurement of LV function with normals ranging 10-20 mmHg. PCWP reflects the LA pressure and is used to assess LV filling pressures with normals ranging from 4-12 mmHg.
Measure cardiac output/cardiac index and perform hemodynamic measurements every 1-4 hours.	Directly measures the volume of cardiac output in L/min, and gives calculated information regarding preload and afterload. Normal CO should range from 4-8 L/min and CI from 2.5-4 L/min/m^2. SVR which represents afterload should range between 900-1400 dynes/sec/cm^5.
Monitor for malfunction of IAB and IABP and correct problems rapidly. Manually flutter IAB prn pump failure.	Improper timing of balloon can promote complications and worsen condition. Early inflation leads to regurgitation into the left ventricle or premature closing of the valve, and increases afterload. Late inflation decreases augmentation and reduces coronary perfusion. Early deflation allows the pressure to rise to normal end-diastolic levels preceding systole which does not reduce af-

INTERVENTIONS	RATIONALES
	terload. Late deflation encroaches on the next systole and increases afterload. IAB cannot be left in patient longer than 30 minutes without movement of balloon due to thrombus formation on the IAB.
Provide adequate amounts of gas (CO_2 or helium) in IAB; refill IAB every 2 hours or more often if fever present.	Underinflation of IAB can result in subtherapeutic effects from minimizing blood displacement. Increased body temperature increases the normal loss of gas from the balloon.
Notify MD if augmentation cannot be maintained, afterload is not reduced, or if reddish-brown fluid noted in tubing of IAB.	Signals problems with catheter pump, or patient requiring immediate attention. Discoloration in IAB tubing signifies that a fracture in the catheter has occurred and the fluid is actually blood. At this point, prepare for removal of the catheter.
Determine level of consciousness, mental changes, neurological deficits.	Mental changes will result as tissue perfusion to brain decreases.
Monitor urine output every hour. Notify MD if < 30 cc/hr, or > 200 cc/hr in the absence of diuretics or fluid challenge.	Low cardiac output will cause decreased tissue perfusion to kidneys and oliguria. Migration of the IAB can partially or totally occlude the renal arteries leading to oliguria or anuria. Increased urine may indicate problems with other body systems, such as SIADH.
Monitor presence and equality of peripheral pulses, extremity color, temperature, and sensations. Notify MD of problems.	Decreased or absent pulses may indicate migration of IAB and possible occlusion of arteries.
Elevate head of bed no more than 30 degrees. Do not flex involved leg.	Flexion greater than this may cause catheter to kink and fracture.
Assist with ROM to uninvolved leg as needed, and with flexion/extension of involved foot.	Reduces complications from immobility.

INTERVENTIONS	RATIONALES
Monitor general chemistry, renal profile, and CBC.	Provides information about potential blood loss and infection; chemistry profiles provide information about impending hepatic or renal insufficiency.

Information, Instruction, Demonstration

INTERVENTIONS	RATIONALES
Instruct patient/family on procedure, benefits, risks, post-procedure care.	Provides knowledge and allows patient to make an informed choice.
Instruct/demonstrate ROM to uninvolved leg, and flexion/extension to foot of involved leg.	Provides activity as tolerated while on IABP.
Prepare patient/family for placement on IABP, post-procedure care.	IABP may be necessary to increase cardiac output, and decrease afterload and preload in order to decrease the workload on the damaged heart.

Discharge or Maintenance Evaluation

- Patient/family will be able to verbalize correct information regarding care, risks, and benefits.

- Patient will have optimum perfusion to all body systems.

- Cardiac output will be within normal limits.

- Patient will be able to accurately demonstrate exercises.

- Patient will report no episodes of chest pain or shortness of breath.

- Hemodynamic parameters and vital signs will be within normal limits.

- Lung sounds will be clear and free of adventitious breath sounds with optimal oxygenation.

- Urinary output will be within normal limits.

- Minimal activity will be tolerated without shortness of breath or extreme fatigue.

- Medications will be administered with no undesirable effects.

Risk for infection

Related to: invasive lines, catheters, puncture wounds, invasive procedures, environmental exposure from devices left in place for extended periods of time

Defining characteristics: disruption of skin surfaces, redness, drainage, elevated temperature

Outcome Criteria

Patient will be free of infection with no fever or chills.

All invasive lines will be free of erythema, edema, and drainage.

INTERVENTIONS	RATIONALES
Inspect all invasive lines for signs of infection and/or bleeding.	Invasive lines provide entry route for pathogens.
Change site dressing using sterile technique every day. Notify MD for signs of infection.	Insertion site provides a direct route for infection, and must be monitored to prevent complications.
Monitor temperature every 2-4 hours. Obtain cultures of urine, sputum, and blood for evaluation as warranted.	Sudden temperature increases may indicate infective process. Cultures can isolate the specific pathogen so as to enable specific antibiotic therapy to be ordered.
Change IV tubing/arterial line tubing per protocol, using aseptic technique. Change peripheral lines every 3 days and prn.	Decreases the incidence of infection. Bacteria begins to grow within 24 hours in IV solution. Replacement of IV lines prevents phlebitis and risks of infective complications.

Instruction, Information, Demonstration

INTERVENTIONS	RATIONALES
Inform patient of need for changing peripheral lines, solutions, and care to sites.	Facilitates knowledge and patient comprehension and compliance with treatment.
Instruct patient to notify nurse for pain to invasive sites, or other symptoms of infection.	May indicate infection.

Discharge or Maintenance Evaluation

- Patient will have no signs of infection to invasive line sites.

- Peripheral lines will be changed within 3 days to avoid risk of infection.

- Patient will have no signs of systemic infection.

Risk for fluid volume deficit

Related to: potential blood loss from oozing/draining sites of invasive lines

Defining characteristics: bleeding from puncture sites and wounds, actual blood loss as measured by hemoglobin/hematocrit, hypotension, tachycardia

Outcome Criteria

Patient will have no significant blood loss from invasive lines.

INTERVENTIONS	RATIONALES
Measure all sources of intake and output.	Provides information to evaluate fluid status.
Weigh daily.	Weight gain over 24 hours usually indicates fluid gain. Fluid imbalance can be approximated as 1 lb = 500 cc fluid.
Monitor vital signs and hemodynamic pressures.	Tachycardia, hypotension, and changes in hemodynamics may indicate volume depletion.

INTERVENTIONS	RATIONALES
Test all body fluids for presence of occult blood.	Anticoagulation may place patient at risk for bleeding.
Monitor insertion site for bleeding, hemorrhage, or hematoma. Apply pressure dressing if warranted, and notify MD for sustained bleeding from site.	Bleeding tendencies are increased due to concomitent use of systemic anticoagulants and patient is at risk for bleeding.
Monitor PT, PTT, platelets, and CBC.	PT, PTT, and platelets provide information about coagulation; CBC provides information about potential blood loss.
Administer IV solutions and volume expanders as indicated.	IV solutions and volume expanders may be required to treat rapidly decreasing circulating volume due to exsanguination.
Administer packed RBCs, blood, or platelets as warranted.	Hemorrhagic volume losses may be life-threatening. Replacement of platelets may be necessary to provide normal coagulation.
Administer vitamin K or protamine sulfate if warranted.	May be required to return coagulation times to normal or reverse effects of heparin.

Instruction, Information, Demonstration

INTERVENTIONS	RATIONALES
Instruct patient to report any noted bleeding or oozing on body.	Prompt observation of complications can result in prompt treatment.
Instruct patient to avoid any activity that may promote bleeding.	Prevents accidental injury and decreases chance of hemorrhage.

Discharge or Maintenance Evaluation

• Patient will be able to verbalize signs/symptoms of bleeding to report.

• Patient will be compliant in avoidance of safety concerns.

• Patient will have stable hemodynamic status with no over hemorrhage from any site.

Pacemakers

Artificial cardiac pacemakers are used to provide an electrical stimulus to depolarize the heart and cause a contraction to occur at a controlled rate. The function of the pacemaker, or pacer, is to maintain the heart rate when the patient's own intrinsic system is unable to do so. The stimulus is produced by a pulse generator and delivered via electrodes/leads that are implanted in the epicardium or endocardium. The electrodes may be unipolar or bipolar and the proximal end attaches to the pulse generator. In the unipolar electrode, one wire, positioned in the heart, senses and stimulates the electrical heart activity and is connected with the negative terminal on the pulse generator. The other electrode, or ground, is attached to the positive terminal on the pulse generator. This type of lead usually requires a lower threshold of stimulation. The bipolar electrode has both the sensing and ground electrode in the catheter, and provides better contact with the heart muscle. In the event that one of the bipolar wires malfunctions, it can still be used as a unipolar lead. The pacemaker will produce a pacer spike on the EKG prior to the depolarized waveform and this indicates pacemaker capture. Continuous observation for problems with the pacemaker should be performed to ensure that failure to pace, failure to capture, and failure to sense are treated promptly.

The pacemaker rate is set depending on the patient's requirements. The optimal setting is one in which the lowest rate that controls the particular dysrhythmia and provides for adequate cardiac output. The stimulation threshold is the minimal amount of electrical energy required to stimulate the heart to produce a 1:1 capture, and is measured in milliamperes (mA). The sensitivity control reflects the size of the wave that is sensed by the pacemaker and is measured in millivolts (mV), with the smaller number relating to the most sensitivity. Pacemakers are used for varying degrees of heart block, sick sinus syndrome, sinus node dysfunction, overriding of some cardiac dysrhythmias, prophylactically during diagnostic testing, myocardial infarctions, congestive heart failure due to rhythm disturbances, after open heart surgery or in congenital anomalies of the heart.

Temporary pacers are used when the duration of need is short and permanent pacers are placed for life-long use. Temporary pacemakers can be placed via a transthoracic approach during open heart surgery, transvenous approach into the right atrium or right ventricle, or transcutaneously (external pacer) with skin electrodes while awaiting placement of an internal pacemaker.

Placement of the temporary pacemaker can be performed at the bedside in cases of emergency, but use of fluoroscopy is recommended when feasible to ensure proper placement. External pacemaker electrodes can either be placed on the chest, or one to the anterior and one posterior to the chest.

Synchronous pacing, known as demand pacing, is commonly used because the pacer is able to sense the patient's heart impulse. If the patient's rate falls below the rate set on the pacer, the pacer is able to sense this and send an impulse to the desired chamber of the heart and cause the rate to remain at the preset level. Dual chamber synchronous pacing, or AV sequential, is the closest to normal physiologic function and facilitates the atrial kick.

Asynchronous, or fixed-rate, pacing provides impulses to the atrium, ventricle, or both regardless of the patient's intrinsic rate. This should be used solely for those occasions when no electrical activity is present to avoid potential lethal competitive dysrhythmias.

Pacemakers are classified by a 5-letter code developed by the Inter-Society Commission for Heart Disease in which letters are used to denote the chamber paced, the chamber sensed, response to sensing, programmable functions and antitachy-dysrhythmia functions.

Several complications may occur as a result of pacemakers—pneumothorax, hemothorax, myocardial perforation, hematoma, bleeding, dysrhythmias, pulmonary embolism, electrical microshock, cardiac tamponade, coronary artery laceration, failure to pace, failure to sense, and failure to capture.

MEDICAL CARE

Chest x-ray: used to evaluate placement of lead wires

Electrocardiography: used to monitor for heart rhythm problems, dysrhythmias, and for function/malfunction of pacemakers

Surgery: for placement of permanent pacemakers

NURSING CARE PLANS

Alteration in tissue perfusion: cardiopulmonary, cerebral

Related to: cardiac dysrhythmias, heart blocks, tachydysrhythmias, decreased blood pressure, decreased cardiac output

Defining characteristics: decreased blood pressure, decreased heart rate, decreased cardiac output, changes in level of consciousness, mental changes, cold clammy skin, cardiopulmonary arrest

Outcome Criteria

Patient will be free of dysrhythmias with adequate cardiac output to perfuse all body organs.

INTERVENTIONS	RATIONALES
Monitor EKG for changes in rhythm, rate, and presence of dysrhythmias. Treat as indicated.	Observation for pacemaker malfunction promotes prompt treatment. Pacer electrodes may irritate ventricle and promote ventricular ectopy.
Keep monitor alarms on at all times, with rate limits set 2-5 beats above and below set rate.	Provides for immediate detection of pacemaker failure or malfunction.
Obtain and observe rhythm strip every 4 hours and prn. Notify MD for abnormalities.	Identifies proper functioning of pacemaker, with appropriate capture and sensing.
Monitor vital signs every 15 minutes until stable, then every 2 hours.	Assures adequate perfusion and cardiac output.
Monitor for signs of failure to capture and correct problem.	Potential causes are low voltage, battery failure, faulty connections, catheter or wire fracture, improper placement of catheter, or fibrosis at tip of catheter.
Monitor for signs of failure to sense patient's own rhythm and correct problem.	Potential causes are lead dislodgment, battery failure, low sensitivity, catheter wire fracture, or improper placement of catheter.
Monitor for signs of failure to pace and correct problem.	Potential causes are battery failure, lead dislodgment, disconnection, or catheter lead fracture.
Ensure that all electrical equipment is grounded. Avoid touching equipment and patient at same time. Patients should not use radios, shavers, etc.	Prevents potential for microshock and accidental electrocution. Electric current seeks the path of least resistance, and the potential for stray current to travel through the electrode into the patient's heart may precipitate ventricular fibrillation.

INTERVENTIONS	RATIONALES
Place a dry rubber glove over exposed terminals or leads. Wear rubber gloves when handling the electrodes, terminals, etc.	Provides insulation to prevent stray current contact. Static electricity may pass from person to person through the leads.
Pacemaker batteries should not be changed while the pacer is in use. In cases of hardship, batteries should be changed as quickly as possible, wearing rubber gloves, and using utmost caution to avoid touching the battery terminals.	Patients may be totally dependent on the pacemaker for their rhythm and cardiac output and loss of time incurred to change the battery may result in life-threatening consequences.
Monitor for muscle twitching or hiccoughs.	May indicate lead has dislodged and migrated to chest wall or diaphragm after perforation of heart.
Monitor for sudden complaints of chest pain, and auscultate for pericardial friction rub or muffled heart tones. Observe for JVD and pulsus paradoxus.	May indicate perforation of the pericardial sac, and impending cardiac tamponade.
Monitor for dizziness, syncope, weakness, pronounced fatigue, edema, chest pain, palpitations, pulsations in neck veins, or dyspnea.	During ventricular pacing, AV synchrony may cease and cause a sudden decrease in cardiac output. May indicate "pacemaker syndrome" or failure of the pacer to function which results in decreased perfusion.
Limit movement of the extremity involved near insertion site.	Prevents accidental disconnection and dislodgment of lead wires.
If pacemaker is used concurrently with pulmonary artery catheter obtain wedge pressure only as MD orders.	Inflation of pulmonary artery catheter balloon for capillary wedge pressures may dislodge pacer lead wires and cause pacemaker malfunction.
Monitor patient for low blood sugar levels, use of glucocorticoids or sympathomimetics, mineralocorticoids, or anesthetics.	May impair the pacemaker stimulation thresholds.

INTERVENTIONS	RATIONALES
Protect patient from microwave ovens, radar, diathermy, electrocautery, TENS units, etc.	Environmental electromagnetic interference may impair demand pacemaker function by disrupting the electrical stimulus.
If the patient experiences cardiopulmonary arrest, the pacemaker should be turned off and disconnected from the patient for ventricular fibrillation. After defibrillation, the pacemaker should be reconnected, turned on, and output should be raised to 20 mA, rate above 60.	Disconnection prior to DC countershock prevents pacer damage and potential of diversion of electrical current.

Information, Instruction, Demonstration

INTERVENTIONS	RATIONALES
Instruct on need for pacemaker, procedures involved, expected outcomes, etc.	Provides knowledge, decreases fear and anxiety, and provides baseline for further instruction.
Instruct in checking pulse rate every day for 1 month, then every week, and to notify MD if rate varies more than 5 beats/minute.	Provides patient with some control over situation. Assists in promoting a sense of security. Allows for prompt recognition of deviations from preset rate and potential pacemaker failure.
Instruct on activity limitations: avoid excessive bending, stretching, lifting more than 5 pounds, strenuous activities, or contact sports.	Full range of motion can be recovered in approximately 2 months after fibrosis stabilizes the pacemaker lead. Excessive activity may cause lead dislodgment.
Instruct to avoid shoulder-strap purses, suspenders, or firing rifle resting over generator site.	May promote irritation over implanted generator site.
Instruct to wear a medic-alert bracelet with information about the type of pacemaker and rate.	Provides information about the patient, his condition, and pacemaker should he be incapacitated and cannot speak for himself.

INTERVENTIONS	RATIONALES
Instruct to notify MD if radiation therapy is needed and to wear a lead shield.	Therapy can cause failure of the silicone chip in the pacer with repeated radiation.
Instruct to avoid electromagnetic fields, magnetic resonance imaging, radio transmitters, arc welding equipment, large running motors, or large ungrounded power tools. If patient notices dizziness or palpitations, he should try to move away from the area, and if symptoms persist, to seek medical attention. Late model microwave ovens are no longer thought to be a threat due to tighter seals preventing leakage of energy.	May affect the function of the pacemaker and alter the programmed settings. Sometimes these magnetic fields will affect the pacemaker function only if direct contact is made and once distance is placed between the patient and the equipment, normal function of the pacemaker resumes. If programmed settings are altered the pacer will require reprogramming. Hyperbaric oxygen chambers may also affect pacer function.

Discharge or Maintenance Evaluation

• Patient will be free of dysrhythmias and able to maintain cardiac output within normal limits.

• Patient will be able to recall accurately all instructions given.

• Patient will be able to recall and adhere to all activity restrictions.

• Permanent pacemaker function will be without complication, with no lead dislodgment or competitive rhythms noted.

Alteration in skin integrity

Related to: insertion of temporary or permanent pacemaker, alteration in activity

Defining characteristics: disruption of skin tissue, insertion sites

Outcome Criteria

Patient will have healed wound sites without signs/symptoms of infection.

INTERVENTIONS	RATIONALES
Inspect pacemaker insertion site for erythema, edema, warmth, drainage, or tenderness.	Prompt detection of problems promotes prompt treatment.
Change dressing daily, or per hospital protocol, using sterile technique.	Allows for observation of site and detection of inflammation or infection. Sterile technique is recommended due to the close proximity of the portal to the heart increasing the potential for systemic infection.
Pacemaker lead wires should be coiled and taped securely to patient; pulse generator should be secured to avoid pulling.	Avoids potential for accidentally disconnecting pacemaker from generator, or dislodging leads from heart.

Information, Instruction, Demonstration

INTERVENTIONS	RATIONALES
Instruct on wound care to pacer site; to avoid taking showers for 2 weeks after pacer insertion.	Promotes compliance with care to decrease potential for infection. Moisture can promote bacterial growth.
Instruct to observe for and report to MD the following symptoms: redness, drainage, temperature greater than 100 degrees, pain or tenderness to site, or swelling at site.	Provides for prompt recognition of complications and facilitates prompt treatment.
Instruct to avoid constrictive clothing until site has healed.	May cause discomfort at incision site from pressure and rubbing against skin.
Instruct on need for pacemaker removal/replacement.	Pulse generators may require removal for battery replacement, fracture of lead wires, pacemaker failure, etc.

Discharge or Maintenance Evaluation

- Patient will have well-healed incision with no signs/symptoms of infection.

- Patient will be able to recall accurately all instructions given.

- Patient will be able to demonstrate appropriate wound care prior to discharge.

Potential for injury

Related to: pacemaker failure, hemothorax or pneumothorax after insertion, bleeding, lead migration, heart perforation

Defining characteristics: decreased cardiac output, hemorrhage, diaphoresis, hypotension, restlessness, dyspnea, cyanosis, chest pain, muscle twitching, hiccoughs, muffled heart sounds, jugular vein distention, pulsus paradoxus

Outcome Criteria

Patient will be free of any complications that may be associated with pacemaker insertion.

INTERVENTIONS	RATIONALES
Monitor for bleeding at pacer site. Apply pressure dressings as warranted.	Bleeding at incisional site may occur based on the patient's coagulation status. Pressure dressings or manual pressure may be required to control bleeding.
Monitor for pulse presence at site distal to pacer insertion.	Hemorrhage may promote tissue edema and compression to arterial blood flow resulting in diminished or absent pulses.
Monitor for hypotension, diaphoresis, dyspnea, and restlessness.	May indicate puncture of the subclavian vasculature and potential hemothorax.

INTERVENTIONS	RATIONALES
Monitor for dyspnea, chest pain, pallor, cyanosis, absent or diminished breath sounds, tracheal deviation, and feeling of impending doom.	May indicate puncture of the lung and pneumothorax.
Monitor for muscle twitching and hiccoughs. Notify MD.	May indicate perforation of the heart with pacing to the chest wall or diaphragm.
Observe for signs/symptoms of cardiac tamponade—pericardial friction rub, pulsus paradoxus, muffled heart tones, JVD.	May indicate perforation of the pericardial sac and impending cardiac tamponade.

Discharge or Maintenance Evaluation

- Patient will have no complications associated with pacemaker insertion.

- Patient will have clear breath sounds, with no inadequacy of oxygenation.

- Patient will be free of infection or hemorrhage.

Alteration in comfort
[See MI]

Related to: pacemaker insertion or transcutaneous pacing

Defining characteristics: communication of pain, facial grimacing, restlessness, changes in pulse and blood pressure

Anxiety
[See MI]

Related to: change in health status, fear of death, threat to body image, threat to role functioning, pain

Defining characteristics: restlessness, insomnia, anorexia, increased respirations, increased heart rate, increased blood pressure, difficulty concentrating, dry mouth, poor eye contact, decreased energy, irritability, crying, feelings of helplessness

Impaired physical mobility

Related to: pain, limb immobilization

Defining characteristics: inability to move as desired, imposed restrictions on activity, decreased muscle strength and coordination, limited range of motion

Outcome Criteria

Patient will regain optimal mobility within limitations of disease process, and will have increased strength and function of limbs.

INTERVENTIONS	RATIONALES
Evaluate patient's perception of degree of immobility.	Psychological and physical immobility are interrelated. Psychological immobility is used as a defense mechanism when they have no control over their body, and this can lead to disproportionate fear and concern. Changes in body image promote psychological immobility and may result in emotional handicaps.
Maintain bedrest for 24-48 hours after permanent pacer inserted.	Provides time for stabilization of leads and decreases potential for dislodgment.
Immobilize extremity proximal to pacer insertion site with arm board, sling, etc.	Prevents potential for dislodgment of lead due to movement.
Resume range of motion exercises 5 days after permanent pacer insertion to affected extremity. Provide ROM to unaffected extremity as warranted.	Promotes gradual increase of activity. Stretching should be avoided until lead wire has been secured in heart by fibrotic changes. ROM prevents stiffness of shoulders and joint immobility.
Encourage extension/dorsiflexion exercises to feet every 1-2 hours.	Promotes venous return, prevents venous stasis, and decreases potential for thrombophlebitis.

INTERVENTIONS	RATIONALES
Monitor for progression and improvement in stiffness/pain.	Physical therapy may be required if immobility results are severe.
Apply trapeze bar to bed.	Allows for easier movement by allowing patient to assist with movement in bed.
Reposition every 2 hours and prn.	Prevents potential for immobility hazards such as pressure areas and atelectasis.

Information, Instruction, Demonstration

INTERVENTIONS	RATIONALES
Encourage deep breathing exercises every 1-2 hours; avoid forceful coughing.	Facilitates lung expansion and decreases potential for atelectasis. Coughing may dislodge pacemaker lead.

Discharge or Maintenance Evaluation

• Patient will regain optimal mobility of all joints with no signs or symptoms of complications.

• Patient will be able to demonstrate and recall instructions regarding deep breathing and range of motion exercises.

Disturbance of body image

Related to: presence of pulse generator, loss of control of heart function, disease process

Defining characteristics: fear of rejection, fear of reaction from others, negative feelings about body, refusal to participate in care, refusal to look at wound

Outcome Criteria

Patient will accept change in body image and deal constructively with situation.

INTERVENTIONS	RATIONALES
Evaluate level of patient's knowledge about disease process, treatment, and anxiety.	May identify extent of problem and interventions that will be required.
Evaluate the extent of loss to the patient/family, and what it means to them.	Depending on the time frame for patient teaching prior to the insertion of the pacemaker, the patient may not have received adequate information, and may have difficulty dealing with changes in his body appearance as well as generalized health condition and loss of control.
Evaluate stage of grieving.	Provides recognition of appropriate versus inappropriate behavior. Prolonged grief may require further care.
Observe for withdrawal, manipulation, noninvolvement with care, or increased dependency. Set limits on dysfunctional behavior and help patient to seek positive behaviors that will assist with recovery.	May suggest problems with adjustment to health condition, grief response to the loss of function, or worry about others accepting patient's new body status. Patients may deal with crises in the same manner as previously dealt and may need redirection in behaviors to facilitate recovery and acceptance.
Provide positive reinforcement during care and with instruction and setting goals. Do not give false reassurance.	Promotes trust and establishes rapport with patient as well as provides an opportunity to plan for the future based on reality of situation.
Provide opportunity for patient to take active role in wound care.	Promotes self-esteem and facilitates feelings of control of body and health.
Provide reassurance that pacemaker will not alter sexual activity.	Promotes knowledge and decreases fear.

Information, Instruction, Demonstration

INTERVENTIONS	RATIONALES
Discuss potential for mood changes, anger, grief, etc. after discharge, and to seek help if persisting for lengthy time.	Facilitates identification that feelings are not unusual and must be recognized in order to effectively deal with them.
Identify support groups for patient/family to contact.	Provides ongoing support for patient and family and allows for ventilation of feelings.
Consult counselor/therapist as warranted.	May require further interventions to resolve emotional or psychological problems.

Discharge or Maintenance Evaluation

- Patient will be able to effectively deal with body image disturbances in present situation.

- Patient will be able to talk with family, therapist, or others about emotional or psychological problems.

- Patient will be able to problem-solve and identify short- and long-term goals within reasonable expectations of clinical situation.

Knowledge deficit
[See MI]

Related to: lack of understanding, lack of understanding of medical condition, lack of recall, new health crisis

Defining characteristics: questions regarding problems, inadequate follow-up on instructions given, misconceptions, lack of improvement of previous regimen, development of preventable complications

PACEMAKERS

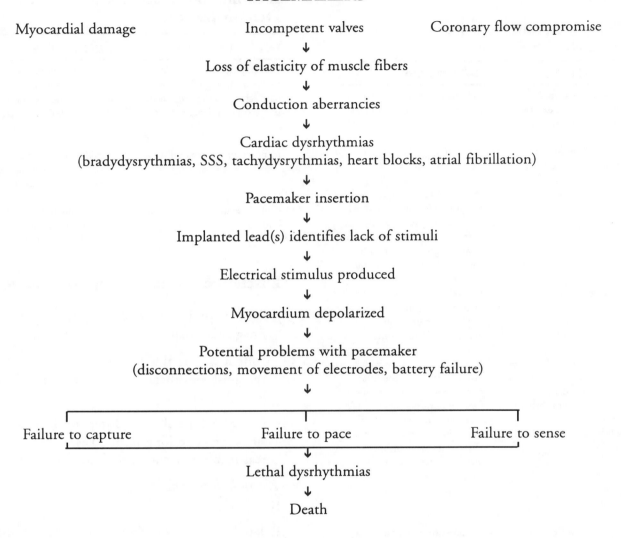

Myocardial damage   Incompetent valves   Coronary flow compromise
                                                  ↓
                              Loss of elasticity of muscle fibers
                                                  ↓
                                   Conduction aberrancies
                                                  ↓
                                   Cardiac dysrhythmias
(bradydysrythmias, SSS, tachydysrythmias, heart blocks, atrial fibrillation)
                                                  ↓
                                   Pacemaker insertion
                                                  ↓
                      Implanted lead(s) identifies lack of stimuli
                                                  ↓
                             Electrical stimulus produced
                                                  ↓
                             Myocardium depolarized
                                                  ↓
                        Potential problems with pacemaker
       (disconnections, movement of electrodes, battery failure)
                                                  ↓

Failure to capture   Failure to pace   Failure to sense
                                                  ↓
                             Lethal dysrhythmias
                                                  ↓
                                        Death

Cardiac Surgery

Coronary artery disease treatment requires the maximization of cardiac output and this can be accomplished by improvement in heart muscle function and increase of blood flow through coronary artery bypass grafting and/or valvular replacements. Open heart surgery is commonly performed for three-vessel disease, valve dysfunction and congenital heart defects and requires blood to be diverted from the heart and lungs to facilitate a bloodless operative field.

In coronary artery bypass graft (CABG) surgery, a graft from the arms or legs is anastomosed to the aorta with the distal portion to the involved coronary artery to bypass the diseased obstruction and supply adequate blood flow to the heart. The internal mammary artery is also being utilized for CABG surgery because the patency rate is 90-95% over a 5-10 year time period, and there are less problems with differences in lumen size since an artery is then anastomosed to an artery without the need for routing from the aorta. In valvular surgery, incompetent or leaking valves are replaced with prosthetic ones.

Not all patients with coronary artery disease are candidates for CABG surgery. It is usually recommended for those patients with intractable angina, signs of ischemia, or an increased risk of coronary ischemia/infarction as a result of angiographical studies. Complications may occur in almost every body system and may be a result of the disease process or defect, the surgery, or the use of cardiopulmonary bypass, and so the decision for surgery is a multi-faceted one.

One of the most important factors in the decision of candidacy for CABG surgery is the ejection fraction. This is the ratio of stroke volume compared to the end-diastolic volume and an ejection fraction greater than 55 reflects a good operative risk. Ejection fraction less than 25% is usually considered inoperable because of the high mortality associated with it.

The surgery is performed via a median sternotomy incision which provides exposure of the heart and avoids the pleural spaces. A cannula is placed in a vein and an artery and then attached to the cardiopulmonary bypass machine whereby the diverted blood is mechanically oxygenated and circulated to the other parts of the body. The machine, which is operated by a trained perfusionist, substitutes for left ventricular pumping and creates a blood-gas exchange. After the patient's body temperature has been cooled to around 86 degrees, the aorta is cross-clamped and a cold cardioplegic solution, usually containing dextrose, potassium, magnesium and inderal, is placed around the heart and injected into the coronary arteries. This causes an electromechanical arrest and provides an inert operative site. Cross-clamp durations longer than 3 hours usually result in severe complications for the patient. After the grafts have been completed or valves replaced, perfusion is slowly discontinued and cannulas are removed when arterial blood pressure and cardiac functioning are adequate. Two atrial and ventricular pacing wires are placed, as well as arterial lines, pulmonary artery catheter, left atrial line, and mediastinal or pleural chest tubes.

Common complications associated with CABG surgery include perioperative MI, vein graft closure, hemorrhage, blood trauma, complement activation, coagulation abnormalities, fluid shifts, increased catecholamine levels, fat emboli, microemboli, dysrhythmias, pericarditis, postpericardiotomy syndrome, embolism, pneumonia, atelectasis, hemothorax, pneumothorax, and post-cardiotomy delirium. Other complications that are seen less often include stress ulcer, renal failure, respiratory failure, cardiac tamponade, cardiogenic shock, endocarditis, gastrointestinal bleeding, mediastinitis, and paralytic ileus.

MEDICAL CARE

Pulmonary function studies: used to ascertain baseline pulmonary function

Laboratory: hemoglobin/hematocrit used to monitor oxygen-carrying capability, need for blood replacement, and to monitor for dehydration status; electrolytes used to monitor for imbalances which can affect cardiac function; BUN and creatinine used to monitor renal function; liver profile used to monitor liver function and perfusion; glucose used to monitor for presence of diabetes, nutritional alterations, or organ dysfunction; cardiac enzymes and isoenzymes used to monitor for presence of acute or perioperative myocardial infarction; coagulation profiles used to determine baseline and monitor for coagulation problems; antibody or complement levels used to monitor for postpericardiotomy syndrome or Dressler's syndrome; type and crossmatch for blood to have available blood products on hand in case of hemorrhage; ACT used to monitor heparinization

Arterial blood gases: used to monitor oxygenation and assess acid-base balance and ability to wean off mechanical ventilation

Electrocardiography: used to observe for changes in cardiac function, presence of conduction problems, dysrhythmias, or ischemic changes

Echocardiography: used to evaluate wall motion of the heart

Chest x-ray: used to identify heart size and position, pulmonary vasculature, pulmonary changes, verifies position of endotracheal tube, pacing wires, and hemodynamic catheters; monitors for barotrauma

Cardiac catheterization: used to evaluate abnormal pressures preop, to assess for pressure gradients across the valves, and to locate and measure coronary lesions

NURSING CARE PLANS

Risk for decreased cardiac output

Related to: myocardial depression, dysrhythmias, electrolyte imbalances, hypovolemia, hypervolemia, myocardial infarction, coronary artery spasm, vasoconstriction, impaired contractility, alteration in preload, alteration in afterload, hypoperfusion, microemboli, hypoxia, damaged myocardium, use of PEEP while on ventilatory support

Defining characteristics: elevated blood pressure, elevated mean arterial pressure greater than 120 mmHg, elevated systemic vascular resistance greater than 1400 dyne-seconds/cm^5, cardiac output less than 5 L/min or cardiac index less than 2.7 L/min/m^2, tachycardia greater than 110, cold, pale extremities, absent or decreased peripheral pulses, EKG changes, hypotension, S_3 or S_4 gallops, decreased urinary output, diaphoresis, orthopnea, dyspnea, crackles (rales), jugular vein distention, edema, chest pain

Outcome Criteria

Vital signs and hemodynamic parameters will be within normal limits for patient, with no dysrhythmias noted.

INTERVENTIONS	RATIONALES
Monitor vital signs, especially heart rate and blood pressure. Notify MD of abnormalities. Blood pressure should be taken/monitored every 15 minutes until stable, or every 5 minutes during active titration.	Tachycardia may occur as a response to pain, anxiety, blood and fluid deficit, and stress, but rates over 130 increases myocardial oxygen consumption and workload on the heart, decreasing cardiac output. Increased blood pressure may promote alterations in heart pressures and increase the risk of complications, as well as placing pressure on suture lines of new grafts. Hypotension may result from fluid deficit, dysrhythmias, and cardiac failure, as well as predispose peripheral vein grafts to close.
Evaluate hypotension that is not responsive to fluid bolus, tachycardia, and distant heart sounds.	May indicate cardiac tamponade in a heart that is unable to fill adequately to maintain cardiac output. Tamponade usually occurs immediately post-op but may occur later during recovery period.
Monitor hemodynamic pressures every 1 hour and prn. Maintain pressures with titration of vasoactive drugs per MD ordered parameters.	Assists with recognition of complications and allows for manipulation of cardiac pressures by use of fluids and medications. Vasoconstriction is the cause of elevated SVR, and with increases in SVR, may indicate left ventricular dysfunction. Cardiac output then becomes dependent on outflow resistance.
Measure cardiac output/cardiac index every 1-2 hours immediately post-op.	Cardiac output is a measurement that is equal to the product of the stroke volume and the heart rate. Cardiac indexes above 3.0 $L/min/m^2$ are usually adequate except in cases of septic shock. Adequate cardiac output relates to the adequacy of function of other body organs. After CABG surgery, most patients require an increase in CO to meet the stress imposed by the operation and the accompanying increase in oxygen consumption.

INTERVENTIONS	RATIONALES
Measure left atrial pressure and pulmonary artery wedge pressures.	Determines the left ventricular end-diastolic volume; increases in pressure may indicate congestive heart failure or pulmonary edema, and decreases may indicate low blood volume. Trends and changes in values are of more importance than single readings. Left ventricular dysfunction can elevate left heart filling pressures without a rise in right heart pressures.
Monitor urine output hourly and notify MD if less than 30 cc/hr.	Urine output is an indication of adequate cardiac output and renal perfusion.
Observe for decreased peripheral pulses, cool or cold moist skin, or cyanosis.	May indicate low cardiac output.
Monitor for changes in level of consciousness, mental status changes, restlessness, or confusion.	Cerebral perfusion is dependent on adequate cardiac output. Hypoperfusion or microemboli may result in CNS deficits.
Monitor for JVD, peripheral edema, and pulmonary congestion. Auscultate for crackles (rales).	May indicate present or impending congestive heart failure.
Observe for shortness of breath, decreases in oximetry, or dyspnea.	May indicate hypoxia and decreased cardiac output.
Monitor EKG for cardiac conduction disturbances, dysrhythmias, or changes in rate/rhythm.	Lethal dysrhythmias may occur as a result of electrolyte imbalances, myocardial ischemia or infarction, or problems with electrical conduction, with an associated drop in cardiac output.
Monitor for complaints of severe chest pain.	May indicate a perioperative or postoperative myocardial infarction.
Provide for uninterrupted rest periods and assist with care as needed.	Prevents fatigue and increased workload on the heart leading to decrease in cardiac output and perfusion.

INTERVENTIONS	RATIONALES
Administer IV fluids as ordered.	Maintains fluid status and hydration, as well as provides access for emergency medications.
Administer blood products as ordered.	Blood or packed red cells may be required to maintain adequate oxygen-carrying capability, and adequate circulating volume for cellular activity. Platelet function and count is decreased with use of cardiopulmonary bypass and proportional to the duration of bypass and depth of hypothermia during surgery.

Information, Instruction, Demonstration

INTERVENTIONS	RATIONALES
Attempt to reverse any contributing factor such as untreated DKA or endocrine dysfunction.	These may precipitate a low CO state.
Prepare patient for placement on IABP.	Promotes knowledge and decreases fear.

Discharge or Maintenance Evaluation

* Patient will have maximal cardiac output and stable hemodynamic pressures.

* Patient will have adequate perfusion of all body systems.

* Patient will be able to recall instructions correctly.

Alteration in comfort

Related to: mediastinal, leg, or arm incisions, myocardial infarction, angina, inflammation, tissue damage

Defining characteristics: communication of discomfort or pain, restlessness, irritability, increased heart rate, increased blood pressure

Outcome Criteria

Patient will be free of pain or pain will be controlled to patient's satisfaction.

INTERVENTIONS	RATIONALES
Evaluate complaints of pain—type, location, intensity based on 0-10 scale. Compare preoperative pain perceptions with postoperative pain.	Pain may be perceived in different ways by each individual and is important to differentiate incisional pain from other types of chest pain. CABG patients usually do not have severe discomfort to the chest incision but may have increased discomfort with donor site pain. Severe pain should be investigated for possibility of complications.
Monitor vital signs.	Heart rates usually increase with pain but bradycardia may occur especially in severely damaged myocardium. Blood pressure may be increased with incisional pain, but can also be labile or decreased when chest pain is severe or if myocardial ischemia/necrosis occurs.
Evaluate complaints of pain in legs or abdomen, or vague non-specific complaints, especially if associated with changes in mental status or vital signs.	May be indicative of development of thrombophlebitis, infection or GI dysfunction.
Monitor for complaints of pain and/or paresthesia to ulnar area of the hand, and possibly pain to shoulders and arms.	May result from stretching of the brachial plexus during positioning of the arms during surgery and generally resolves over time without specific treatment.
Observe for anxiety, irritability, crying, restlessness, or insomnia.	Nonverbal cues may indicate the presence of pain.
Administer analgesics as soon as discomfort is noticed, or prophylactically prior to painful procedures.	Pain results in muscle tension, which can decrease circulation and intensify pain perception. Medication given prior to procedures known to cause pain may facilitate cooperation with pro-

INTERVENTIONS	RATIONALES
	cedures and allow for easier chest movement with respiratory therapy.
Provide back rubs, position changes, and diversionary activities.	Promotes relaxation and helps to redirect attention away from discomfort, thereby reducing the amount of analgesic required.
Encourage deep breathing, visualization, or guided imagery.	Promotes decrease in stress and may reduce analgesic need.

Information, Instruction, Demonstration

INTERVENTIONS	RATIONALES
Instruct on methods to reduce strain on muscles when positioning.	Supporting extremities and the maintenance of good body alignment reduce muscle tension and provide comfort.

Discharge or Maintenance Evaluation

- Patient will be comfortable, pain-free, and be able to recall methods for stress reduction and pain control accurately.

- Patient will be able to identify differences between postoperative and preoperative chest pain.

- Patient will be able to maintain optimal body alignment and minimize muscle tension.

Risk for ineffective breathing pattern/impaired gas exchange

Related to: inadequate ventilation, ventilation/perfusion mismatching, abnormal ABGs, pain, blood loss, atelectasis, pneumothorax, hemothorax, increased pulmonary vascular resistance, increased capillary permeability, chemical mediators, decrease in surfactant

Defining characteristics: dyspnea, tachypnea, apnea, ventilation/perfusion mismatching, abnormal ABGs, pain, increased hemodynamic pressures, oxygen saturation less than 90%, adventitious breath sounds, hypoxia, hypoxemia

Outcome Criteria

Patient will be eupneic with clear breath sounds, and have no evidence of hypoxia/hypoxemia.

INTERVENTIONS	RATIONALES
Monitor respiratory rate and depth, presence of dyspnea, use of accessory muscles, nasal flaring, and increasing respiratory work effort.	Respiratory rates may be increased by pain, fever, blood loss, fluid loss, anxiety, hypoxia, or gastric distention. Decreases in rate may occur with use of narcotic analgesics. Prompt recognition of potential complications can promote prompt treatment.
Auscultate lung fields for diminished or absent breath sounds or for adventitious sounds.	Breath sounds are frequently diminished immediately post-op as a result of atelectasis. Loss of breath sounds in a previously ventilated lung may indicate a partial or total lung collapse, especially when chest tubes have recently been discontinued. Adventitious breath sounds may indicate fluid or secretions have accumulated in the interstitial spaces or airways resulting in a partial occlusion of the airway.
Evaluate chest expansion for symmetry.	Unilateral incomplete chest expansion may indicate that air or fluid is preventing complete expansion of the pleural space, possibly a pneumothorax.
Administer oxygen by cannula or mask as warranted.	Provides supplemental oxygen to decrease the workload on the heart and to maximize oxygen delivery to under-perfused tissues.

INTERVENTIONS	RATIONALES
Observe for pallor or cyanosis, especially to mucous membranes.	Cyanosis of lips, nailbeds, or earlobes, or generalized duskiness may indicate hypoxia as a result of heart failure or pulmonary dysfunction. Pallor is frequently noted immediately postoperatively due to blood loss or insufficient blood replacement.
Observe for presence of cough and sputum character.	Endotracheal tube intubation may promote throat irritation which can result in coughing, but cough may also indicate impending pulmonary congestion or infection. Purulent sputum may reflect pneumonia.
Encourage deep breathing exercises, inspiratory spirometer, or coughing exercises.	Promotes expansion/re-expansion of airways. Adventitious breath sounds may indicate presence of secretions or fluid in lungs.
Observe for signs of respiratory distress, tachycardia, extreme restlessness and feeling of impending doom.	May indicate impending pneumothorax or hemothorax, expecially after chest tube removal. May require reinsertion of chest tubes.
Monitor respiratory status and ventilatory settings every 1-2 hours while on ventilator.	CABG patients are placed on mechanical ventilation support until awake from anesthesia. FIO_2 is initially 100% and then gradually decreased, while maintaining an adequate PaO_2 above 90. FIO_2 should be decreased to .50 as rapidly as possible to prevent actual pulmonary changes that occur with high levels of oxygen. Tidal volumes are usually maintained between 10-15 cc/Kg of ideal body weight to allow for less interference with venous return.
Assist with weaning from ventilatory support. Monitor for hemodynamic instability and decreasing oxygen saturation. Monitor ABGs as ordered.	Weaning is usually performed by reducing the rate and then a trial on a T-bar or CPAP mode. Patients who have a history of smoking or COPD often have prolonged need for ventilatory sup-

INTERVENTIONS	RATIONALES
	port post-CABG due to their mechanism of breathing. Ventilators provide controlled amounts of oxygen and tidal volumes, and COPD patients have their inert drive to breathe removed by the use of ventilation. Occasionally with use of the cold cardioplegic solution, the phrenic nerve is injured resulting in a loss of function of the diaphragm which is necessary for 60% of the spontaneous tidal volume for the patient.
Suction patient every 2-4 hours and prn. Use pulmonary toilette and hyperoxygenate prior to and after suctioning.	Removes mucous that may occlude airways. Saline instillation helps to liquefy secretions to facilitate easier removal. Oxygen concentration drops drastically with suctioning procedures and leaves the patient compromised with an increased oxygen consumption.
Auscultate breath sounds pre- and post-suctioning.	Provides for comparison of breath sounds to evaluate for improvement. Occasionally, suctioning will move secretions up the bronchial tree and may cause a partial or total occlusion of an airway. Decreases in previously ventilated lung fields may indicate this phenomenon has occurred.
Monitor use of amiodarone and protamine sulfate. Observe for respiratory impingement.	Some drugs can exacerbate pulmonary problems by their method of action.

Information, Instruction, Demonstration

INTERVENTIONS	RATIONALES
Prepare patient for placement on mechanical ventilation if warranted.	Lengthy instruction may not be prudent or possible depending on the severity of the situation. If oxygenation cannot be maintained with the use of supplemental oxygen, the only alternative is intubation/ventilation.
Prepare patient for insertion of tracheostomy after 10 days of ETT intubation/ventilation.	Prolonged endotracheal intubation may result in tracheal or nasal necrosis or rupture of cuff. Tracheostomy is considered to prevent ulceration into arteries or other vital tissues, but may need to be avoided due to potential for contamination of sternotomy wound from secretions.
Instruct patient on need for ambulation, movement, change in position.	Promotes lung expansion and prevents pulmonary congestion.
Instruct on need for respiratory treatments, coughing, deep breathing.	Reassures patient that complying with aggressive pulmonary regimen will not cause injury to surgical sites.
Prepare patient for reinsertion of chest tubes as warranted.	Promotes re-expansion of lung by removing accumulated fluid, blood, or air, and restores normal negative pressure in the pleural cavity.

Discharge or Maintenance Evaluation

- Patient will be free of dyspnea with adequate ABGs and oxygenation, and without evidence of cyanosis or pallor.

- Patient will have clear breath sounds to all lung fields with no lung collapse.

- Patient will be compliant with respiratory regimen, and will be able to recall all instructions accurately.

Alteration in skin integrity

Related to: insertion of temporary or permanent pacemaker, alteration in activity, surgical incisions, puncture wounds, drains

Defining characteristics: disruption of skin tissue, insertion sites

Outcome Criteria

Patient will have healed wound sites without signs/symptoms of infection.

INTERVENTIONS	RATIONALES
Inspect pacemaker insertion site for erythema, edema, warmth, drainage, or tenderness.	Prompt detection of problems promotes prompt treatment.
Observe all incisions for healing and progress. Notify MD for incisional areas that are not healing, areas that have reopened or dehisced, edematous and erythematous tissues, bloody or purulent drainage, or hot painful areas.	Chest incisions usually heal first due to minimal amounts of muscle tissue involved. Donor sites have more muscle tissue, usually are more lengthy incisions and have poorer circulation thereby requiring a longer healing process. Signs may indicate a failure to heal, or the development of complications that require further intervention.
Culture drainage from wound as warranted.	Identifies causative organism that may result in local or systemic infection, and allows for identification of suitable antimicrobial therapy.
Change dressings daily, or per hospital protocol, using sterile technique.	Allows for observation of site and detection of inflammation or infection. Sterile technique is recommended due to the close proximity of the portal to the heart increasing the potential for systemic infection.

INTERVENTIONS	RATIONALES
Utilize steri-strips to support incisions when sutures are removed.	Maintains approximation of healing wound edges to facilitate healing of skin tissues.
Provide adequate nutritional and fluid intake.	Maintains adequate circulating volume, assists to meet energy requirements to facilitate tissue healing and perfusion.

Information, Instruction, Demonstration

INTERVENTIONS	RATIONALES
Instruct on wound care to wound sites.	Promotes compliance with care to decrease potential for infection. Moisture can promote bacterial growth.
Instruct to observe for and report to MD the following symptoms: redness, drainage, temperature greater than 100 degrees, pain or tenderness to site, or swelling at site.	Provides for prompt recognition of complications and facilitates prompt treatment.
Instruct to avoid constrictive clothing until site has healed.	May cause discomfort at incision site from pressure and rubbing against skin.
Instruct to avoid tub baths until allowed by MD.	Effort needed to get in and out of tub requires use of pectoral and arm muscles which may contribute to placing undue stress on suture lines of sternotomy.

Discharge or Maintenance Evaluation

- Patient will have well-healed incision with no signs/symptoms of infection.

- Patient will be able to recall accurately all instructions given.

- Patient will be able to demonstrate appropriate wound care prior to discharge.

Potential for injury
[See Pacemakers]

Related to: pacemaker failure, hemothorax or pneumothorax after insertion, bleeding, lead migration, heart perforation

Defining characteristics: decreased cardiac output, hemorrhage, diaphoresis, hypotension, restlessness, dyspnea, cyanosis, chest pain, muscle twitching, hiccoughs, muffled heart sounds, jugular vein distention, pulsus paradoxus

Anxiety
[See MI]

Related to: change in health status, fear of death, threat to body image, threat to role functioning, pain

Defining characteristics: restlessness, insomnia, anorexia, increased respirations, increased heart rate, increased blood pressure, difficulty concentrating, dry mouth, poor eye contact, decreased energy, irritability, crying, feelings of helplessness

Knowledge deficit
[See MI]

Related to: lack of understanding, lack of understanding of medical condition, lack of recall

Defining characteristics: questions regarding problems, inadequate follow-up on instructions given, misconceptions, lack of improvement of previous regimen, development of preventable complications

Impaired physical mobility
[See Pacemakers]

Related to: pain, limb immobilization

Defining characteristics: inability to move as desired, imposed restrictions on activity, decreased muscle strength and coordination, limited range of motion

Disturbance of body image
[See Pacemakers]

Related to: presence of pulse generator, loss of control of heart function, disease process, presence of scars/wounds

Defining characteristics: fear of rejection, fear of reaction from others, negative feelings about body, refusal to participate in care, refusal to look at wound

Aortic Aneurysm

An aneurysm is a localized dilation of an artery that may occur as a congenital anomaly or as a result of arteriosclerosis and high blood pressure. There are three types of aneurysms found—saccular in which the vessel distention protrudes from one side; fusiform in which the distention involves the entire circumference of the vessel; and dissecting in which a tear occurs in the intimal layer of the artery and with pressure, blood splits the wall producing a hematoma that separates the medial layers of the aortic wall. In dissecting aneurysms, generally the separation of the layers does not completely encircle the lumen but may run the entire length of the vessel.

Factors that may precipitate aneurysm formation include atherosclerosis, hypertension, syphilis, Marfan's syndrome, cystic medial necrosis, trauma, congenital abnormalities, and pregnancy.

Aneurysms that result from Marfan's syndrome usually involve the first portion of the aorta, and result in aortic insufficiency. Syphilitic aneurysms usually occur in the ascending thoracic aorta.

Abdominal aortic aneurysms (AAA) usually involve that part of the aorta between the renal and iliac arteries, and thoracic aortic aneurysms (TAA) occur mainly in the ascending, transverse or descending aorta with a prevalence toward men between 60 and 70 years of age. Mycotic aneurysms occur as a result of weakness in the vessel from an infective process, such as endocarditis, and usually involve the peripheral arteries, but have been known to affect the aorta.

AAA as a result of arteriosclerosis may be asymptomatic until they become large enough to palpate, large enough to cause pressure and pain, or until leaking or rupture occurs. Frequently, rupture of the AAA leads to vascular collapse and shock, and ultimately, death if not treated.

The goal for treatment is to remove or repair the aneurysm and restore vascular circulation. Aneurysms are generally monitored until their size reaches 6 cm or greater, and then surgical intervention is indicated to prevent complications such as rupture, stroke, or organ ischemia. Dacron grafts are used to help establish blood flow.

MEDICAL CARE

Oxygen: to increase available oxygen supply

Electrocardiography: used to monitor heart rhythm and rate for changes associated with decreases in perfusion, dysrhythmias, and for signs of left ventricular hypertrophy

Chest x-ray: used to observe for increase in aortic diameter, right tracheal deviation, and pleural effusions

Abdominal x-ray: used to visualize aneurysm

CT scans: used to visualize vessel wall thickness, lumen size, length of the aneurysm, and any mural thrombi

Angio-aortography: used to visualize lumen, extent of disease, extent of collateral circulation, arteriovenous fistulas, extent of dissection, and double lumens

Ultrasound: used to visualize the vessels and aneurysm non-invasively, amount of blood flow, and velocity of blood flow

Laboratory: CBC used to monitor for decreases in hemoglobin and hematocrit and for increases in leukocytes; BUN and creatinine used to monitor for renal dysfunction; urinalysis used to monitor hematuria and proteinuria to detect renal compromise

Surgery: necessary to replace aneurysm with dacron graft and/or repair the aneurysm

NURSING CARE PLANS

Alteration in tissue perfusion: cardiopulmonary, cerebral, gastrointestinal, peripheral, renal

Related to: arterial occlusion, aneurysm, dissecting aneurysm, or operative complications

Defining characteristics: pulsating mass, bruits, thrills, abdominal pain, low back pain, nausea/vomiting, syncope, chest pain, cough, hoarseness, dysphagia, dyspnea, shortness of breath, pallor, loss of pulses, paresthesias, paralysis

Outcome Criteria

Patient will achieve and maintain hemodynamic stability, with all body systems adequately perfused, and in the absence of pain.

INTERVENTIONS	RATIONALES
Monitor blood pressure in upper and lower extremities.	Normally systolic BP in thigh is greater than in the arm, but is reversed much of the time with abdominal aneurysms.
Monitor other vital signs and hemodynamic parameters.	Hypertension may exacerbate cardiac and peripheral perfusion instability.
Monitor pulses in both wrists as well as in both legs.	Pulse differences may be noted between wrists and between legs if the aneurysm interferes with circulation to that particular extremity.
Observe for the 5 P's—pain to extremity, pallor, pulselessness, paresthesia, and paralysis. Notify MD.	These may be associated with thrombosis of the AAA.

INTERVENTIONS	RATIONALES
Monitor for pain especially onset of sudden sharp pain, and notify MD.	Abrupt severe tearing pain in chest radiating to shoulders, neck, back, and abdomen is indicative of aortic dissection and requires prompt intervention. Low back pain may indicate impending rupture.
Observe for dysphagia.	Aneurysm may exert pressure on esophagus.
Observe for voice weakness, hoarseness, paroxysmal cough, or dyspnea.	Aneurysm may exert pressure on laryngeal nerve or on the trachea.
Auscultate for bruits over arteries; observe and palpate gently for thrill over abdomen. Auscultate for cardiac murmurs.	Indicates diminished blood flow indicative of aneurysm. A large aneurysm will have a palpable mass and thrill. An aortic murmur will be present if the aneurysm involves the aortic ring.
Administer antihypertensives as ordered to maintain BP within acceptible parameters.	Hypertension may exacerbate decreased tissue perfusion and compromise cardiovascular status.
Prepare patient for surgery as indicated.	Surgical intervention may be mandatory if circulation is compromised.

Information, Instruction, Demonstration

INTERVENTIONS	RATIONALES
Instruct on disease process, need for surgery, postoperative care.	Reduces anxiety and promotes knowledge and compliance.
Monitor vital signs and hemodynamic parameters. Maintain blood pressure at MD-ordered parameters.	Hypertension may exacerbate bleeding due to pressure on suture lines, and hypotension may not provide enough blood flow to keep graft open. Hypotension, tachycardia, and decreased hemodynamic pressures may indicate hypovolemia or hemorrhage.

INTERVENTIONS	RATIONALES
Auscultate lung fields for adventitious breath sounds. Assist patient with cough, deep breathing exercises, incentive spirometry.	Bedrest promotes atelectasis and decreased lung expansion which may lead to pneumonia.
Monitor oxygen saturation by oximetry. Administer oxygen as ordered.	Maintenance of adequate oxygenation necessary for adequate tissue perfusion.
Monitor peripheral pulses every hour for 24 hours, then every 4 hours, for color, temperature, capillary refill, and presence of pulses. Notify MD if absent.	Pulselessness indicates decreased or no blood flow. Occlusion of peripheral arteries leads to ischemia and necrosis.
Measure circumference of abdomen or legs and notify MD of significant changes.	Significant differences between extremities or from day to day may indicate hemorrhage.
Monitor EKG for changes and dysrhythmias.	Decreases in tissue perfusion may cause cardiac decompensation, MIs, and dysrhythmias.
Monitor I&O every hour and notify MD if < 30 cc/hr.	Surgical procedures may result in decreased renal blood flow due to length of cross clamp time during aneurysm repair.
Do not elevate head of bed > 30-45 degrees.	Higher flexion may cause flexion at femoral artery site and may impede blood flow.
Auscultate abdomen for bowel sounds. Monitor NG aspirate for amount and characteristics.	Most major thoracoabdominal surgical patients develop an ileus and require decompression of bowel with nasogastric tube.
Monitor patient for diarrheal stools and notify MD.	May indicate bowel ischemia due to length of surgical procedure and decreased perfusion to gut.
Observe for mental changes, confusion, restlessness, and headache.	May be due to repair of ascending and thoracic aortic aneurysms.

Discharge or Maintenance Evaluation

- Patient will have stable vital signs and hemodynamic pressures.

- Patient will be pain free.

- Patient will be alert, oriented, and able to verbalize instructions accurately.

- Patient will have adequate perfusion to all body systems.

- Lung fields will be clear and patient eupneic.

Alteration in comfort

Related to: pressure exerted on various structures by aneurysm, infringement on nerves, surgical procedures

Defining characteristics: pain to abdomen, lower back, hips, scrotum, chest, shoulders, neck, and back; nausea/vomiting, increases in blood pressure, increased heart rate, facial grimacing, moaning, shortness of breath

Outcome Criteria

Patient will be free of pain, with no associated deviations of vital signs.

INTERVENTIONS	RATIONALES
Monitor vital signs, and notify MD for unstable vital signs that do not change with analgesia.	Pain may increase heart rate, increase blood pressure or decrease blood pressure, but instability may occur from a variety of other causes.
Assess for dull abdominal pain, lower backache, lower back pain.	May indicate impending rupture of abdominal aortic aneurysm.
Assess for sudden severe pain to abdomen that may radiate to back, hips, or scrotum, and is associated with nausea, vomiting, and hypotension.	May indicate aortic dissection or rupture of AAA and requires immediate surgical intervention. MI should also be ruled out.

INTERVENTIONS	RATIONALES
Assess for sudden tearing-type of pain to chest that may radiate to shoulders, neck, and back.	May indicate thoracic aortic aneurysm.
Observe for difficulty in swallowing or talking. Assess for voice hoarseness or cough. Observe for shortness of breath.	May indicate that aneurysm is placing pressure against esophagus, laryngeal nerve, or trachea.
Assess for pain to extremities, with mottling/cyanosis/pallor, pulselessness, or paralysis.	May indicate claudication of peripheral arteries as a result of enlarged aneurysm placing pressure on vasculature. Paralysis may indicate acute thrombosis of the AAA.
Assess for complaints of pain that are vague or involve unrelated areas of body.	May be an early sign of impending complications, such as thrombophlebitis or ulcer.
Administer analgesics as ordered. Medicate prior to painful procedures as warranted.	Provides pain relief/reduction, decreases anxiety, and reduces the workload on the heart and vasculature. Comfort and cooperation with painful procedures may be enhanced by prior medication administration.
Maintain bedrest with position of comfort.	Reduces oxygen consumption and demand.
Maintain relaxing environment to promote calmness.	Reduces competing stimuli which reduces anxiety and assists with pain relief.
Provide back rubs, repositioning every 2 hours and prn, and encourage diversionary activity.	Promotes relaxation and may redirect attention from pain. Analgesics may be reduced in dosage and frequency by minimizing pain level.

Information, Instruction, Demonstration

INTERVENTIONS	RATIONALES
Instruct in relaxation techniques, deep breathing, guided imagery, visualization, etc.	Helps to decrease pain and anxiety and provides distraction from pain.
Instruct in activity alterations and limitations.	Decreases myocardial oxygen demand and workload.
Instruct in medication effects, side effects, contraindications, and symptoms to report.	Promotes knowledge and compliance with therapeutic regimen. Alleviates fear.
Instruct patient to request pain medication when pain becomes noticeable and not to wait until pain is severe.	Pain promotes muscle tension, and may impair circulatory status and impair healing process.
Instruct in methods of splinting abdomen when coughing or deep breathing.	Supports surgical incision to allow patient to expand lungs to prevent atelectasis, and minimizes pain level.
Instruct in using pillows to maintain body alignment and support extremities.	Promotes comfort and reduces muscle tension and strain.

Discharge or Maintenance Evaluation

- Patient will report pain being absent or relieved with medication administration.

- Medication will be administered prior to pain becoming severe.

- Patient will be able to recall instructions on medications accurately.

- Activity will be modified in such a way as to prevent increased pain.

Risk for impaired skin integrity
[See Thrombophlebitis]

Related to: edema, bedrest, surgery, pressure, altered circulation and blood flow, altered metabolic states

Defining characteristics: skin surface disruptions, incisions, ulcerations, wounds that do not heal

Knowledge deficit
[See MI]

Related to: lack of understanding, lack of understanding of medical condition, lack of recall

Defining characteristics: questions regarding problems, inadequate follow-up on instructions given, misconceptions, lack of improvement of previous regimen, development of preventable complications

AORTIC ANEURYSM

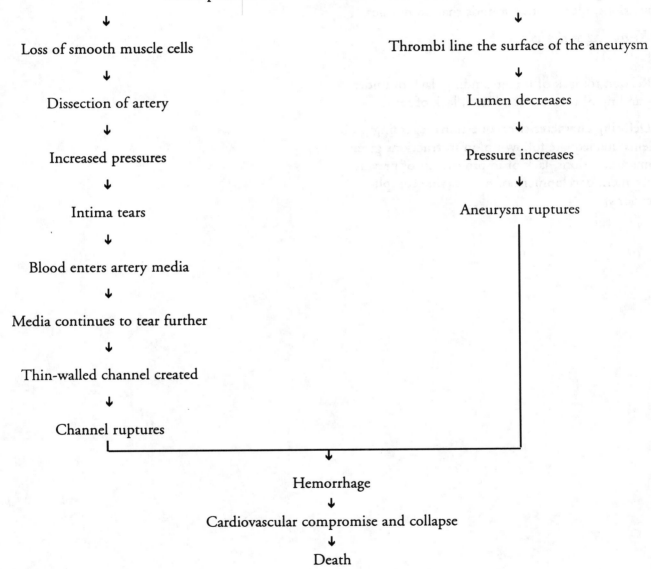

Degeneration of artery
↓
Weakening of arterial wall
↓
Blood pressure increases tension and weakened areas

↓   ↓

Loss of smooth muscle cells   Thrombi line the surface of the aneurysm
↓   ↓
Dissection of artery   Lumen decreases
↓   ↓
Increased pressures   Pressure increases
↓   ↓
Intima tears   Aneurysm ruptures
↓
Blood enters artery media
↓
Media continues to tear further
↓
Thin-walled channel created
↓
Channel ruptures

Hemorrhage
↓
Cardiovascular compromise and collapse
↓
Death

RESPIRATORY SYSTEM

Adult Respiratory Distress Syndrome (ARDS)

Chronic Obstructive Pulmonary Disease (COPD)

Pulmonary Embolism

Pneumonia

Pneumothorax

Status Asthmaticus

Mechanical Ventilation

Adult Respiratory Distress Syndrome (ARDS)

Adult respiratory distress syndrome (ARDS) is also known as shock lung, wet lung, white lung, or acute respiratory distress syndrome, and occurs frequently after an acute or traumatic injury or illness involving the respiratory system. The body responds to the injury with life-threatening respiratory failure and hypoxemia.

ARDS is usually noted 12-24 hours after the initial insult or 5-10 days after sepsis occurs. Dyspnea with hyperventilation and hypoxemia are usually the first clinical symptoms. Adventitious breath sounds frequently are not present initially.

Some of the most common precipitating factors are trauma, aspiration, pneumonia, near-drowning, toxic gas inhalation, sepsis, shock, DIC, oxygen toxicity, coronary artery bypass, pancreatitis, fat or amniotic embolism, radiation, head injury, heroin use, massive hemorrhage, smoke inhalation, drug overdose, or uremia. Mortality is high (60-70%) despite treatment and often, patients who do survive, may have chronic residual lung disease. In some cases, patients may have normal pulmonary function after recovery.

The latent phase of ARDS begins when the pulmonary capillary and alveolar endothelium become injured. The insult causes complement to be activated, as well as granulocytes, platelets, and the coagulation cascade. Free oxygen radicals, arachidonic acid metabolites and proteases are released into the system. Humoral substances, such as serotonin, histamine and bradykinin, are released. This results in red blood cell and high plasma protein leakage into the interstitial spaces, due to increased capillary permeability and increased pulmonary hydrostatic pressure. Initially, there may be little evidence of respiratory

problems, and chest x-rays may be normal or show minimal diffuse haziness. The fluid leakage increases and lymphatic flow increases with the acute phases with widespread damage to pulmonary capillary membranes and inflammation. Increases in intra-alveolar edema leads to capillary congestion and collagen formation. Surfactant production and activity decreases, which causes decreased functional residual capacity, increased pulmonary shunting with widening A-a gradients, decreased pulmonary compliance, and ventilation/perfusion mismatching results. Chest x-rays will then show the ground glass appearance and finally a complete white-out of the lung.

The chronic phases occurs when the endothelium thickens; Type I cells, which are the gas-exchange pneumocytes, are replaced by Type II cells, which are responsible for producing surfactant, and along with fibrin, fluid and other cellular material form a hyaline membrane in place of the normal alveoli.

The goals of treatment are to improve ventilation and perfusion, to treat the underlying disease process that caused the lung injury, and to prevent progression of potentially fatal complications. Oxygen therapy with high levels of oxygen, mechanical ventilatory support with PEEP, and fluid and drug management are required.

MEDICAL CARE

Laboratory: cultures to identify causative organisms when bacterial infection is present and to identify proper antimicrobial agent; C5A levels increase with disease process; fibrin split products increase; platelets decrease; lactic acid levels increase

Chest x-ray: used to evaluate lung fields; early x-rays may be normal or have diffuse infiltrates; later x-rays will show bilateral ground glass appearance or complete whiting-out of lung fields; assists with differentiation between ARDS and cardiogenic pulmonary edema since heart size is normal in ARDS

Oxygen: to correct hypoxia and hypoxemia

Arterial blood gases: to identify acid-base problems, hypocapnia, hypercapnia, and hypoxemia, and to evaluate progress of disease process and effectiveness of oxygen therapy

Ventilation: to provide adequate oxygenation and ventilation in patients who are unable to maintain even minimal levels

Pulmonary function studies: used to evaluate lung compliance and volumes which are normally decreased; physiologic dead space is increased and alveolar ventilation is compromised

NURSING CARE PLANS

Ineffective breathing pattern
[See Mechanical Ventilation]

Related to: decreased lung compliance, pulmonary edema, increased lung density, decreased surfactant

Defining characteristics: use of accessory muscles, dyspnea, tachypnea, bradypnea, altered ABGs

Impaired gas exchange
[See Mechanical Ventilation]

Related to: intra-alveolar edema, atelectasis, ventilation/perfusion mismatching, decreased arterial PO_2, decreased amount and activity of surfactant, alveolar hypoventilation, formation of hyaline membranes, alveolar collapse, decreased diffusing capacity, shunting

Defining characteristics: tachypnea, cyanosis, use of accessory muscles, tachycardia, restlessness, mental changes, abnormal arterial blood gases, intrapulmonary shunting increased, A-a gradient changes, hypoxemia, increased dead space

Ineffective airway clearance
[See Mechanical Ventilation]

Related to: interstitial edema, increased airway resistance, decreased lung compliance, pulmonary secretions

Defining characteristics: dyspnea, tachypnea, cyanosis, use of accessory muscles, cough with or without production, anxiety, restlessness, feelings of impending doom

Anxiety
[See Mechanical Ventilation]

Related to: health crisis, effects of hypoxemia, fear of death, change in health status, change in environment

Defining characteristics: apprehension, restlessness, fear, verbalized concern

Knowledge deficit
[See Mechanical Ventilation]

Related to: lack of information, inability to process information, lack of recall

Defining characteristics: verbalized concerns and questions

Decreased cardiac output

Related to: increased positive airway pressures, sepsis, dysrhythmias, increased intrapulmonary edema, left ventricular failure

Defining characteristics: tachycardia, cardiac output less than 4 L/min, cardiac index less than 2.5 L/min/m², cold clammy skin, decreased blood pressure

Outcome Criteria

Patient will be hemodynamically stable.

INTERVENTIONS	RATIONALES
Monitor vital signs every 1-2 hours, and prn.	Mechanical ventilation and the use of PEEP increase the intrathoracic pressures which results in compression of the large vessels in the chest and this causes decreased venous return to the heart and decreased blood pressure.
Obtain PA pressures every hour, cardiac output/index every 4 hours, and calculate other hemo-dynamic values.	PA pressures will be elevated but wedge pressure will be normal. This is the classic marker to differentiate between cardiogenic and non-cardiogenic pulmonary edema. Most ARDS patients have adequate cardiac function at least initially, unless decreases in CO/CI are due to PEEP.
Monitor for mental changes, decreased peripheral pulses, cold or clammy skin.	May indicate decreased cardiac output and decreased perfusion.

Discharge or Maintenance Evaluation

• Patient will have adequate perfusion and cardiac output/index within normal limits for physio-logic condition.

• Patient will have no mental status changes or peripheral perfusion impairment.

Risk for fluid volume excess

Related to: interstitial edema, increased pulmonary fluid with normal intravascular volume, transfusions, resuscitative fluids

Defining characteristics: edema, dyspnea, orthop-nea, rales, wheezing

Outcome Criteria

Patient will be hemodynamically stable, with no signs of pulmonary edema.

INTERVENTIONS	RATIONALES
Monitor for peripheral or depen-dent edema, or distended neck veins.	May indicate fluid excess that results in venous congestion and leads to respiratory failure.
Auscultate lung fields for adven-titious breath sounds.	Bronchovesicular sounds heard over entire lung fields result when lung density increases. Crackles and rhonchi may be auscultated in pulmonary edema.
Monitor intake and output every hour. Notify MD if urine less than 30 cc/hr.	Identifies fluid imbalances and possible sources.
Weigh every day.	Weight gains of > 2 lbs./day or 5 lbs./week indicate fluid reten-tion.
Monitor for vocal fremitus.	May be present due to increased lung density resulting from pul-monary edema.
Monitor vital signs.	Tachycardia and elevated blood pressure may result from fluid excess and heart failure.
Restrict fluids as warranted.	May be required to help with fluid balance regulation.

Discharge or Maintenance Evaluation

• Patient will have no edema or weight gain.

• Patient will be eupneic with no adventitious breath sounds to auscultation.

Risk for fluid volume deficit

Related to: fluid shifts, diuretics, hemorrhage

Defining characteristics: decreased blood pressure, oliguria, anuria, low pulmonary artery wedge pres-sures

Outcome Criteria

Patient will achieve and maintain a normal and balanced fluid volume status and be hemodynami-cally stable.

INTERVENTIONS	RATIONALES
Monitor vital signs every 1–2 hours, and prn.	Tachycardia, hypotension and decreases in pulse quality may indicate fluid shifting has resulted in volume depletion. Temperature elevations with diaphoresis may result in increased insensible fluid loss.
Monitor intake and ouput every hour, and notify MD of significant fluid imbalances.	Continuing negative balances may result in volume depletion.
Weigh daily.	Changes in weight from day to day may correlate to fluid shifts that may occur.
Observe skin turgor and hydration status.	Decreases in skin turgor, tenting of skin, and dry mucous membranes may indicate fluid volume deficits.
Administer IV fluids as ordered.	Replaces fluids and maintains circulating volume.
Monitor labwork for sodium and potassium levels.	Diuretic therapy may result in hypokalemia and hyponatremia.

Discharge or Maintenance Evaluation

- Patient will achieve normal fluid balance.

- Patient will be hemodynamically stable, with no weight change.

- Patient will have urine output within normal limits.

ADULT RESPIRATORY DISTRESS SYNDROME (ARDS)

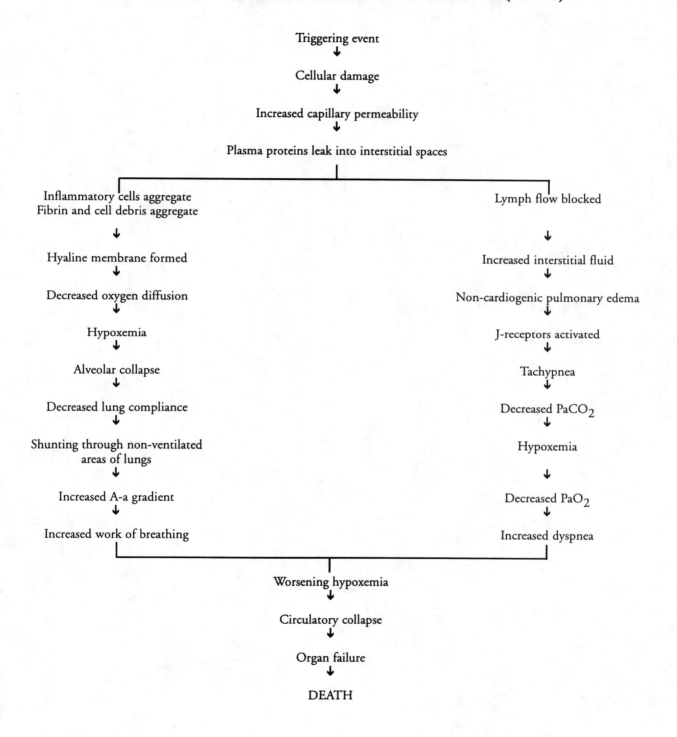

Triggering event
↓
Cellular damage
↓
Increased capillary permeability
↓
Plasma proteins leak into interstitial spaces

Inflammatory cells aggregate
Fibrin and cell debris aggregate
↓
Hyaline membrane formed
↓
Decreased oxygen diffusion
↓
Hypoxemia
↓
Alveolar collapse
↓
Decreased lung compliance
↓
Shunting through non-ventilated areas of lungs
↓
Increased A-a gradient
↓
Increased work of breathing

Lymph flow blocked
↓
Increased interstitial fluid
↓
Non-cardiogenic pulmonary edema
↓
J-receptors activated
↓
Tachypnea
↓
Decreased $PaCO_2$
↓
Hypoxemia
↓
Decreased PaO_2
↓
Increased dyspnea

Worsening hypoxemia
↓
Circulatory collapse
↓
Organ failure
↓
DEATH

Chronic Obstructive Pulmonary Disease (C O P D)

Chronic obstructive pulmonary disease (COPD) is irreversible condition in which airways become obstructed and resistance to air flow is increased during expiration when airways collapse. COPD is usually further subdivided into other diseases such as bronchitis and emphysema, and actually COPD refers to these simultaneous disease entities.

Emphysematous changes include enlarging of the air spaces distally to the terminal bronchioles, and concurrent changes in alveolar walls. Capillary numbers decrease in the remaining walls and may sclerose. Gas exchange is decreased due to the reduction in available alveolar surfaces as well as decreased perfusion to non-ventilated areas. Ventilation/perfusion mismatching occurs and functional residual capacity is increased. The anteroposterior diameter of the chest is often enlarged due to the loss of elasticity and increased air trapping in the airway supportive structures. These type A patients are often called "pink puffers" because of the increased response to hypoxemia. Symptoms include dyspnea and increase in breathing effort, which result in a well-oxygenated, or pink, patient who displays overt dyspnea, or puffing.

Bronchitis is usually associated with prolonged exposure to lung irritants, which results in inflammatory changes and thickening of bronchial walls, and increases in mucous production. The patient exhibits a chronic productive cough due in part to the increase in size of mucous glands and decrease in cilia. These type B patients are often called "blue bloaters" because their response to hypoxemia is reduced, with increasing $PaCO_2$ levels and cyanosis. These patients frequently have bouts of cor pulmonale, or right-sided heart failure, resulting in peripheral edema.

The most common precipitating factors for COPD include cigarette smoking, air or environmental pollution, allergic response, autoimmunity, and genetic predisposition. Treatment is aimed at avoidance of respiratory allergens and irritants, controlling bronchospasms, and improving airway clearance.

MEDICAL CARE

Laboratory: cultures used to identify causative organisms and determine appropriate antimicrobial therapy; CBC used to identify presence of infection with elevated white blood cell count, and to monitor for increases in RBCs and hematocrit as the body tries to compensate for oxygen transport requirements; alpha$_1$-antitrypsin levels used to identify deficiency that may be present if patient has heredity predisposition; theophylline levels used to monitor for therapeutic levels and/or toxicity

Pulmonary function studies: used to evaluate pulmonary status and function, and to identify airway obstruction, increased residual volume, total lung capacity, compliance, decreased vital capacity, diffusing capacity, and expiratory volumes with emphysema patients; increased residual volume, decreased vital capacity and forced expiratory volumes with normal static compliance and diffusion capacity with bronchitis patients

Chest x-ray: used to identify hyperinflation of lungs, flattened diaphragm, or pulmonary hypertension; used to identify barotrauma that may occur, increased antero-posterior chest diameter, large retrosternal air spaces, or secondary cardiovascular complications with right-sided heart failure

Electrocardiography: used to identify dysrhythmias associated with this disease; tall p waves in inferior leads, vertical QRS axis, atrial dysrhythmias, right ventricular hypertrophy, sinus tachycardia, and right axis deviation

Oxygen: used to improve hypoxemia; liter flow should be low in order to maintain the patient's respiratory drive; PaO_2 may be acceptable at 55-60 mmHg to avoid hypoventilation and maintain function

IV fluids: used to maintain hydration and for administration of medical therapeutics

Bronchodilators: xanthines and sympathomimetics are used to relieve bronchospasms and help to promote clearance of mucoid secretions

Antibiotics: used to treat respiratory infections

Arterial blood gases: used to identify acid-base disturbances, presence of hypoxemia and hypercapnia, and to evaluate responses to therapies

Chest physiotherapy: percussion and postural drainage are used to facilitate mobilization of secretions and promote clearance of airways

Corticosteroids: used to decrease secretions and reduce inflammation in the lungs; use of steroids is controversial

Psychological treatment: use of anti-anxiety agents to decrease fear and anxiety related to dyspnea, without sedation to depress the respiratory drive; psychotherapy may be required to enable patients to cope with their ongoing disease process

NURSING CARE PLANS

Ineffective airway clearance
[See Mechanical Ventilation]

Related to: bronchospasm, fatigue, increased work of breathing, increased mucous production, thick secretions, infection

Defining characteristics: dyspnea, tachypnea, bradypnea, bronchospasms, increased work of breathing, use of accessory muscles, increased mucous production, cough with or without productivity, adventitious breath sounds

Ineffective breathing pattern
[See Mechanical Ventilation]

Related to: pain, increased lung compliance, decreased lung expansion, fear, obstruction, decreased elasticity/recoil

Defining characteristics: dyspnea, tachypnea, use of accessory muscles, cough with or without productivity, adventitious breath sounds, prolongation of expiratory time, increased mucous production, abnormal arterial blood gases

Impaired gas exchange
[See Mechanical Ventilation]

Related to: obstruction of airways, bronchospasm, air-trapping, right-to-left shunting, ventilation/perfusion mismatching, inability to move secretions, hypoventilation

Defining characteristics: hypoxemia, hypercapnia, mental changes, confusion, restlessness, dyspnea, vital sign changes, inability to tolerate activity, respiratory acidosis

Anxiety
[See Mechanical Ventilation]

Related to: threat of death, change in health status, life-threatening crises

Defining characteristics: fear, restlessness, muscle tension, helplessness, communication of uncertainty and apprehension, feeling of suffocation

Activity intolerance

Related to: fatigue, weakness, increased effort and work of breathing, inadequate rest, hypoxia, hypoxemia

Defining characteristics: dyspnea, decreased oxygen saturation levels with movement or activity, increased heart rate and blood pressure with movement or activity, feelings of tiredness and weakness

Outcome Criteria

Patient will be able to tolerate minimal activity without respiratory compromise.

INTERVENTIONS	RATIONALES
Monitor for patient's response to activity changes.	Identifies patient's ability to compensate for increases in activity and provides baseline date from which to plan care.
Monitor vital signs before, during, and after increased activity levels.	Increases in heart rate greater than 10/minute or respiratory rate greater than 32 may indicate that patient has reached his maximal activity limit and further activity may result in circulatory/respiratory dysfunction.
Plan activities to ensure patient obtains adequate amounts of rest and sleep.	Decreases potential for dyspnea and provides rest to prevent excessive fatigue.
Assist patient with activities as warranted.	Conserves energy and decreases oxygen consumption and dyspnea.
Increase activity gradually and encourage patient participation.	Gradual increases facilitate increased tolerance to activity by balancing oxygen supply and demand, and patient cooperation may facilitate feelings of self-worth and adequacy.
Administer inhalers as ordered prior to activities.	Helps prevent dyspnea by performing activities at peak time of medication effects.

Information, Instruction, Demonstration

INTERVENTIONS	RATIONALES
Instruct on techniques to save energy expenditure: shower stools, arm and leg rests, gathering required articles and placement within reach, etc.	Helps to decrease energy expenditure and fatigue, which may result in increased dyspnea.
Provide patient with exercise regimen protocol.	Promotes independence and self-worth; increases tolerance to exercises.
Instruct on breathing exercises to be performed with activity.	Promotes effective respiratory patterns during exertion.

Discharge or Maintenance Evaluation

- Patient will be able to tolerate activity without excessive dyspnea or hemodynamic instability.

- Patient will be able to perform ADLs within limits of disease process.

- Patient will be able to recall information accurately, and will be able to utilize relaxation and breathing techniques effectively.

- Patient will be compliant with prescribed exercise regimens.

Ineffective individual/family coping
[See Mechanical Ventilation]

Related to: changes in lifestyle and health status, sensory overload, fear of death, physical limitations, inadequate support system, inadequate coping mechanisms, continual dyspnea

Defining characteristics: inability to meet role expectations, inability to meet basic needs, constant worry, apprehension, fear, inability to problem-solve, anger, hostility, aggression, inappropriate defense mechanisms, low self-esteem, insomnia, depression, destructive behaviors, vacillation when choices are required, delayed decision-making, muscle tension, fatigue

Risk for infection

Related to: disease process, inability to move secretions, decreased cilia function, immunosuppression, poor nutrition

Defining characteristics: increased temperature, chills, elevated white blood cell count, inability to move secretions

INTERVENTIONS	RATIONALES
Monitor for increased dyspnea, sputum color and character changes, cough, and temperature elevation.	Yellow or green sputum, with increased viscosity usually indicates infection. Prompt recognition facilitates prompt treatment.
Obtain sputum specimen for culture and sensitivity as ordered.	Identifies the causative organism and provides information regarding appropriate antimicrobial agent required.
Administer antibiotics as ordered.	Controls and clears the infection and any secondary infections in the bronchial tree. Improvement should be noted within 24–48 hours after antimicrobial agent has begun.
Monitor for abrupt changes in other body systems; cardiac abnormalities and alteration in heart sounds, increasing pain, changes in mental status, recurring temperature elevations.	May indicate presence of secondary infection or resistance to ordered antibiotics. Superinfections, systemic bacteremia, inflammatory cardiac conditions, meningitis or encephalitis may occur.
Provide adequate rest time for patient.	Helps to facilitate healing and natural immunity.

Discharge or Maintenance Evaluation

• Patient will exhibit no signs/symptoms of secondary infection.

Altered nutrition: less than body requirements
[See Mechanical Ventilation]

Related to: dyspnea, inability to take in sufficient food, increased metabolism due to disease process, decreased level of consciousness, fatigue, increased sputum, medication side effects

Defining characteristics: actual inadequate food intake, altered taste, altered smell sensation, weight loss, anorexia, absent bowel sounds, decreased peristalsis, muscle mass loss, changes in bowel habits, abdominal distention, nausea, vomiting

Knowledge deficit

Related to: lack of information, lack of recall of information, cognitive limitations

Defining characteristics: request for information, statement of misconception, statement of concerns, development of preventable complications, inaccurate follow-through with instructions

Outcome Criteria

Patient will be able to recall information accurately and will follow through with all instructions.

INTERVENTIONS	RATIONALES
Assess knowledge of COPD disease process, medications, and treatments.	Identifies level of knowledge and provides baseline from which to plan teaching.
Instruct on medication effects, side effects, contraindications, and signs/symptoms to report.	Promotes knowledge and compliance with treatment regimen.
Instruct in proper technique for using and cleaning inhalers.	Proper technique, including appropriate time intervals between puffs, facilitates effective delivery and therapeutic effect.
Instruct on need to avoid smoking and other respiratory irritants.	May initiate and exacerbate bronchial irritation which can result in increased mucous production and airway obstruction.
Instruct on effective coughing	Effective coughing reduces

INTERVENTIONS	RATIONALES
techniques; postural drainage, chest physiotherapy, etc.	fatigue and facilitates removal of secretions. Percussion and postural drainage help to mobilize tenacious secretions.
Instruct to drink 10-12 glasses of water per day.	Maintains hydration and promotes easier mobilization of secretions.
Instruct on use of supplemental oxygen at low flow rates, and reasons to avoid increasing flow indiscriminately.	COPD patients will rarely require more than 2–3 L/min to maintain their optimum oxygenation levels. Increasing flow rates will increase their PaO_2 but may decrease their respiratory drive and may result in drowsiness and confusion.
Instruct on oxygen safety: avoiding flammable objects, use of vaseline or other petroleum products, and ambulation with tubing.	Promotes physical and environmental safety.
Instruct on avoiding sedative or antianxiety drugs as warranted.	Sedative may result in respiratory depression and impair cough reflexes.
Instruct on avoiding people with infections; encourage patient to obtain influenza and pneumonia vaccinations as warranted.	Prevents exposure to other infections, and decreases potential for incidence of upper respiratory infections.
Instruct on activity limitations, methods to conserve energy and promote rest, pursed-lip breathing, etc.	Helps decrease fatigue, optimizes activity level within range of disease process, and reduces dyspnea and oxygen consumption.
Instruct on signs/symptoms to notify MD: increased temperature, change in sputum color or character, increasing dyspnea.	Provides for prompt recognition of infection to facilitate prompt intervention prior to respiratory failure.
Instruct to continue with follow-up medical care.	Provides for monitoring of progression of disease, presence of complications, or exacerbations, and facilitates changes in medical regimen to concur with current medical condition.
Provide patient/family with information regarding support groups, such as the American Lung Association, etc.	Support groups may be required to provide emotional assistance and respite for caregiver(s).

INTERVENTIONS	RATIONALES
Assist patient/family to set realistic goals for long- and short-term.	Provides a plan for patient and facilitates self-involvement with realistic goals and methods to meet them. Fosters independence and reduces anxiety.

Discharge or Maintenance Evaluation

- Patient will be able to recall information regarding disease process and treatment regimen.

- Patient will be able to recall accurately the signs/symptoms for which to notify MD, the effects and side effects of medications, and proper procedure for using inhalers.

- Patient will be able to demonstrate accurately proper cough techniques, pursed-lip breathing, and proper positioning to facilitate breathing.

- Patient/family will be able to access support systems effectively.

CHRONIC OBSTRUCTIVE PULMONARY DISEASE (C O P D)

(smoking, pollution, infection)
↓
Inflammation
↓
Alpha$_1$-antitrypsin inhibited
↓
Elastase production
↓
Lung elastin broken down

EMPHYSEMA
(Pink Puffers)

Increased response to hypoxemia
↓
Terminal air spaces enlarged
↓
Destruction of alveolar walls
↓
Loss of elastic recoil
↓
Increased air trapping
↓
Airways collapse, decreasing gas exchange surface
↓
Decreased resistance to lung expansion
Increased lung volumes
↓
Ventilation/perfusion mismatching
↓
Air sacs replaced by bullae
↓
Increased dyspnea and work of breathing

CHRONIC BRONCHITIS
(Blue Bloaters)

Decreased response to hypoxemia
↓
Hypertrophy and hyperplasia of mucus glands
↓
Goblet cell metaplasia
↓
Increased mucus production and viscosity
↓
Mucus plugs in airways decrease airway size
↓
Bronchial wall thickening increased
↓
Increased airway resistance, decrease
in vital capacity and expiratory flow rates
↓
Hypoxemia
↓
Increased PaCO$_2$
↓
Increased pulmonary constriction

Hypoxia
↓
Further pulmonary constriction
Increased pulmonary artery pressures
↓
(See Next Page)

C O P D continued

Pulmonary hypertension

↓

Right ventricular strain

↓

Right ventricular hypertrophy

↓

Right ventricular failure
Cor Pulmonale

↓

Left ventricular failure

↓

Circulatory collapse

↓

Death

Pulmonary Embolism

A pulmonary embolus (PE) usually results after a deep vein thrombus partially or totally dislodges from the pelvis, thigh, or calf. The clot then lodges in one or more of the pulmonary arteries and obstructs forward blood flow and oxygen supply to the lung parenchyma. Pressure is backed up and results in increased pulmonary artery pressures and vascular resistance, right ventricular failure, tachycardia, and shock. Alveolar dead space is increased which results in ventilation/perfusion mismatching and decreased PaO_2. The embolus releases chemicals that decrease surfactant and increase bronchoconstriction. Hyperventilation due to carbon dioxide retention results in decreased $PaCO_2$. Fat embolism, septic embolism, or amniotic fluid embolism are rarely causes of PE and when they are, usually occlude smaller arterioles or capillaries. A pulmonary embolus is classified as being massive when more than half the pulmonary artery circulation is occluded.

Infarction of the pulmonary circulation occurs less than 10 per cent of the time and usually results when the patient has an underlying chronic cardiac or pulmonary disease. Pulmonary infarcts may be reabsorbed and fibrosis may cause scar tissue formation. Usually collateral pulmonary circulation maintains lung tissue viability.

The main risk factors that may predispose pulmonary embolism formation are bedrest, immobility, cardiac disease, venous disease, pregnancy, malignancy, fractures, estrogen contraceptives, obesity, burns, blood dyscrasias, surgery, and trauma. Thrombus formation occurs with blood flow stasis, coagulopathy alterations, and damage to the endothelium of the vessel walls, and these three factors are known as Virchow's triad.

The most common signs/symptoms are dyspnea, chest pain, and cough with hemoptysis. Other symptoms may be present, such as lightheadedness, diaphoresis, cyanosis, pleural friction rubs, S_2 split, tachypnea, tachycardia, anxiety, mental changes, gallops, dysrhythmias, rales, and hypotension, but are dependent on the size of the embolus and presence of infarction or complications.

MEDICAL CARE

Laboratory: PTTs done daily to monitor heparin therapy; LDH may be elevated in pulmonary embolus, but other diagnoses must be ruled out; fibrin split products usually increase consistently with PE; CBC may show increased hematocrit due to hemoconcentration, and increased RBCs

Chest x-ray: used to rule out other pulmonary diseases; shows atelectasis, elevated diaphragm and pleural effusions, prominence of pulmonary artery, and occasionally, a wedge-shaped infiltrate commonly seen in pulmonary embolism

Nuclear radiographic testing: lung scans are used to show perfusion defects beyond occluded vasculature; xenon ventilation scans are used to differentiate between pulmonary embolism and COPD, and together with perfusion scans, will reveal ventilation/perfusion mismatches

Pulmonary angiography: used as a definitive test when other tests do not ensure the diagnosis in high-risk patients; identifies intra-arterial filling defects and obstruction of pulmonary artery branches

Electrocardiography: used to reveal right axis deviation, right-sided heart strain, right bundle branch block, tall peaked P waves, ST segment depression and T wave inversion, as well as supraventricular tachydysrhythmias

Phlebography: used to identify deep vein thrombosis in legs

Oxygen: to provide supplemental oxygen to maintain oxygenation

Pulmonary artery catheterization: used to place catheter to enable hemodynamic monitoring and to assess response to therapies

Arterial blood gases: used to assess for hypoxemia and acid-base imbalances

Thoracentesis: may be used to rule out empyema if pleural effusion is noted on chest x-ray

Beta-blockers: used in pulmonary hypertension to dilate the pulmonary vasculature to increase tissue perfusion

Cardiac glycosides: used only if absolutely mandatory during the acute hypoxemia phase due to the potential for lethal dysrhythmias or cardiac failure

Analgesics: used to alleviate pain and discomfort

Anticoagulants: heparin is used initially in the treatment of PE, with change to coumadin/warfarin PO for 3-6 months

Thrombolytics: streptokinase or urokinase enhances conversion of plasminogen to plasmin to prevent venous thrombus

Antiplatelet drugs: aspirin and dipyridamole used to prevent venous thromboembolism

Surgery: embolectomy may be performed to remove the clot; umbrella filter may be placed or surgical interruption of the inferior vena cava may be performed to prevent migration of clots into the pulmonary vasculature

NURSING CARE PLANS

Ineffective breathing pattern

Related to: increase in alveolar dead space, physiologic lung changes due to embolism, bleeding, increased secretions, decreased lung expansion, inflammation

Defining characteristics: dyspnea, use of accessory muscles, shallow respirations, tachypnea, increased work of breathing, decreased chest expansion on involved side, cough with or without productivity, adventitious breath sounds

Outcome Criteria

Patient will be eupneic with clear lung fields and arterial blood gases within normal limits.

INTERVENTIONS	RATIONALES
Monitor respiratory status for changes in rate and depth, use of accessory muscles, increased work of breathing, nasal flaring, and symmetrical chest expansion.	In PE, respiratory rate is usually increased. The effort of breathing is increased and dyspnea is often the first sign of PE. Depending on the severity and location of the PE, depth of respirations may vary. Chest expansion may be decreased on the affected side due to atelectasis or pain.
Provide supplemental oxygen via nasal cannula or mask.	Provides oxygen and may decrease work of breathing.
Monitor for presence of cough and character of sputum.	Bloody secretions may result from pulmonary infarction or abnormal anticoagulation. A dry cough may result with alveolar congestion.
Auscultate lung fields for adventitious breath sounds and/or rubs.	Breath sounds may be diminished or absent if airway is obstructed due to bleeding, clotting, or collapse. Rhonchi or wheezing may result in conjunction with obstruction.
Auscultate heart sounds.	Splitting of S_2 may occur with pulmonary embolus.
Encourage deep breathing and effective coughing exercises.	Improves lung expansion and helps to remove secretions which may be increased with PE.

Information, Instruction, Demonstration

INTERVENTIONS	RATIONALES
Prepare patient/family for placement on mechanical ventilation.	May be required if respiratory distress is severe.
Instruct on avoiding shallow respirations and splinting.	Eupnea decreases potential for atelectasis and improves venous return.
Prepare patient/family for bronchoscopy as warranted.	May be required to remove mucous plugs and/or clots in order to clear airways.

Discharge or Maintenance Evaluation

• Patient will be able to maintain his own respirations without mechanical assistance.

• Patient will be eupneic, with no adventitious lung or heart sounds.

• Patient will be able to recall all information accurately.

Impaired gas exchange
[See Mechanical Ventilation]

Related to: atelectasis, airway obstruction, alveolar collapse, pulmonary edema, increased secretions, active bleeding, altered blood flow to lung, shunting

Defining characteristics: dyspnea, restlessness, anxiety, apprehension, cyanosis, arterial blood gas changes, hypoxemia, hypoxia, hypercapnia, decreased oxygen saturation

Risk for decreased cardiac output
[See Heart Failure]

Related to: dysrhythmias, cardiogenic shock, heart failure

Defining characteristics: elevated blood pressure, elevated mean arterial blood pressure, elevated systemic vascular resistance, cardiac output less than

4 L/min or cardiac index less than 2.7 L/min/m_2, cold, pale extremities, EKG changes, hypotension, S_2 split sounds, S_3 or S_4 gallops, dyspnea, crackles (rales), chest pain

Risk for altered tissue perfusion: cardiopulmonary, peripheral, cerebral

Related to: impaired blood flow, alveolar perfusion and gas exchange impairment, occlusion of the pulmonary artery, migration of embolus, hypoxemia, increased cardiac workload

Defining characteristics: dyspnea, chest pain, tachycardia, dysrhythmias, productive cough, hemoptysis, edema, cyanosis, syncope, jugular vein distention, weak pulses, hypotension, convulsions, loss of consciousness, restlessness, hemiplegia, coma

Outcome Criteria

Patient will be hemodynamically stable, eupneic, with no alterations in perfusion to any body system.

INTERVENTIONS	RATIONALES
Monitor vital signs and notify MD for significant changes.	Hypoxemia will result in increased heart rate as the body tries to compensate for the decrease in perfusion.
Monitor EKG for rhythm disturbances and treat as indicated.	Hypoxemia, right-sided heart strain, and electrolyte imbalances may induce dysrhythmias.
Auscultate for S_3 or S_4 heart sounds.	Increases in heart workload may result in heart strain and failure as perfusion decreases, and may result in gallop rhythm.
Monitor for presence of peripheral pulses and notify MD for significant changes.	Presence of deep vein thrombus may occlude the circulation and result in diminished or absent pulses.
Assess for Homan's and Pratt's signs.	Presence of these signs may or may not be related to PE.

INTERVENTIONS	RATIONALES
Assess skin color, temperature and capillary refill.	Impairment of blood flow may induce pallor or cyanosis to the skin or mucous membranes. Cool clammy skin or mottling may indicate peripheral vasoconstriction/shock.
Monitor for restlessness or changes in mental status or level of consciousness.	May indicate occlusion, impaired cerebral blood flow, hypoxia, or development of stroke.

Information, Instruction, Demonstration

INTERVENTIONS	RATIONALES
Prepare patient for insertion of pulmonary artery catheter.	May be required to monitor hemodynamic status and assess response to therapy.
Prepare patient for surgery as warranted.	Surgical intervention may be required if patient develops recurrent emboli in spite of treatment, or if anticoagulant therapy cannot be given. Ligation of the vena cava or insertion of an umbrella filter may be necessary.
Instruct on thrombolytic agents as warranted.	Streptokinase, urokinase, or alteplase (t-PA) may be required if the pulmonary embolus is massive and compromises hemodynamic stability.

Discharge or Maintenance Evaluation

- Patient will have adequate tissue perfusion to all body systems.

- Patient will have stable hemodynamic parameters and vital signs will be within normal limits.

- Oxygenation will be optimal as evidenced by pulse oximetry greater than 90% and adequate ABGs.

PULMONARY EMBOLISM

Embolus obstructs blood flow
↓

Chemicals released
↓
Bronchoconstriction
↓
Decreased PaO$_2$

Pulmonary pressures increased
↓
Pulmonary vasoconstriction
Pulmonary hypertension
↓
Right ventricular failure
↓

Alveolar dead space increased
↓
Ventilation perfusion
mismatch
↓
Increased airway resistance
Decreased lung compliance
↓

Decreased cardiac output

Hypotension
↓

Pulmonary vasoconstriction
↓

Decreased tissue perfusion ← Decreased PaO$_2$
↓
Cardiopulmonary collapse
↓
Death

Pneumonia

Pneumonia is an acute infection of the lung's terminal alveolar spaces and/or the interstitial tissues which results in gas exchange problems. The major challenge is identification of the source of the infection. Pneumonia ranks as the sixth most common cause of death in the United States.

When the infection is limited to a portion of the lung, it is known as segmental or lobular pneumonia; when the alveoli adjacent to the bronchioles are involved, it is known as bronchopneumonia, and when the entire lobe of the lung is involved, it is known as lobar pneumonia.

Pneumonia may be caused by bacteria, viruses, mycoplasma, rickettsias, or fungi. The causative organism gains entry by aspiration of oropharyngeal or gastric contents, inhalation of respiratory droplets, from others who are infected, by way of the blood stream, or directly with surgery or trauma.

Viral types are more common in some areas, but identification of causative organisms may be difficult with limited technology.

Patients who develop bacterial pneumonia usually are immunosuppressed or compromised by a chronic disease, or have had a recent viral illness. The most common type of bacterial pneumonia is pneumococcal pneumonia, in which the organism reaches the lungs via the respiratory passageways and result in the collapse of alveoli. The inflammatory response that this generates causes protein-rich fluid to migrate into the alveolar spaces and provides culture media for the organism to proliferate and spread.

Frequently pneumonia is predisposed by upper respiratory infections, chronic illness, cancer, surgery, atelectasis, chronic obstructive pulmonary disease, asthma, cystic fibrosis, bronchiectasis,

influenza, malnutrition, smoking, alcoholism, immunosuppressive therapy, aspiration, sickle cell disease, head injury or coma.

Aspiration pneumonia occurs after aspiration of gastric or oropharyngeal contents, or other chemical irritants into the trachea and lungs. Stomach acid damages the respiratory endothelium and may result in non-cardiogenic pulmonary edema, hemorrhage, destruction of surfactant-producing cells, and hypoxemia. The pH of the aspirated material determines the severity of the injury with pH less than 2.5 causing severe damage. Morbidity is high even with treatment.

In pneumonia's early stages, pulmonary vessels dilate and erythrocytes spread into the alveoli and cause a reddish, liver-like appearance, or red hepatization, in the lung consolidation area. Polymorphonuclear cells then enter the alveolar spaces and the consolidation increases to a grey hepatization. The leukocytes trap bacteria against the alveolar walls or other leukocytes so that more organisms are found in the increasing margins of the consolidation. The macrophage reaction occurs when mononuclear cells advance into the alveoli and phagocytize the exudate debris.

Diagnosis may be assisted with the observation of sputum characteristics, with bacterial pneumonia having mucopurulent sputum, viral and mycoplasmic pneumonias having more watery secretions, pneumococcal pneumonia having rust-colored sputum, and Klebsiella noting dark red mucoid secretions.

The initial signs/symptoms are sudden onset of shaking chills, fever, purulent sputum, pleuritic chest pain that is worsened with respiration or coughing, tachycardia, tachypnea, and use of accessory muscles.

Staphylococcal pneumonia is frequently noted after influenza or in hospitalized patients with a nosocomial superinfection following surgery, trauma, or immunosuppression. Pleural pain, dyspnea, cyanosis, and productive coughing with copious pink secretions are common symptoms. Streptococcal pneumonia occurs rarely with the exception as a complication after measles or influenza. Klebsiella pneumonia is virulent and necrotizing, and is usually seen with alcoholic or severely debilitated patients. Pneumonia that is caused by Hemophilus influenzae occurs after viral upper respiratory infections, or concurrently with bronchopneumonia, bronchitis, and bronchiolitis. Sputum is usually yellow or green, and patients have fever, cough, cyanosis, and arthralgias. Viral pneumonia may be caused by influenza, adenoviruses, respiratory syncytial virus, rhinoviruses, cytomegalovirus, herpes simplex virus, and childhood diseases; it is usually milder. Symptoms include headache, anorexia, and occasionally mucopurulent sputum that is bloody.

MEDICAL CARE

Laboratory: white blood cell count may be normal or low but usually is elevated with polymorphonuclear neutrophils; cultures of sputum, blood, and CSF may be obtained to identify the causative organism and antimicrobial agent best suited for eradication; electrolytes may show decreased sodium and chloride levels; serology and cold agglutinins may be done for identification of viral titers; sedimentation rate is usually elevated

Pulmonary function studies: used to evaluate ventilation/perfusion problems; volumes may be decreased due to alveolar collapse; airway pressures may be increased; lung compliance may be decreased

Arterial blood gases: to evaluate adequacy of oxygen and respiratory therapies, as well as to identify acid-base imbalances and acidotic/alkalotic states

Chest x-ray: used to demonstrate small effusions and abscesses, pulmonary consolidations, and empyema; may be clear with mycoplasma pneumonia

Oxygen: used to supplement room air, and to treat hypoxemia that may occur

Antibiotics: used in the treatment after culture results are obtained to eradicate the infective organism

Thoracentesis: used to remove fluid if pleural fluid is present; assists in the diagnosis of pleural empyema

Surgery: may be required for open lung biopsy or treatment of effusions and empyema; bronchoscopy with bronchial brushings may be indicated for progressive pneumonias that are unresponsive to medical treatment

Nerve blocks: intercostal blocks may be required to control pleuritic pain

NURSING CARE PLANS

Ineffective airway clearance

Related to: inflammation, edema, increased secretions, fatigue

Defining characteristics: adventitious breath sounds, use of accessory muscles, cyanosis, dyspnea, cough with or without production

Outcome Criteria

Patient will maintain patency of airway, have clear breath sounds, and will be able to effectively clear secretions.

INTERVENTIONS	RATIONALES
Monitor respiratory status for changes, increased work of breathing, use of accessory muscles, and nasal flaring.	Tachypnea and hyperpnea are frequently noted with pneumonia.
Observe for symmetrical chest expansion.	Unilateral pneumonia will result in asymmetrical chest movement due to decreased lung compliance on the affected side and because of pleuritic pain.
Observe for cyanosis and/or mental status changes.	May indicate impending or present hypoxemia.
Assess vocal fremitus.	Increased fremitus is noted over consolidated areas in pneumonia. Decreased or absent fremitus may indicate that a foreign body is obstructing a large bronchus.
Percuss chest for changes.	Percussion may be dull over consolidated areas or in areas of atelectasis.
Auscultate lung fields.	Fine crackles or bronchial breath sounds are noted in lobar pneumonia; in other types of pneumonia, bronchial sounds are rarely heard. Wheezes may indicate aspiration of a solid object. Inspiratory stridor may indicate the presence of an obstruction to a large bronchus.
Assist with bronchoscopy as warranted.	May be required to remove mucous plugs and prevent or improve atelectasis.
Assist with thoracentesis as warranted.	May be required to drain purulent fluid.

Impaired gas exchange
[See Mechanical Ventilation]

Related to: inflammation, infection, ventilation/perfusion mismatching, fever, changes in oxyhemoglobin dissociation curve

Defining characteristics: dyspnea, tachycardia, cyanosis, hypoxia, hypoxemia, abnormal arterial blood gases

Alteration in comfort
[See MI]

Related to: inflammation, dyspnea, fever, coughing

Defining characteristics: pleuritic chest pain worsened with respiration or cough, muscle aches, joint pain, restlessness, communication of pain/discomfort

Risk for altered nutrition: less than body requirements
[See Mechanical Ventilation]

Related to: increased metabolic demands, fever, infection, abnormal taste sensation, anorexia, abdominal distention, nausea, vomiting

Defining characteristics: actual inadequate food intake, altered taste, altered smell sensation, weight loss, anorexia, nausea, vomiting, abdominal distention, decreased muscle mass and tone

Risk for fluid volume deficit
[See ARDS]

Related to: fluid loss from fever, diaphoresis, or vomiting, decreased fluid intake

Defining characteristics: decreased blood pressure, oliguria, anuria, low pulmonary artery wedge pressures

Risk for fluid volume excess
[See ARDS]

Related to: inflammatory response, pulmonary edema

Defining characteristics: rales, crackles, wheezing, pink frothy sputum, abnormal arterial blood gases

Knowledge deficit

Related to: lack of information, competing stimuli, misinterpretation of information

Defining characteristics: request for information, failure to improve, development of preventable complications

Outcome Criteria

Patient will be able to verbalize and demonstrate understanding of information.

INTERVENTIONS	RATIONALES
Instruct on need for vaccines for influenza and pneumonia.	Influenza increases the chance of secondary pneumonia infection; vaccinations help to prevent the occurrence and spread of infective process.
Instruct in continued need for coughing and deep breathing.	Patient is at risk for recurrence of pneumonia for 6-8 weeks following discharge.
Instruct in importance of continuing with follow-up medical care.	Helps prevent complications and recurrence of pneumonia.
Instruct in need to quit or avoid smoking.	Smoking destroys the action of the cilia and impairs the lungs' first line of defense against infection.

Discharge or Maintenance Evaluation

- Patient will be able to accurately verbalize understanding of all instructions.

- Patient will be compliant in avoiding smoking.

- Patient will not have preventable complications from illness.

PNEUMONIA

Airborne pathogenic or direct contact spread

Defect in defense and immunity　　　Virulent microorganisms　　　Overwhelming exposure

Infectious organism lodges in bronchioles

Alveolar collapse

Inflammation of interstitial
tissues of lungs

Vascular engorgement of alveoli with fluid

RBCs and fibrin move into alveoli

Fibrin accumulates
Disintegration of RBCs and fibrin

Exudate digested by enzymes

Action provides excellent culture media to increase spread of organisms

Consolidation

Removal of pathogenic mucus by
coughing, suctioning, or macrophagic action

RESOLUTION

Continued infection despite use of
antimicrobial therapy

Abscess formation

Necrosis of pulmonary tissues

Overwhelming sepsis

DEATH

Pneumothorax

A pneumothorax occurs when free air accumulates in the pleural cavity between the visceral and parietal areas, and causes a portion or the complete lung to collapse. Pressure in the pleural space is normally less than that of atmospheric pressure but following a penetration injury, air can enter the cavity from the outside changing the pressure within the lung cavity and causing it to collapse. Air can also migrate to the area when the esophagus is perforated or a bronchus ruptures, leaking air into the mediastinum (pneumomediastinum). Barotrauma related to mechanical ventilatory support using high levels of PEEP leads to alveoli rupture and collapse. Gas formation from gas-forming organisms can also result in pneumothorax.

Pneumothorax may occur spontaneously in cases where a subpleural bleb or emphysematous bulla ruptures due to chronic obstructive pulmonary disease, tuberculosis, cancer, or infection and this is the most common reason in otherwise healthy individuals. A tension pneumothorax is a life-threatening emergency and occurs when air is permitted into the pleural cavity but not allowed to escape, resulting in increased intrathoracic pressure and complete collapse of the lung. It compromises the opposite lung because of increasing pleural pressures and causes a mediastinal shift which interferes with ventilation and venous return. Severe shortness of breath, hypotension, and shock ensues, and emergent treatment of needle thoracentesis must be performed to relieve the pressure until a chest tube can be placed.

A hemothorax occurs when the lung collapse is due to accumulation of blood. Blood accumulations usually occur from the pulmonary vasculature, the intercostal and internal mammary arteries, the mediastinum, the spleen or the liver.

A hemothorax not only results in cardiopulmonary effects, but also may involve problems with hemorrhagic shock. The rate at which shock may occur depends on the source and rapidity of bleeding.

The severity of a pneumothorax, no matter what the origin, relates to the degree of collapse. A small partial pneumothorax may resolve by itself when the air is reabsorbed. In cases where collapse is more than 20-30 percent, a closed, water-seal drainage system and insertion of a chest tube via a lateral intercostal space is required. In cases where rapid re-expansion is desired, 15-25 cm H_2O suction may be added to the drain system.

A pneumothorax may result spontaneously or with trauma, such as a penetrating chest wound, gunshot wound, knife wound, or after a procedure such as insertion of a centrally placed venous catheter line. Some symptoms of pneumothorax include abrupt onset of pleuritic chest pain, shortness of breath, decreased or absent breath sounds, tachycardia, tachypnea, hyperresonant percussion, shock, and hypotension.

MEDICAL CARE

Laboratory: hemoglobin and hematocrit may be decreased with blood loss

Chest x-ray: used to evaluate air or fluid accumulations, collapse of lungs, or mediastinal shifts; a visceral pleural line may be visualized

Arterial blood gases: vary depending on the severity of the pneumothorax; oxygen saturation usually decreases, PaO_2 is usually normal or decreased, and $PaCO_2$ is occasionally increased

Chest tube: placement required to facilitate re-expansion of the collapsed lung and to permit drainage of fluid from lung

Thoracentesis: needle thoracentesis is required for

the immediate management of a tension pneumothorax to relieve the pressure in the pleura by removing air and/or fluid

Surgery: thoracotomy with excision or oversewing of the bullae may be required if the patient develops 2 or more pneumothorax on one side

NURSING CARE PLANS

Ineffective breathing pattern

Related to: air and/or fluid accumulations, pain, decreased lung expansion

Defining characteristics: dyspnea, tachypnea, use of accessory muscles, nasal flaring, decreased chest expansion, cyanosis, abnormal arterial blood gases

Outcome Criteria

Patient will be eupneic, with adequate oxygenation, and will maintain adequate ABGs.

INTERVENTIONS	RATIONALES
Monitor respiratory status for increase in rate, decrease in depth, dyspnea, or cyanosis.	Physiologic changes that result from the lung collapse may cause respiratory distress and may lead to hypoxia.
Auscultate breath sounds.	Breath sounds may be absent in areas where atelectasis occurs, and may be decreased with partially collapsed lung fields.
Observe for symmetrical chest expansion.	Moderate to severe pneumothorax will result in asymmetrical chest expansion until the lung is fully re-expanded.
Observe for position of trachea.	Tracheal deviation away from the affected lung occurs in tension pneumothorax.
Listen for sucking sounds with inspiration; if present, apply occlusive dressing over wound while patient performs valsalva maneuver.	Indicates an open pneumothorax which impairs ventilation. During inspiration air moves into the pleural space and collapses lung; with expiration, air moves out of the pleural space.

INTERVENTIONS	RATIONALES
	Application of a dressing seals the chest wall defect, while the valsalva maneuver helps to expand the lung.
Observe for paradoxical movements of the chest during respiration; if present, stabilize the flail area with a sandbag or pressure dressing, and turn to the affected side.	May indicate flail chest and impaired ventilation. Procedures help to stabilize the area to facilitate improved respiratory exchange.
Place patient in semi-sitting position.	Promotes lung expansion and improves ventilatory efforts.
Prepare patient for and assist with insertion of chest tube.	Intercostal tube placement is required when a pneumothorax is greater than 20–30% in order to facilitate re-expansion of the lung. Instruction, when feasible, reduces patient anxiety and improves cooperation.
Once chest tube is inserted, ensure that connections are tightened and taped securely per hospital protocol.	Prevents air leaks and disconnections at the connector sites.
Monitor water-seal drainage bottles to ensure fluid level is above drain tube.	Fluid must be maintained above the end of the tube to prevent air from being sucked into lung and resulting in further collapse.
Maintain prescribed level of suction to drainage system.	Usually 15–25 cm H_2O pressure suction is sufficient to maintain intrapleural negative pressure and facilitate fluid drainage and re-expansion of the lung.
Observe the water-seal drainage system for bubbling.	Bubbling should occur during expiration and demonstrates that the pneumothorax is vented through the system. Bubbling should diminish and finally cease as the lung re-expands. If no bubbling is present in system, this may indicate either complete re-expansion of the lung or obstruction in the chest tube/drainage system.
Monitor drainage system for continuous bubbling and ascertain if the problem is patient- or	Continuous bubbling may result from a large pneumothorax or from air leaks in the drainage

INTERVENTIONS	RATIONALES
system-centered. Clamp chest tube near the patient's chest.	system. When the tube is clamped as described and bubbling ceases, the problem is patient-centered with potential air leak at the insertion site or within the patient. If the bubbling continues, the leak is within the drainage system.
If patient has insertion site air leak, apply vaseline–impregnated gauze around site, and reassess the problem.	Provides a seal and corrects the air leak problem.
If patient has drainage system air leak, ascertain the location by clamping the tube downward toward the system by increments. Secure connections.	Determines the location of the problem and corrects air leaks at the connectors.
Observe for fluid tidaling.	Fluctuation of the fluid within the tubing, or tidaling, demonstrates pressure changes during inspiration and expiration, and is normally 2–10 cm during inspiration. Increases may occur during coughing or forceful expiration but continuous increases in tidaling may indicate a large pneumothorax or airway obstruction.
Monitor fluid drainage for character and amount, and notify MD if drainage is greater than 100 cc/hr for more than 2 hours.	Provides for prompt detection of hemorrhage and prompt intervention. Some drainage systems have the potential for auto-transfusion, and this should be done per hospital policy.
Strip chest tubes gently, if at all, per hospital protocol.	Some facilities and physicians avoid milking, or stripping, of the tubes due to the potential for suction to draw lung tissue into the orifice of the tube and damage the tissue, as well as rupturing of small blood vessels. The procedure changes intrathoracic pressure which may result in chest pain or coughing. Stripping may be required to maintain drainage when large blood clots or fibrin strands are present or if the drainage is viscid or purulent.

INTERVENTIONS	RATIONALES
Place chest drainage system below the level of the chest, and coil tubing carefully to avoid kinking.	Promotes drainage of air and fluid, and prevents kinking and occlusion of tubing.
Obtain chest x-rays daily.	Identifies the presence of pneumothorax and resolution or deterioration.
If chest tube is accidentally removed, apply vaseline-impregnated gauze and pressure dressing, and notify MD.	Provides a seal over chest wound to prevent pneumothorax from recurring or worsening. Prompt treatment may prevent cardiopulmonary impairment.
If chest tube becomes accidentally disconnected from tubing, reconnect as cleanly and quickly as possible.	Disconnection may result in atmospheric air entering the pleural space and worsening or causing pneumothorax.
Observe dressing over chest tube insertion site for drainage and notify MD for significant drainage.	Excessive drainage on dressing may indicate malposition of the chest tube, infection, or other problem.
Assure that chest tube clamps (2 for each tube) are present in patient's room and are taken with patient when transported out of unit.	Provides for emergencies which may require clamping of the tube.
Assist with removal of chest tube as warranted, and apply vaseline-impregnated gauze and dry sterile dressing over site, and change per hospital protocol.	Once lung is re-expanded and fluid drainage has ceased, chest tubes are removed. Gauze provides a seal over the open wound to prevent recurrence of pneumothorax.
Monitor patient for changes in respiratory status, oxygenation, chest pain, dyspnea, or presence of subcutaneous emphysema.	May indicate recurrent pneumothorax and requires prompt intervention and reinsertion of intercostal tube.

Information, Instruction, Demonstration

INTERVENTIONS	RATIONALES
Instruct on function of chest tube/drainage system.	Provides knowledge and decreases patient anxiety.
Instruct patient to avoid pulling or lying on tubing.	Prevents obstruction of tube and facilitates drainage.

INTERVENTIONS	RATIONALES
Instruct on signs/symptoms to report to nurse: dyspnea, chest pain, changes in sounds of bubbling from drainage system.	Promotes prompt recognition of problems that may require prompt intervention.

Discharge or Maintenance Evaluation

• Patient will be eupneic with no adventitious breath sounds.

• Patient will have symmetrical chest expansion and midline tracheal placement with no episodes of dyspnea.

• Patient will achieve and maintain re-expansion of lung with no recurrence or complications.

PNEUMOTHORAX

Air enters pleural cavity
↓
Pleural pressure increased above atmospheric pressure
↓
Lung collapses
↓
High pressure gradient between alveolus and adjacent vascular sheet
↓
Decreased PaO_2
Increased $PaCO_2$
↓
Air moves along pulmonary vessels to mediastinum
↓
Mediastinal shifting
↓
Interference with ventilation and venous return
↓
Increased pulmonary pressures
Low PCWP, high CVP
↓
Shock
↓
Cardiovascular collapse
↓
DEATH

Status Asthmaticus

Status asthmaticus is a critical emergency that requires prompt intervention to avoid acute and possibly fatal, respiratory failure. In this condition, the asthmatic attacks are unresponsive to medical therapeutics, with severe bronchospasms creating decreased oxygenation and perfusion.

During an acute asthmatic attack, the individual may demonstrate varying degrees of respiratory distress depending on the duration of the attack, and the severity of spasm. The underlying cause of asthma is still as yet unknown, but is thought to be due to imbalances in adrenergic and cholinergic control of the airways, and their response to the allergens, infections, or emotional factors with which they come in contact. Intrinsic asthma occurs when the triggering factors are irritation, infection, or emotions, and extrinsic asthma occurs when precipitated by allergic or complement-mediated factors. Asthma may be drug-induced by aspirin, indomethacin, tartrazine, propranolol, and timolol.

In asthma, the airways are narrowed due to the bronchial muscle spasms, edema, inflammation of the bronchioles, and thick, tenacious mucous production. The narrowing leads to areas of obstruction and these become hypoventilated and hypoperfused. Eventually a ventilation/perfusion mismatch occurs and may lead to hypoxemia and an increasing A-a gradient. When $PaCO_2$ rises to the point of respiratory acidosis, the patient is then considered to be in respiratory failure.

The three most common causes of status asthmaticus are allergen exposure, noncompliance with medication regime, and respiratory infection exposure. Environmental factors, such as excessively hot, cold, or dusty areas, may initiate status asthmaticus because of the effect they have on the air that is breathed.

Wheezing may occur not only with asthma, but with chronic obstructive pulmonary disease, congestive heart failure, pulmonary embolism, and tuberculosis, and these diagnoses should be ruled out.

Patients who have status asthmaticus suffer pronounced fatigue due to the continuous efforts of breathing, and they easily become dehydrated due to the hyperpnea. The patient usually has dyspnea, tachypnea, wheezing, tachycardia, pulsus paradoxus, and severe anxiety. The goals of treatment include ventilatory support and maintenance of adequate airways, and the prevention of respiratory failure or barotrauma.

MEDICAL CARE

Laboratory: CBC and sputum specimens usually show eosinophilia

Chest x-ray: used to observe for infiltrates or hyperinflation to the lungs; may be used to visualize pneumothorax, hemothorax, or pneumomediastinum

Arterial blood gases: to identify problems with oxygenation and acid-base balance

Spirometry: to provide information about severity of an attack, and to assess for improvement with therapy; FEV_1 is the forced expiratory volume for 1 second and is usually < 1500 cc during an asthmatic attack and will increase 500 cc or more if treatment is successful

Oxygen: to provide supplemental available oxygen

Bronchodilators: used to relax bronchial smooth muscle to dilate bronchial tree to facilitate air exchange

Beta-adrenergic agents: ephedrine, epinephrine, isoproterenol, metaproterenol, terbutaline; used to relax bronchial smooth muscle

Corticosteroids: used to decrease inflammatory response and decrease edema

Antibiotics: used when infective process is documented; usually bacterial infection is not a common precipitating factor

Mechanical ventilation: necessary when respiratory failure is present and hypoxemia persists despite medical therapy

IPPB: used to assist the patient with deep inspiration to facilitate more productive coughing of thick mucous and to deliver medication by an aerosol route

NURSING CARE PLANS

Ineffective airway clearance

Related to: airway obstruction, edema of bronchioles, inability to cough or to cough effectively, excessive mucous production

Defining characteristics: adventitious breath sounds, dyspnea, tachypnea, shallow respirations, cough with or without productivity, cyanosis, anxiety, restlessness

Outcome Criteria

Patient will maintain patency of airway and will be able to effectively clear secretions.

INTERVENTIONS	RATIONALES
Administer bronchodilators as ordered.	Nebulizers are usually the first line treatment for asthma. Aminophylline is frequently prescribed to relax bronchial smooth muscle and mediates histamine release and cAMP degradation, which facilitates improved air flow.
Monitor lab levels for attainment	Therapeutic levels range between

INTERVENTIONS	RATIONALES
and maintenance of therapeutic levels. Observe patient for anorexia, nausea, vomiting, abdominal pain, nervousness, restlessness, and tachycardia.	10-20 mcg/ml. Symptoms may indicate theophylline toxicity, which will require titration of the drug dosage.
Administer sympathomimetics as ordered.	Epinephrine is usually given SQ every 20-30 minutes for 3 doses as needed to relieve bronchoconstriction. Terbutaline is usually not the first drug of choice in acute situations due to the delayed onset of action, but is frequently used after the patient shows improvement.
Assist/administer inhalation therapy as ordered.	Nebulizers and intermittent positive pressure breathing treatments may be used in mild to moderate episodes but should not be used during acute attacks because of the potential for bronchospasm in response to the aerosol agent.

Information, Instruction, Demonstration

INTERVENTIONS	RATIONALES
Monitor for side effects, such as tachycardias, tremors, nausea, vomiting, or bronchospasm.	May occur as adverse reactions from medications. May require change in specific drug used.

Discharge or Maintenance Evaluation

- Patient will maintain patent airway and be able to cough and clear own secretions.

- Patient will have clear breath sounds with no adventitious sounds or airway compromise.

- Patient will have adequate oxygenation.

Impaired gas exchange
[See Mechanical Ventilation]

Related to: bronchospasm, inflammation to bronchi, hypoxemia, fatigue

Defining characteristics: dyspnea, tachypnea, hypoxia, hypoxemia, hypercapnia, restlessness, anxiety, abnormal ABGs, dysrhythmias, decreased oxygen saturation

Anxiety
[See Mechanical Ventilation]

Related to: dyspnea, change in health status, threat of death

Defining characteristics: fear, restlessness, muscle tension, apprehension, helplessness, sense of impending doom

STATUS ASTHMATICUS

Hyperactive airways
↓
Mucosal edema + bronchial muscle constriction/spasm
↓
Mucus plugs
↓
Inflammatory response
↓

Decreased PaO_2
Hypoxia
↓
Increased airway resistance
Increased work of breathing

Dehydration CO_2 retention   Tachypnea
↓   ↓   Wheezing
Increased mucus plugs   Increased oxygen demand   Decreased $PaCO_2$
↓   ↓   ↓
Hypoxia   Increased CO_2 production   Respiratory alkalosis
↓   ↓   ↓
Decreased PaO_2 Respiratory acidosis   Hypoxemia
↓
Right ventricular strain

Reactive pulmonary hypertension
↓
Ventricular failure
↓
Cardiac dysrhythmias

Cardiovascular compromise
↓
Cardiopulmonary collapse
↓

DEATH

Mechanical Ventilation

Mechanical ventilation is used as an artificial adjunct to maintain and optimize ventilation and oxygenation in those patients that are unable to do so on their own for whatever the reason. It is utilized when other adjuncts are ineffective to regulate oxygen and carbon dioxide levels and provide for an adequate acid-base balance.

Major types of ventilators include negative external pressure and positive pressure ventilators. The external type is very rarely seen today, such as the "iron lung" used for the treatment of polio and the chest ventilator used for home treatment of neuromuscular diseases. These ventilators apply pressure against the thorax that is less than room air, in order to accomplish ventilation by changes in lung pressures. There are no requirements for artificial airways and are fairly easy to use. The patient must remain in or under the unit and, as such, activity is limited, and the negative pressure exerted may result in venous pooling and decreased cardiac output.

Positive pressure ventilators are further subclassified according to the factor that initiates the inspiratory phase, and what factor causes the inspiratory phase to cease. Pressure-cycled ventilators use oxygen or compressed air valves to deliver a gas volume until a preset pressure limit is achieved. As the lung compliance and airway resistance changes, inspired tidal volumes, alveolar ventilation and FIO_2 changes also. The alarm systems for this ventilator are sometimes inadequate and the ventilator cannot compensate for leaks that may occur in the system.

Volume-cycled ventilators, currently the most common found in intensive care settings, deliver a preset gas volume to the patient regardless of airway resistance or compliance. Most have safety features to limit excessive airway pressures, and

FIO_2 and exhaled tidal volumes are more accurate.

High-frequency ventilation is used when other methods have not been successful in oxygenation and ventilation of the patient. It uses lower tidal volumes and increased respiratory rates to decrease the incidence of barotrauma and cardiac decompensation. Frequencies range from 60-200 times/min, and in high-frequency oscillation, movement of air to and from the airway is performed at 600-3000 cycles/min.

PEEP, or positive end-expiratory pressure, is used to improve oxygen exchange in persistent hypoxemia when increases in FIO_2 have not improved the situation. PEEP produces an increased functional residual capacity (FRC) which increases the available lung alveoli surface for oxygenation by maintaining the alveoli in an open position. High levels of PEEP may contribute to the incidence of barotrauma and hemodynamic compromise, and is most effective when maintained for lengthy periods of time. To this end, a special PEEP ambu bag must be used to maintain the pressure in order to maintain the beneficial effects.

MEDICAL CARE

Laboratory: CBC, transferrin, albumin, prealbumin, electrolytes used to monitor infection, imbalance, and nutritional status; cultures done to identify infective organism and specify antimicrobial agent required for eradication

Intubation: artificial airway is required for mechanical ventilation

Arterial blood gases: used to determine levels of oxygen, carbon dioxide, and pH to identify acid-base disturbances, hypoxemia, and to monitor for changes in respiratory status

Respiratory treatments: used to instill varied agents into the lungs to reduce spasm, increase hydration and liquification of secretions, and to facilitate removal of secretions

Ventilatory management: ventilator settings are changed periodically based on patient condition and arterial blood gas analysis to ensure optimum ventilation and oxygenation

Tracheostomy: performed when nasal or oral intubation is impossible, or after significant time of nasal/oral intubation on a prolonged ventilator patient

NURSING CARE PLANS

Ineffective airway clearance

Related to: thick tenacious secretions, airway obstruction, edema of bronchioles, inability to cough or to cough effectively, presence of artificial airway

Defining characteristics: adventitious breath sounds, dyspnea, tachypnea, shallow respirations, cough with or without productivity, cyanosis, fever, anxiety, restlessness

Outcome Criteria

Patient will maintain patency of airway, have clear breath sounds, and will be able to effectively clear secretions.

INTERVENTIONS	RATIONALES
Monitor airway for patency and provide artificial airways as warranted. Prepare for mechanical ventilation.	Artificial airways will be required if patient cannot maintain patency. Oropharyngeal airways hold tongue anteriorly but may precipitate vomiting if length is not accurately measured. Nasopharyngeal airways are more easily tolerated in conscious patients but may cause nosebleeds and may easily become occluded. Esophageal
	obturator airways are useful only in emergency situations and must be replaced as quickly as possible. These are easier to insert than endotracheal tubes, but stimulate vomiting and cannot be used in conscious patients. The trachea may accidentally be intubated and the esophagus may be perforated. Endotracheal intubation requires advanced training and skill, and may be accidentally placed in the esophagus, develop leaks that may decrease oxygenation, and over time, may necrotize tissues. Artificial airways may become occluded by mucous, blood, or other secretions; endotracheal tubes may become twisted or compressed, or severe spasms may occlude airway.
Monitor tube placement for migration; place marking on tube and note length and position at least every 8 hours; tube should be adequately secured to maintain placement.	Tube migration may occur with coughing, re-taping, or accidentally, with the potential for improper placement resulting in hypoxia. Comparison of previous placement guidelines will provide prompt recognition of differences and changes, and facilitate prompt intervention.
Prepare for placement on mechanical ventilation as warranted.	If routine medical therapeutics are not effective in controlling the spasms, hypoxemia, and hypoxia, respiratory failure will ensue, and mechanical ventilation will be required to assure adequate oxygenation and perfusion.
Auscultate lung fields for presence of breath sounds, changes in character, and presence to all lobes; observe for symmetrical chest expansion.	Proper tube placement will result in equal bilateral breath sounds and symmetrical chest expansion. Adventitious breath sounds, such as rhonchi and wheezes, may indicate airflow has been obstructed by occlusion of the tube or migration into an inappropriate position. Absence of breath sounds to left lung fields

INTERVENTIONS	RATIONALES
	may indicate intubation of the right main stem bronchus.
Suction patient every 2-4 hours and prn, being sure to hyperoxygenate patient prior to, during, and after procedure; limit active suctioning to 15 seconds or less at a time; use pulmonary toilette instillation as needed.	Patients who are intubated frequently have ineffective cough reflexes or are sedated and have some muscular involvement that may impair coughing, and suctioning is required to remove their secretions. Suctioning time should be minimized and hyperoxygenation performed to reduce the potential for hypoxia.
Position patient in high-Fowler's or semi-Fowler's position.	Promotes maximal lung expansion.
Turn patient every 2 hours and prn.	Repositioning promotes drainage of pulmonary secretions and enhances ventilation to decrease potential for atelectasis.
Administer bronchodilators as ordered.	Promotes relaxation of bronchial smooth muscle to decrease spasm, dilates airways to improve ventilation, and maximizes air exchange.

Information, Instruction, Demonstration

INTERVENTIONS	RATIONALES
Instruct on splinting abdomen with pillow during cough efforts.	Promotes increased expiratory pressure and helps to decrease discomfort.
Instruct on alternative types of coughing exercises, such as quad thrusts, if patient has difficulty during coughing.	Minimizes fatigue by assisting patient to increase expiratory pressure and facilitates cough.
Instruct on deep breathing exercises.	Promotes full lung expansion and decreases anxiety.
Perform chest percussion and postural drainage as warranted.	Mobilizes secretions and facilitates ventilation of all lung fields.

Discharge or Maintenance Evaluation

- Patient will maintain patent airway and be able to cough and clear own secretions.

- Patient will have clear breath sounds with no adventitious sounds or airway compromise.

- Patient will not have any aspiration complications.

- Patient will be able to adequately perform coughing.

Impaired gas exchange

Related to: bronchospasm, mucous production, edema, inflammation to bronchial tree, hypoxemia, fatigue

Defining characteristics: dyspnea, tachypnea, hypoxia, hypoxemia, hypercapnia, confusion, restlessness, cyanosis, inability to move secretions, tachycardia, dysrhythmias, abnormal ABGs, decreased oxygen saturation by oximetry

Outcome Criteria

Patient will have arterial blood gases within normal range for patient, with no signs of ventilation/perfusion mismatching.

INTERVENTIONS	RATIONALES
Monitor pulse oximetry for oxygen saturation and notify MD if < 90.	Oximetry readings of 90 correlate with PaO_2 of 60. Levels below 60 do not allow for adequate perfusion to tissues and vital organs. Oximetry uses light waves to identify differences between saturation and reduced hemoglobin of the tissues and may be inaccurate in low blood flow states.
Monitor transcutaneous oxygen tension if available.	Measures the oxygen concentration of the skin, but may cause burns if monitor site is not rotated frequently. Skin, blood flow and temperature may affect these readings.

INTERVENTIONS	RATIONALES
Provide oxygen as ordered.	Provides supplemental oxygen to benefit patient. Low flow oxygen delivery systems use some room air and may be inadequate for patient's needs if their tidal volume is low, respiratory rate is high, or if ventilation status is unstable. Low flow systems should be used in patients with COPD so as to not depress their respiratory drive. High levels of oxygen may cause severe damage to tissues, oxygen toxicity, increases in A-a gradients, microatelectasis, and ARDS.
Monitor for changes in mental status, restlessness, anxiety, headache, confusion, dysrhythmias, hypotension, tachycardia, and cyanosis.	May indicate impending or present hypoxia and hypoxemia.
Monitor ABGs for changes and/or trends.	Provides information on measured levels of oxygen and carbon dioxide as well as acid-base balance. Promotes prompt intervention for deteriorating airway status. PaO_2 alone does not reflect tissue oxygenation; ventilation must be adequate to provide gas exchange.
Administer oxygen as ordered.	Oxygen by itself may not always correct hypoxia of tissues and restore perfusion.
Monitor for signs/symptoms of oxygen toxicity (nausea, vomiting, dyspnea, coughing, retrosternal pain, extremity paresthesias, pronounced fatigue, or restlessness).	Oxygen toxicity may result when oxygen concentrations are greater than 40% for lengthy durations of time, usually 8 to 24 hours, and may cause actual physiologic changes in the lungs. Progressive respiratory distress, cyanosis, and asphyxia are late signs of toxicity. Oxygen concentrations should be maintained as low as possible in order to maintain adequate PaO_2.
Limit PEEP (positive end-expiratory pressures) to 5–20 cm H_2O.	PEEP is used to improve oxygen exchange in persistent hypoxemia

INTERVENTIONS	RATIONALES
Use PEEP ambu bag when suctioning patient.	despite increasing levels of oxygen by producing an increased functional residual capacity which then increases the available lung alveoli surface for oxygenation. PEEP may predispose the patient to barotrauma with elevated levels. Ambu bags that are capable of maintaining PEEP levels are required because short intervals minimize the beneficial effects of PEEP.

Information, Instruction, Demonstration

INTERVENTIONS	RATIONALES
Prepare patient for placement on mechanical ventilation as warranted.	May be necessary to maintain adequate oxygenation and acid-base balance.
Assist with respiratory therapists measurements of oxygen analyzing, lung compliance, vital capacity, and A-a gradients.	Provides information to facilitate early detection of oxygen toxicity.

Discharge or Maintenance Evaluation

- Patient will have arterial blood gases within normal limits for patient.

- Patient will be eupneic with adequate oxygenation and no signs/symptoms of oxygen toxicity.

Ineffective breathing pattern

Related to: fatigue, dyspnea, secretions, inadequate oxygenation, respiratory muscle weakness, respiratory center depression, decreased lung expansion, placement on mechanical ventilation

Defining characteristics: dyspnea, tachypnea, bradypnea, apnea, cough, nasal flaring, cyanosis, shallow respirations, pursed-lip breathing, changes in inspiratory/expiratory ratio, use of accessory muscles, diminished chest expansion, barrel chest, abnormal arterial blood gases, fremitus, anxiety, decreased oxygen saturation

Outcome Criteria

Patient will be eupneic, with adequate oxygenation, and will maintain adequate ABGs within normal limits.

INTERVENTIONS	RATIONALES
Prepare patient for placement on mechanical ventilation and intubation procedures.	Promotes knowledge and reduces fear. May promote cooperation.
Assist with intubation of patient; auscultate all lung fields for breath sounds.	Placement of an artificial airway (endotracheal tube [ETT] or tracheostomy) is required for mechanical ventilation support. Nasotracheal intubation may be preferred to prevent oral discomfort and necrosis, but is associated with a high incidence of sinus disease.
Hyperoxygenate patient and auscultate for bilateral breath sounds and observe for bilateral symmetrical chest expansion.	Prolonged difficulty in placement of the tube may result in hypoxia. If symmetrical chest expansion is not observed, or if breath sounds cannot be heard bilaterally, this may indicate improper placement of the tube into the right main bronchus or esophagus, and correction of this problem must be addressed promptly.
Utilize low pressure endotracheal tubes for intubation.	High pressure cuffed tubes may promote tracheal necrosis or result in a tracheal fistula.
Maintain airway; secure tube with tape or other securing device.	Artificial airways may become occluded by mucous or other secretory fluids, may develop a cuff leak resulting in inability to maintain pressures sufficient for ventilation, or may migrate to a position whereby adequate oxygenation is impaired. Tubes should be adequately secured to prevent movement, loss of airway, and tracheal damage.
Obtain chest x-ray after ETT is inserted.	Radiographic confirmation of tube placement is mandatory;

INTERVENTIONS	RATIONALES
	the tube should be 2-3 cm above the carina.
If ETT is placed orally, daily changes from side to side of mouth should be routinely performed.	Prevents tissue necrosis from pressure of tube against teeth, lips, and other tissues. Oral tubes promote saliva formation, cause nausea and vomiting if movement of tube stimulates retching, and prevents the patient from closing his mouth without biting down on the tube.
Suction patient as needed, making sure to hyperoxygenate before, during, and after procedure. Utilize sterile normal saline for pulmonary toilette instillation prior to suctioning procedures as warranted/ordered.	Suctioning is required to remove secretions because the patient is unable to do so on his own. Effective coughing is decreased because of the inability to increase intrathoracic pressure when the glottis is restricted from air. Suctioning places patient at risk for inadequate oxygenation and decreased perfusion. Hyper-oxygenation helps to limit this sudden decrease in available oxygen. Mucous production is usually increased with placement of ETT due to ciliary movement being impaired and the body's response to the foreign tube. Pulmonary toilette is controversial but may be helpful to liquefy secretions to facilitate easier removal.
Restrain patient as warranted and as per hospital protocol.	Prevents accidental extubation in sedated or confused patients.
Monitor ventilator settings at least every 2-4 hours and prn; FIO_2 should be analyzed periodically to ensure correct amount is being maintained; tidal volume should ideally be 10–15 cc/Kg body weight; airway pressures (peak inspiratory pressure and plateau pressure) should be noted for identification of trends; inspiratory and expiratory ratio; sigh volume and rate.	Ventilator settings are adjusted based on the disease process and patient's condition to maintain optimal oxygenation and ventilation while the patient is unable to do so on his own. Oxygen percentages may not be completely accurate and analysis must be performed to ensure proper amounts are being delivered. Exhaled tidal volumes should be monitored and changes may indicate changes in lung compliance or problems with delivering specific volumes.

INTERVENTIONS	RATIONALES	INTERVENTIONS	RATIONALES
	Increases in airway pressures may indicate bronchospasm, presence of mucoid and other secretions, obstruction of the airway, pneumothorax, or ARDS with high pressure levels and disconnection of tubing, inadequate cuff pressure or non-synchronous breathing with low pressure levels. I:E ratio should be 1:2 but may be altered to improve gas exchange. Sighs, when used, are commonly 1 1/2 times the volume of a normal breath, 2-6 times per hour to facilitate expansion of alveoli to reduce the potential for atelectasis. Ventilator settings may be inadvertently changed, or due to forgetfulness, increased oxygenation used for suctioning procedure may not be turned down to ordered amounts. This may result in oxygen toxicity or inadequate ventilation.		Increasing volumes of air required to maintain ventilatory pressures, or increasing cuff pressures may indicate cuff leak and will require replacement of airway to maintain oxygenation.
		Auscultate for adventitious breath sounds, subcutaneous emphysema, or localized wheezing.	May indicate migration of airway tube. Movement from trachea into tissue may cause mediastinal or subcutaneous emphysema and/or pneumothorax. Intubation of the bronchus may result in decreased unilateral chest expansion with decreased breath sounds, and localized wheezing. Movement of the tube to the level of the carina may result in excessive coughing, diminished breath sounds, and inability to insert suction catheter.
Observe for temperature of ventilator circuitry; drain tubing away from the patient as warranted.	Intubation bypasses the body's natural warming/humidifying action, and requires increased temperature and moisturizing of the delivered oxygen. The temperature of the ventilator circuitry (and the delivered oxygen) should be maintained at approximately body temperature to avoid hyperthermic reactions. Temperature increases and humidification promote condensation of water in tubing which may restrict adequate volume delivery. Drainage of fluid toward the patient or toward the reservoir may promote bacterial infestations.	Monitor ABGs for trends, and change ventilator settings as ordered.	Maintains adequate oxygenation and acid-base balance.
		Observe breathing patterns and note if patient has spontaneous breaths in addition to ventilatory breaths.	Increased or decreased ventilation may be experienced by ventilator patients who may try to compensate by competing with ventilatory breaths. Tachypnea may result in respiratory alkalosis; bradypnea may result in acidosis with increased $PaCO_2$.
Monitor airway cuff for leakage, noting amount of air volume in cuff and cuff pressures at least every 4–8 hours and prn.	Proper cuff inflation is done with the least amount of air to ensure a minimal leak with maintenance of adequate ventilatory pressures and tidal volumes. Cuff pressures should be less than 25 cm H_2O to prevent tracheal necrosis.	Observe patient for non-synchronous respirations with ventilator ("fighting the ventilator"). Administer sedation or sedation/neuromuscular blockade, as ordered.	Asynchrony with the ventilator decreases alveolar ventilation, increases intrathoracic pressures, and decreases venous return and cardiac output. Pavulon paralyzes all muscles in body to facilitate synchrony with ventilation support. Patients may be completely alert when paralyzed, so sedation is MANDATORY prior to administration of Pavulon. Often, a sedation cocktail of narcotics and/or benzodiazepines may be titrated with better results to achieve adequate sedation.

Information, Instruction, Demonstration

INTERVENTIONS	RATIONALES
Prepare patient for placement of tracheostomy as warranted.	Prolonged ventilatory support via nasal or oral endotracheal tube may lead to necrosis of tissues due to pressure exerted by the tube. Tracheostomy is more comfortable for the patient, decreases the airway resistance, and may reduce the amount of dead space.
Observe for pulsation of tracheostomy with neck vein pulsation and notify MD.	May indicate close proximity to innominate vessels that may lead to necrosis and erosion into vessels and result in hemorrhage.
Assess for cuff leakage and change/notify MD for change of airway.	Cuffs which have leaks that enable a patient to have the ability to speak, in which air may be felt at the nose and/or mouth, changing pressures with ventilation, and/or decreased exhaled volumes require change in order to maintain adequate oxygenation and ventilation.
Obtain chest x-rays every day and prn while patient is intubated.	Facilitates recognition of tube migration, atelectatic changes, presence of pneumothorax, or other significant changes.
Insure that neostigmine bromide or edrophonium chloride is available.	These reverse effects of pancuronium.

Discharge or Maintenance Evaluation

- Patient will be able to maintain own airway and expectorate sputum.

- Patient will have arterial blood gases within normal limits of patient disease process.

- Patient will be eupneic with no adventitious breath sounds.

- Patient will have artificial airway intact with no signs/symptoms of complications.

Impaired verbal communication

Related to: intubation, artificial airway, muscular paralysis

Defining characteristics: inability to speak, inability to communicate needs, inability to make sounds

Outcome Criteria

Patient will achieve a method to communicate his needs.

INTERVENTIONS	RATIONALES
Evaluate patient's ability to speak or communicate by other means.	Patient may be fluent in sign language, or able to communicate in writing to make needs known.
Ensure that call light is placed within easy reach of patient at all times, and that the light system is flagged to denote patient's impairment.	Provides patient with concrete evidence that he may call for assistance and that the nurse will be available to meet his needs. Flagging system ensures that personnel not familiar with the patient will be alerted to his inability to speak.
Make eye contact with patient at all times; ask questions that may be answered by nodding of the head; provide paper and writing utensils, magic slate, or communication board for communication.	Communication may be possible if patient is able to nod head yes or no, or blink eyes in sequence. Writing may be illegible due to disease process or sedation, and may frustrate and fatigue patient.

Information, Instruction, Demonstration

INTERVENTIONS	RATIONALES
Instruct patient in using tongue to make clicking noise, or in tapping table or side rails to gain nurse's attention as a secondary means of calling for assistance.	Provides alternate method to communicate with nurse and helps to allay fear of abandonment.

INTERVENTIONS	RATIONALES
Instruct family members in talking with patient to provide information about issues of concern to patient, and help them to deal with the awkwardness of a one-sided conversation.	Promotes understanding for the family and assists in incorporating family into the patient's care to maintain contact with reality.

Discharge or Maintenance Evaluation

• Patient will be able to speak or make needs known.

• Patient will develop an adequate alternative means of communication and be able to utilize communication to make needs known.

• Patient's family will be able to recognize their own contribution to the patient's recovery.

Anxiety

Related to: ventilatory support, threat of death, change in health status, change in environment, life-threatening crises

Defining characteristics: fear, restlessness, muscle tension, apprehension, helplessness, communication of uncertainty, sense of impending doom, worry

Outcome Criteria

Patient will have decreased anxiety and be able to function at acceptable levels with anxiety-producing stimuli.

INTERVENTIONS	RATIONALES
Evaluate patient's perception of crisis or threat to self.	Identifies problem base and facilitates plan for intervention.
Monitor for changes in vital signs, restlessness, or facial tension.	May indicate patient's level of response to stressors and level of anxiety.
Encourage patient to express fears and concerns and provide information pertinent to those	Promotes verbalization of concerns, and allows time for identification of fears to progres-

INTERVENTIONS	RATIONALES
concerns. Do not give false reassurance.	sively begin work on emotional barriers. False reassurance tends to minimize patient's feelings resulting in impaired trust and increased anxiety.
Provide support and encouragement to family members and assist them in dealing with their own fears/concerns.	Family's anxiety may be communicated to the patient and result in increased anxiety levels.
Discuss safety precautions involved with ventilatory support; emergency power source, emergency oxygen and equipment, alarm systems, etc.	Provides concrete answers to help decrease anxiety and fear of the unknown, and to relay emergency plans for patient.
Ensure that patient's call light is placed within easy reach at all times, and that alternative methods of summoning assistance have been discussed.	Provides reassurance that nurses will be available to assist with patient's needs, and decreases anxiety.
Administer antianxiety medications as ordered.	Helps to reduce anxiety to a manageable level when other techniques have failed.

Information, Instruction, Demonstration

INTERVENTIONS	RATIONALES
Instruct in use of relaxation techniques and guided imagery.	Promotes reduction in stress and anxiety, and provides opportunity for patient to control his situation.
Consult psychiatrist, psychologist, or counselor as warranted.	Patient may require further intervention for dealing with emotional problems.

Discharge or Maintenance Evaluation

• Patient will be able to verbalize concerns and fears and be able to rationally deal with them in appropriate ways.

• Patient will be able to function with anxiety reduced at a manageable level.

- Patient will be able to utilize methods to reduce anxiety.

Ineffective individual/family coping

Related to: change in health status, change in ability to communicate, sensory overload, change in environment, fear of death, physical limitations, inadequate support system, inadequate coping mechanisms, threat to self, pain

Defining characteristics: inability to meet role expectations, inability to meet basic needs, worry, apprehension, fear, inability to problem solve, hostility, aggression, inappropriate defense mechanisms, low self-esteem, insomnia, depression, destructive behaviors, vacillation when choices are required, delayed decision making, muscle tension, headaches, pain

Outcome Criteria

Patient will be able to recognize problems with coping and be able to problem-solve adequately.

INTERVENTIONS	RATIONALES
Evaluate patient's/family's coping skills and ability to verbalize problems.	Provides baseline information to establish interventions best suited to the patient/family/situation. Coping abilities that the patient has utilized previously may be used in the current crisis to provide a sense of control.
Discuss concerns and fears of loss of control with patient, and provide feedback.	Identifies needs for intervention and helps to establish a trusting relationship.
Monitor for dependence on others, inability to make decisions, inability to involve self in care, or inability to express concerns/questions.	May indicate patient's need to depend on others to allow time to regain ability for coping with crises, and promotes feeling of safety. Patient may be afraid to make any decision in which his tenuous condition could be compromised.

INTERVENTIONS	RATIONALES
Provide opportunities for patient to make decisions regarding his care, when feasible.	Provides opportunity to gain some sense of control of his life, decreasing anxiety, and assisting in coping skills.
Discuss current problems and assist with problem-solving to find solutions.	Identifies actual problems and assists patient/family to find real solutions to facilitate increasing self-control and self-esteem.
Discuss feelings of blame, either on self, or on others.	Blaming oneself or others prolongs inability to cope and increases feelings of hopelessness.
Remain non-judgmental of choices patient/family may make. Adopt a non-threatened attitude when anger and hostility are expressed. Set limits on unacceptable behaviors.	Anger and hostile feelings may promote resolution of stages of grief and loss, and should be regarded as an important step in that process. Limits must be set to prevent destructive behavior that will impair patient's self-esteem.
Discuss feelings of anger at God, religious alienation, lack of meaning to life, etc.	Spiritual beliefs are questioned when threats of death occur, and may affect patient's ability to cope with and problem-solve during crises.

Information, Instruction, Demonstration

INTERVENTIONS	RATIONALES
Assess rapport of family members with patient. Involve the family members in the care of the patient when feasible.	Actions of the family may be helpful, but the patient may perceive these as being over-protective or smothering. Helping with patient's care may enhance the family's feelings of importance and control of the situation.
Provide information to the patient and family regarding other agencies and personnel who may assist them with their crisis.	Identifies opportunities for other resources that may be available, and provides means of control over situation.

Discharge or Maintenance Evaluation

- Patient/family will be able to recognize ineffective coping behavior and regain emotional equilibrium.

- Patient/family will be able to adequately problem-solve during crises.

- Patient/family will be able to recognize options and resources for use post-hospitalization.

- Patient/family will be able to make appropriate, informed decisions and be satisfied with choices.

Potential for infection

Related to: intubation, disease process, immuno-suppression, compromised defense mechanisms

Defining characteristics: increased temperature, chills, elevated white blood cell count, purulent sputum

Outcome Criteria

Patient will have no evidence of infective process.

INTERVENTIONS	RATIONALES
Evaluate risk factors that would predispose patient to infection.	Intubation and prolonged mechanical ventilation predispose patient to nosocomial infection. Age, nutritional status, chronic disease progression and invasive procedures and lines also predispose patient to infection.
Monitor sputum for changes in characteristics and color; culture sputum as warranted.	Purulent, malodorous sputum indicates infection. Cultures may be required to identify causative organism and to prescribe appropriate antibiotics.
Monitor tracheostomy site for redness, foul odor, or purulent drainage; culture site as warranted.	Purulent drainage indicates infection. Cultures may be required to identify causative organism and to prescribe appropriate antibiotics.

INTERVENTIONS	RATIONALES
Maintain good handwashing technique and isolation precautions when warranted.	Handwashing is the most important step in preventing nosocomial infection. Patients may require isolation based on their diagnosis to prevent transmission of infection to or from the patient.
Screen visitors who are ill themselves.	Patients are already immuno-compromised and at risk for development of infection.
Maintain sterile technique for all dressing changes and suctioning.	Reduces spread of infection.
Administer antibiotics as ordered.	Required to treat infective organism.

Information, Instruction, Demonstration

INTERVENTIONS	RATIONALES
Instruct patient/family in proper handwashing and disposal of contaminated secretions, tissues, etc.	Reduces risk of transmission of infection to others.
Instruct family to avoid visiting if they have upper respiratory infections.	Patient is already immuno-compromised and is at risk for infection.
Instruct patient/family on antibiotics: effects, side effects, contraindications, and foods/drugs to avoid.	Provides knowledge and enhances cooperation with treatment.

Discharge or Maintenance Evaluation

- Patient will be free of fever, chills, purulent drainage, or other indicators of infective process.

- Patient will be able to recall information accurately regarding antibiotics and infection control procedures.

- Patient/family will be able to recognize risk factors and avoid further compromise of patient.

Altered oral mucous membrane

Related to: oral intubation, increased or decreased saliva, inability to swallow, antibiotic-induced fungal infection

Defining characteristics: oral pain or discomfort, stomatitis, oral lesions, thrush

Outcome Criteria

Patient will be free of oral pain and mucous membranes will remain intact.

INTERVENTIONS	RATIONALES
Observe mouth for missing, loose, or chipped teeth; bleeding, sores, lesions, necrotic areas, or reddened areas.	Teeth may be chipped or knocked out during intubation process and loose teeth may pose a potential for aspiration. Identification of lesions or other problems may facilitate prompt intervention.
Move oral endotracheal tube to other side of mouth at least daily and prn.	Decreases potential for pressure and ultimately, ulceration of lips or mucous membranes.
Provide oral care at least every 8 hours and prn.	Promotes cleanliness, reduces odor, and reduces potential environment for bacterial invasion.
Swab mouth with mouthwash every 4-8 hours and prn.	Removes transient bacteria, reduces odor, and helps to stimulate circulation to oral membranes.
Apply lip balm every 2–4 hours and prn.	Prevents drying and cracking of lips.
Suction patient's oral cavity frequently if patient is unable to handle secretions.	Removes excessive saliva and mucous which may facilitate bacterial growth.
Observe for white patches on tongue and mucous membranes, and notify MD.	May indicate presence of fungal infection (thrush) which will require anti-fungal solution, such as Nystatin.

Information, Instruction, Demonstration

INTERVENTIONS	RATIONALES
Instruct on antifungals as warranted.	Provides knowledge.
Instruct patient in utilizing oral suction equipment when feasible, if patient has copious oral secretions.	Provides a sense of control to the patient, and facilitates removal of excessive secretions.

Discharge or Maintenance Evaluation

• Patient will have intact oral mucous membranes, with no evidence of infection.

• Patient will be able to recall instructions accurately.

• Patient will be able to adequately remove secretions by use of suction equipment.

• Patient will be compliant with performance of oral care.

Altered nutrition: less than body requirements

Related to: intubation, inability to swallow, inability to take in food, increased metabolism due to disease process, surgery, decreased level of consciousness

Defining characteristics: actual inadequate food intake, altered taste, altered smell sensation, weight loss, anorexia, absent bowel sounds, decreased peristalsis, muscle mass loss, decreased muscle tone, changes in bowel habits, nausea, vomiting, abdominal distention

Outcome Criteria

Patient will have adequate nutritional intake with no weight or muscle mass loss.

INTERVENTIONS	RATIONALES
Evaluate ability to eat.	Some patients with tracheostomies are able to eat, while those patients who are endotracheally intubated must be kept NPO due to the positioning of the epiglottis, and will require enteral or parenteral alimentation.
Weigh every day.	Continued weight loss will result in catabolic metabolism and impaired respiratory function.
Observe for muscle wasting.	May indicate muscle stores depletion which can impair respiratory muscle function.
Observe for nausea, vomiting, abdominal distention and palpability, and stool characteristics.	Ventilator patients may develop GI dysfunction from analgesics/sedatives, bedrest, trapped air, and stress, which may result in ileus formation.
Test stools and gastric contents for guaiac.	Stressors of ventilation and presence in ICU may predispose patient to the formation of a stress ulcer resulting in GI bleeding.
Obtain calorie count and assessment of metabolic demands based on disease process.	Establishes imbalances between actual nutritional intake and metabolic needs.
Monitor lab work as warranted; electrolytes, BUN, creatinine, albumin and prealbumin, glucose levels.	Evaluates need for and/or adequacy of nutritional support.
Administer enteral solutions at continual rate by infusion pump as warranted.	Bolus feedings may result in dumping syndrome. Continuous infusion feedings are generally better tolerated and have better absorption. Enteral feeding formulas vary depending on the nutritional needs of the patient. The use of enteral formulas require a functioning GI system.
Determine patency of enteral feeding tubes at least every 8 hours. Flush with 20–30 cc of	Oral or nasal tubes may migrate with coughing, resulting in improper placement and potential for aspiration. Flushing of

INTERVENTIONS	RATIONALES
water every 8 hours, before and after medication administration via the tube, and prn.	tube maintains patency.
Aspirate gastric residuals every 4-8 hours, and decrease or hold feedings per hospital protocol.	Increasing residuals may indicate decreased or absent peristalsis and lack of absorption of required nutrients which may require another form of nutritional support.
Use food coloring to tint feedings. Do not use red coloring.	Helps to identify aspiration of feedings when suctioned. Be aware that the food coloring may cause false readings on occult blood tests on stools. Red coloring should be avoided due to similarity of blood color and this may impair ability to differentiate bleeding problems.
Instill warm cranberry juice, carbonated cola, or mixture of monosodium glutamate and water in enteral tube for signs of occlusion.	Helps to dissolve clogged particulate matter to maintain patency of tube.
Administer antidiarrheal medications as warranted.	Osmolality imbalances may result in diarrhea requiring antidiarrheals for control. Changing strengths or types of feedings may be helpful.
Administer metoclopramide as ordered.	Medication helps to stimulate gastric motility and may be helpful to increase absorption.
Administer parenteral alimentation fluids as warranted via infusion pump.	Provides complete nutritional support without dependence on GI function for absorption. Additives are based upon lab work and patient requirements. Increases in protein and nitrogen may be prescribed for increased metabolic demands of the patient.
Administer intralipids as ordered, if not admixed with TPN solution.	Provides additional caloric benefits as well as a source of essential fatty acids. Lipids may be utilized for respiratory failure to help decrease CO_2 retention.

INTERVENTIONS	RATIONALES
Change solution at least every 24 hours, as well as tubing.	Some additives may be unstable after 24 hours, and prolonged infusion with same solution may promote bacterial growth.
Monitor lab work per hospital protocol; general chemistry, renal profile, CBC, urine or blood glucose levels.	Requirements for electrolyte replacement or alteration in formula may be changed based on this information. High dextrose content in TPN solutions may require additions of insulin to meet metabolic demands if pancreatic disease, hepatic disease, or diabetes are present.
Do not stop TPN abruptly; taper over several days/hours per protocol.	Rebound hypoglycemia may result if dextrose concentrations are abruptly changed.

Information, Instruction, Demonstration

INTERVENTIONS	RATIONALES
Insert nasogastric feeding tube as warranted, utilizing small weighted tube. Obtain chest x-ray or KUB post procedure.	Smaller lumen is less irritating to nasal mucosa, and decreases the incidence of gastroesophageal reflux. Radiographic confirmation of placement is necessary due to the potential for aspiration when patients may have impaired gag reflex.
Maintain elevation of the head of the bed at least 30 degrees at all times.	Helps prevent potential aspiration.
Assist with placement of central venous catheter for TPN administration. Obtain chest x-ray post procedure.	Centrally-placed intravenous lines may enable higher concentrations of amino acids to be utilized. Radiographic confirmation of placement, as well as ruling out hemo- or pneumothorax post procedure, is mandatory.
Instruct in need for supplemental nutritional support, procedures to be performed, and tests that will be required.	Promotes knowledge, decreases fear of the unknown, and facilitates cooperation with procedures. Provides opportunity for patient to make informed choices.

Discharge or Maintenance Evaluation

- Patient will maintain baseline weight with no loss of muscle mass.

- Patient will maintain adequate nutritional status with use of nutritional support, and will experience no complications from support.

- Patient will show no signs of malnutritional status.

- Patient will be able to recall information accurately.

- Patient will maintain a normal nitrogen balance and immunity will not be compromised.

Dysfunctional ventilatory wean response

Related to: fever, pain, muscle fatigue, sedation, anemia, electrolyte imbalance, sleep deprivation, poor nutrition, cardiovascular lability, psychological instability

Defining characteristics: inability to wean, lack or inadequacy of spontaneous respirations, negative inspiratory force or pressure < -20 cm H_2O, PaO_2 < 60 mmHg on FIO_2 > 50%, $PaCO_2$ > 40 mmHg, tidal volume < 5 cc/Kg, vital capacity < 10 cc/Kg, minute ventilation > 10 L/min

Outcome Criteria

Patient will be able to be weaned from ventilatory support successfully with arterial blood gases within normal limits.

INTERVENTIONS	RATIONALES
Monitor vital signs.	Temperature elevations increase metabolism and oxygen demand. Unstable heart rate and rhythm results in increased workload on the heart, increased oxygen consumption and demand. Process of weaning will increase work-

INTERVENTIONS	RATIONALES	INTERVENTIONS	RATIONALES
	load and may compromise an already-stressed body and should not be attempted until these factors have been corrected. Once weaning process has begun, significant changes in heart rate and rhythm, respiratory rate, and blood pressure may indicate a need to slow or discontinue weaning due to respiratory compromise.	Attempt to wean only during the day and after the patient has had a restful sleep period. Avoid activity during weaning.	Crises that may occur with respiratory deterioration and failure to wean may be handled more efficiently when sufficient medical personnel are available, usually during the day. Fatigue may predispose patient to failure due to the need for stamina to withstand the effort of spontaneous breathing. Activity increases oxygen demand and consumption.
Monitor EKG for dysrhythmias and treat as warranted.	Ventilatory support decreases venous return to the heart, increases PVR and SVR. Hypoxemia and pH imbalances may result in dysrhythmias from cardiac compromise.	Evaluate patient's emotional status and ability to cope with weaning.	Weaning process may result in anxiety due to fear of failure to wean and/or ability to breathe spontaneously.
Monitor nutritional status. Evaluate labwork: CBC, transferrin, albumin, prealbumin, electrolytes, etc.	Protein, carbohydrate and fat concentrations can alter the ability to maintain oxygenation. Increased fat concentration prior to weaning may assist in decreasing potential for CO_2 retention and decrease in respiratory drive. Labwork may be used to verify adequacy of nutritive state. Calcium imbalances can decrease the function of the diaphragm, and phosphorus may affect 2, 3-DPG and ATP function, affect respiratory muscle function and red cell membrane stability.	Prior to attempt, assess weaning parameters to ensure patient meets requirements for successful weaning: NIF > -20 cm H_2O, vital capacity > 10-15 cc/Kg, PaO_2 > 60 mmHg on FIO_2 < 40%, resting minute ventilation < 10 L/min, $PaCO_2$ < 40 mmHg, tidal volume > 5 cc/Kg.	Attainment of parameters facilitate best chance for successful weaning and ensures that neuromuscular control is adequate for maintenance of spontaneous ventilation. If carbon dioxide retention is chronic, pH is more indicative of weaning readiness.
		Assess patient for resolution of disease process, absence of inspiratory muscle fatigue, absence of fever, absence of hemodynamic instability, absence of sedative agents or respiratory suppressants, presence of spontaneous respirations, pulmonary shunt < 20%, and adequate hemoglobin and hematocrit.	Factors may promote respiratory insufficiency and compromise which may result in unsuccessful weaning.
Stay with patient until stable, once weaning process has begun. Observe for use of accessory muscles, non-synchronous respiratory pattern, or skin color changes.	Respiratory deterioration may occur rapidly and physical presence is required to observe patient to facilitate prompt intervention. May indicate deterioration in respiratory status, resulting in inability to wean.	Suction patient and perform chest physiotherapy, percussion and postural drainage as warranted prior to disconnection from ventilator.	Removes secretions that may compromise weaning process and promotes improved pulmonary conditions.
Monitor oxygen saturation per oximetry and notify MD if reading less than 90% per pulse oximetry, or sustained reading less than 60% per mixed venous oxygen oximetry; obtain ABGs per protocol.	Oximetry provides identification of tissue oxygen desaturation which usually coincides with decreases in arterial blood gases. Oximetry does not give indication of increased CO_2 levels and these must be verified with ABGs.	Utilize T-bar/T-piece adaptor as ordered. (Usually on T-bar for 10-30 minutes per hour initially.)	Provides oxygen via endotracheal tube or tracheostomy with patient spontaneously breathing.
		Utilize SIMV/IMV mode on ventilator as ordered. (Usually rate decreased by 1-2 breaths/minute every 15-30 minutes.)	Provides ventilatory support to patient with gradually decreasing ventilator breaths and increase of spontaneous breaths. Facilitates gradually increasing respiratory

INTERVENTIONS	RATIONALES
	workload. If weaning is not tolerated, may increase PaCO$_2$ and decrease pH.
Utilize PS (pressure support) as ordered. (Usually 3-5 initially and may increase to 20, with gradual lowering as IMV/SIMV rate lowered.)	Assists patient to overcome airway resistance and support spontaneous breathing by increasing respiratory muscle function.
Utilize CPAP (continuous positive airway pressure) as ordered. (Usually 2-5 cm H$_2$O.)	Patient exhales against continuous positive pressure to prevent atelectasis and improve arterial oxygen tension.
Monitor for MD-set parameters or respiratory rate > 30, increasing PA pressures, heart rate > 110 with new or increased ectopic activity, blood pressure > 20 mmHg from baseline, SaO$_2$ < 90%, tidal volumes < 250 cc; if significant changes occur, place back on ventilator as per protocol.	Alterations in vital signs and hemodynamic may result from insufficient ventilation and respiratory compromise and indicates intolerance of attempts to wean.
Gradually increase time off ventilator with each successful attempt. Once patient is able to tolerate 1-2 hours off of ventilator at a time, weaning may be advanced more rapidly.	The patient's progress will increase as fatigue decreases, respiratory muscle function improves, and patient is emotionally ready to wean.
Determine patient's emotional status and ability to cope with weaning process.	Weaning may result in excessive anxiety due to fear of failure and/or the ability to breathe spontaneously.
Extubate patient when he is able to maintain an airway and his spontaneous respirations are able to maintain oxygenation and ventilatory status per protocol. Intubation equipment should remain at the bedside post-extubation for 4–24 hours or per protocol.	Emergency equipment should be easily available in case reintubation is required due to bronchospasm, laryngospasm, or respiratory deterioration.
To extubate, increase oxygen and suction secretions from trachea, nose and mouth.	Removes secretions that may potentially be aspirated upon removal of tube.
Deflate cuff and remove tube at	Promotes full inflation of the

INTERVENTIONS	RATIONALES
the peak of the inspiratory effort.	lungs so that patient will exhale or cough as tube is removed to prevent aspiration of any secretions that may be remaining after suctioning.
Administer humidified oxygen at prescribed amount.	Provides moisture and oxygen to increase available oxygen, helps to reduce swelling, and facilitates liquification of secretions for easier removal.
Monitor for dyspnea, bronchospasm, laryngospasm, or stridor. Encourage deep breaths and coughing.	May indicate partial obstruction of airway. Deep breathing helps to expand lungs and facilitates movement of secretions.
Monitor for persistent hoarseness and sore throat.	Transient hoarseness and sore throat is normal post-extubation but persistent symptoms may indicate vocal cord paralysis or glottis edema.

Information, Instruction, Demonstration

INTERVENTIONS	RATIONALES
Instruct on weaning process and procedures based on MD protocol.	Decreases fear and anxiety, promotes cooperation, and increases potential for successful weaning attempt.

Knowledge deficit

Related to: change in health status, situational crisis, lack of information, misinterpretation of information, stress, inability to recall information, lack of understanding

Defining characteristics: verbalized questions regarding care, inadequate follow-up on instructions given, misconceptions, lack of improvement, development of preventable complications

Outcome Criteria

Patient will be able to verbalize and demonstrate understanding of information given regarding condition, treatment regimen, and medications.

Information, Instruction, Demonstration

INTERVENTIONS	RATIONALES
Determine patient's baseline of knowledge regarding disease process, normal physiology and function of body systems, and medical treatment regimens.	Provides information regarding patient's understanding of condition as well as a baseline from which to plan teaching.
Monitor patient's readiness to learn and determine best methods to use for teaching. Attempt to incorporate family members in learning process. Reinstruct/ reinforce information as needed.	Patient's physical condition may not facilitate participation in learning, with cognition affected by high stress levels or disease process. Family members may be fearful of equipment and environment which may hamper their ability to learn. Instructions may require repetitive teaching due to competition with other stimuli.
Provide time for individual interaction with patient.	Promotes relationship between patient and nurse, and establishes trust.
Instruct on specific disease process that has required ventilatory support, procedures that may be required, diagnostic tests to be performed, and plans for weaning off ventilator.	Provides knowledge to enable patient to make informed choices, and provides knowledge base on which to build for further teaching.
Instruct on medications pertinent to patient's care.	Provides knowledge and facilitates compliance with regimen.
Discuss potential for ventilator dependence and alterations that may be required in lifestyle. Encourage setting of short- and long-term goals.	Unsuccessful weaning attempts may foster depression and attitude of "giving up." Practical solutions and trouble-shooting problems that may arise, as well as participation in setting of realistic goals may enhance self-worth and self-control.

INTERVENTIONS	RATIONALES
Instruct family on ventilatory support procedures—function of all equipment, how to trouble-shoot problems, and personnel to contact in case of an emergency.	Reduces fear, enables the family to have sense of security about problems that may arise, and assures them that medical assistance can be easily obtained in an emergency.
Instruct family on procedures for suctioning, tracheostomy care, and administration of breathing treatments as ordered.	Promotes knowledge, enhances proper technique for care, and decreases fear.
Instruct family on infection control techniques.	Decreases potential for infection and/or spread of biohazardous materials.
Instruct patient/family on signs/symptoms to notify MD or medical personnel.	Promotes prompt recognition of potentially dangerous problems to facilitate prompt intervention.
Have patient/family perform return demonstration of all tasks instructed.	Provides assurance that care is able to be performed with proper technique, and allows for correction of erroneous methods.
Ensure that prior to discharge, all equipment required will be set up in home.	Reduces anxiety with discharge.
Instruct on all safety concerns; back-up power and equipment.	Promotes sense of security that emergency situations can be handled.

Discharge or Maintenance Evaluation

- Patient/family will be able to accurately recall instructions.

- Patient/family will be able to demonstrate all tasks with appropriate proper methods.

- Patient/family will be able to recall emergency numbers, and signs/symptoms for which to notify medical personnel, and can accurately demonstrate back-up power and equipment.

- Patient/family will be able to follow infection control procedures.

- Patient/family will be able to problem-solve and set realistic goals.

NEUROLOGICAL SYSTEM

CVA

Head Injuries

Spinal Cord Injuries

Guillain-Barré Syndrome

Status Epilepticus

Meningitis

Ventriculostomy/ICP Monitoring

Endarterectomy

CVA

A cerebrovascular accident, or stroke, occurs when a sudden decrease in cerebral blood circulation as a result of thrombosis, embolus, or hemorrhage leads to hypoxia of brain tissues, causing swelling and death. When circulation is impaired or interrupted the small area of the brain becomes infarcted and this changes membrane permeability resulting in increased edema and intracranial pressure (ICP). The clinical symptoms may vary depending on the area and extent of the injury.

Thrombosis of small arteries in the white matter of the brain account for the most common cause of strokes. A history of hypertension, diabetes mellitus, cardiac disease, vascular disease, or atherosclerosis may lead to thrombosis, which causes ischemia to the brain supplied by the vessel involved.

Embolism is the second most common cause of CVA, and happens when a blood vessel is suddenly occluded with blood, air, tumor, fat, or septic particulate. The embolus migrates to the cerebral arteries and obstructs circulation causing edema and necrosis.

When hemorrhage occurs, it is usually the sudden result of ruptured aneurysms, tumors, or AV malformations, or involves problems with hypertension or bleeding dyscrasias. The cerebral bleeding decreases the blood supply and compresses neuronal tissue.

Patients who have strokes frequently have had prior events, such as TIAs (transient ischemic attacks) with reversible focal neurological deficits lasting less than 24 hours or RINDs (reversible ischemic neurological deficits) lasting greater than 24 hours but leaving little, if any, residual neurological impairment.

In addition to the disease processes discussed earlier, cardiac dysrhythmias, alcohol use, cocaine or other recreational drug use, smoking, and the use of oral contraceptives may predispose patients to strokes.

Strokes may cause temporary or permanent losses of motor function, thought processes, memory, speech, or sensory function. Difficulty with swallowing and speaking, hemiplegia, and visual field defects are stations of this disease. Treatment is aimed at supporting vital functions and ensuring adequate cerebral perfusion, and prevention of major complications or permanent disability.

MEDICAL CARE

CT scans: used to identify thrombosis or hemorrhagic stroke, tumors, or hydrocephalus; may not reveal changes immediately

Skull x-rays: may show calcifications of the carotids in the presence of cerebral thrombosis, or partial calcification of an aneurysm in subarachnoid hemorrhage; pineal gland may shift to the opposite side if mass is expanding

Brain scans: used to identify ischemic areas due to CVA but usually are not discernible until up to 2 weeks after injury

Angiography: used to identify site and degree of occlusion or rupture of vessel, assess collateral blood circulation and presence of AV malformations

MRI: used to identify areas of infarction, hemorrhage, and AV malformations

Ultrasound: may be used to gather information regarding flow velocity in the major circulation

Lumbar puncture: performed to evaluate ICP and to identify infection; bloody CSF may indicate a hemorrhagic stroke, and clear fluid with normal pressure may be noted in cerebral thrombosis, embolism, and with TIAs; protein may be elevated if thrombosis results from inflammation

EEG: may be used to help localize area of injury based on brain waves

Laboratory: CBC used to identify blood loss or infection; serum osmolality used to evaluate oncotic pressures and permeability; electrolytes, glucose levels, and urinalysis performed to identify problems and imbalances that may be responsible

Surgery: endarterectomy may be required to remove the occlusion, or microvascular bypass may be performed to bypass the occluded area, such as the carotid artery, aneurysm, or AV malformation

Corticosteroids: used to decrease cerebral edema

Anticonvulsants: used in the treatment and prophylaxis of seizure activity

Analgesics: used for discomfort and pain; aspirin and aspirin-containing products are contraindicated with hemorrhage

TPA: use is controversial because of risks of uncontrolled bleeding

NURSING CARE PLANS

Alteration in tissue perfusion: cerebral

Related to: occlusion, hemorrhage, interruption of cerebral blood flow, vasospasm, edema

Defining characteristics: changes in level of consciousness, mental changes, personality changes, memory loss, restlessness, combativeness, vital sign changes, motor function impairment, sensory impairment

Outcome Criteria

Patient will have improved or normal cerebral perfusion with no mental status changes or complications.

INTERVENTIONS	RATIONALES
Measure blood pressure in both arms.	Cerebral injury may cause variations in blood pressure readings. Hypotension may result from circulatory collapse, and increased ICP may result from edema or clot formation. Differences in readings between arms may indicate a subclavian artery blockage.
Maintain head of bed in elevated position with head in a neutral position.	Helps to improve venous drainage, reduces arterial pressure, and may improve cerebral perfusion.
Provide calm, quiet environment with adequate rest periods between activities.	Bedrest may be required to prevent rebleeding after initial hemorrhage. Activity may increase ICP.
Administer anticoagulants as ordered.	May be warranted to improve blood flow to cerebral tissues and to prevent further clotting and embolus formation. These are contraindicated in hypertension due to the potential for hemorrhage.
Administer antihypertensives as ordered.	Hypertension may be transient when occurring during the CVA, but chronic hypertension will require judicious treatment to prevent further tissue ischemia and damage.
Administer vasodilators as ordered.	Helps to improve collateral circulation and to reduce the incidence of vasospasm.

Information, Instruction, Demonstration

INTERVENTIONS	RATIONALES
Instruct on use of stool softeners and avoidance of straining at stool.	Valsalva maneuvers increase ICP and may result in rebleeding. Stool softeners help to prevent straining.
Prepare patient for surgery as warranted.	May be required to treat problem and prevent further complications.

Impaired verbal communication

Related to: weakness, loss of muscle control, cerebral circulation impairment, neuromuscular impairment

Defining characteristics: inability to speak, inability to identify objects, inability to comprehend language, inability to write, inability to choose and use appropriate words, dysarthria

Outcome Criteria

Patient will be able to communicate normally or will be able to make needs known by some form of communication.

INTERVENTIONS	RATIONALES
Evaluate patient's ability to speak or understand language.	Provides a baseline from which to begin planning intervention. Determination of specific areas of brain injury involvement will preclude what type of assistance will be required.
Assess whether patient suffers from aphasia or dysarthria.	Aphasic patients have difficulty using and interpreting language, comprehending words, and inability to speak or make signs. Dysarthric patients can understand language, but have problems forming or pronouncing words as a result of weakness of paralysis of the oral muscles.

INTERVENTIONS	RATIONALES
Evaluate patient's response to simple commands.	Inability to follow simple commands may indicate receptive aphasia.
Evaluate patient's ability to name objects.	Inability to do so indicates expressive aphasia.
Evaluate patient's ability to write simple sentences or his name.	May indicate patient's disability with receptive and expressive aphasia.
Avoid talking down to patient or making patronizing comments.	Intellect frequently remains unimpaired after injury.
When asking questions, use yes or no type questions initially, and progress as patient is able.	Provides for method of communication without necessity of response to large volumes of information. As patient progresses, the intricacy of questions may increase.
Provide a method of communication for patient, such as a writing board, or communication board to which patient may point.	Allows for communication of needs and allays anxiety.

Information, Instruction, Demonstration

INTERVENTIONS	RATIONALES
Consult with speech therapy.	May be required to identify cognition, function, and plan interventions for recovery.
Assist patient/family to identify and use methods for communication.	Provides method for patient to communicate his needs.

Discharge or Maintenance Evaluation

• Patient will be able to communicate effectively.

• Patient will be able to understand communication problem and access resources to meet needs.

Impaired physical mobility
[See Head Injuries]

Related to: weakness, paralysis, paresthesias, impaired cognition

Defining characteristics: inability to move at will, muscle incoordination, decreased range of motion, decreased muscle strength

Sensory-perceptual alterations: visual, kinesthetic, gustatory, tactile, olfactory

Related to: neurological trauma/deficit, stress, altered reception of stimuli

Defining characteristics: behavior changes, disorientation to time, place, self, and situation, diminished concentration, inability to focus, alteration in thought processes, decreased sensation, paresthesias, paralysis, altered ability to taste and smell, inability to recognize objects, muscle incoordination, muscle weakness, inappropriate communication

Outcome Criteria

Patient will achieve and maintain alertness and orientation with acceptable behavior and motor/sensory function.

INTERVENTIONS	RATIONALES
Assess patient's perceptions and reorient as necessary.	May help decrease distortions of thought and identify reality.
Assess for visual field defects, visual disturbances, or problems with depth perception.	Visual distortion may prevent patient from having realistic perception of his environment.
Assist patient by placing objects in his field of vision.	Allows for recognition of people and objects, and decreases confusion.
Limit amount of stimuli. Avoid excess noise or equipment.	May create sensory overload and confusion.
Observe patient for non-use of extremities. Test for sensation awareness and ability to discern position of body.	May create self-care deficiencies. Loss of sensation or inability to recognize objects may impair

INTERVENTIONS	RATIONALES
	return to function level. Sensory impairment affects balance and positioning.
Evaluate environment for safety hazards, such as temperature extremes.	Promotes safety and decreases potential for injury.

Information, Instruction, Demonstration

INTERVENTIONS	RATIONALES
Instruct patient to observe feet when standing or ambulating, and to make a conscious effort to reposition body parts. Assist with sensory stimulation to non-use side.	Visual and tactile stimulation helps to retrain movement and to experience sensations.

Discharge or Maintenance Evaluation

- Patient will be alert and oriented to all phases.

- Patient will be able to understand changes in functional ability and residual neurological deficits.

- Patient will be able to compensate for dysfunctional abilities.

Risk for impaired swallowing

Related to: neuromuscular impairment

Defining characteristics: inability to swallow effectively, choking, aspiration

Outcome Criteria

Patient will be able to swallow effectively with no incidence of aspiration.

INTERVENTIONS	RATIONALES
Evaluate patient's ability to swallow, extent of any paralysis, ability to maintain airway.	Provides baseline information from which to plan interventions for care.
Maintain head position and support, head of bed elevated at least 30 degrees or more during and after feeding.	Helps to prevent aspiration and facilitates ability to swallow.
Place food in the unaffected side of mouth.	Allows for sensory stimulation and taste, and may assist to trigger swallowing reflexes.
Provide foods that are soft and require little, if any, chewing, or provide thickened liquids.	These types of foods are easier to control and decrease potential for choking or aspiration.
Assist with stimulation of tongue, cheeks, or lips as warranted.	May help to retrain oral muscles and facilitate adequate tongue movement and swallowing.
Monitor intake and output, and caloric intake.	Insufficient nutrient intake orally may result in the need for alternate types of nutritional support.
Administer tube feedings/TPN as warranted/ordered.	May be required if oral intake is insufficient.

Information, Instruction, Demonstration

INTERVENTIONS	RATIONALES
Instruct to use straw for drinking liquids. Maintain swallowing precautions identified by speech therapists.	Helps to strengthen facial and oral muscles to decrease potential for choking.
Encourage family to bring patient's favorite foods.	Familiar foods may increase oral intake.

Discharge or Maintenance Evaluation

- Patient will be able to eat and swallow normally.

- Patient will be able to ingest an adequate amount of nutrients without danger of aspiration.

- Patient will be able to follow instructions and strengthen muscles used for eating/swallowing.

Self-care deficit: bathing, dressing, feeding, toileting

Related to: weakness, decreased muscle strength, muscle incoordination, paralysis, paresthesia, pain, functional impairment

Defining characteristics: inability to perform ADLs, inability to feed self, inability to maintain personal hygiene, inability to dress/undress self, inability to take care of toileting needs

Outcome Criteria

Patient will be able to meet self-care needs within own ability level.

INTERVENTIONS	RATIONALES
Evaluate level of neurological impairment and patient's abilities to perform ADLs.	Provides baseline from which to plan care for patient needs.
Assist patient with ADLs as needed and encourage patient to perform tasks he may be capable of doing.	Assistance may reduce levels of frustration but patient will have more self-esteem with tasks he may complete.
Alter plans of care keeping in mind patient's visual, motor, or sensory deficits.	Assists patient with safety concerns and allows for some degree of independence.
Utilize self-help devices and instruct patient in their use.	Allows patient to perform tasks and improves his self-esteem.
Establish a bowel regime, using stool softeners, suppositories, etc. Offer bedpan or bedside commode at regular intervals.	Medications may be helpful when establishing a bowel regime and to regulate function. Retraining will allow the patient to gain independence and fosters self-esteem.

Information, Instruction, Demonstration

INTERVENTIONS	RATIONALES
Consult physical/occupational therapist.	May be required to assist with development of therapy plan and to identify methods for patient to compensate for neurological deficits.

Discharge or Maintenance Evaluation

- Patient will be able to perform self-care activities by himself or with the assistance of a caregiver.

- Patient will be able to understand and identify methods to facilitate meeting self-care needs.

- Patient will be able to access community resources to meet continuing needs.

CVA

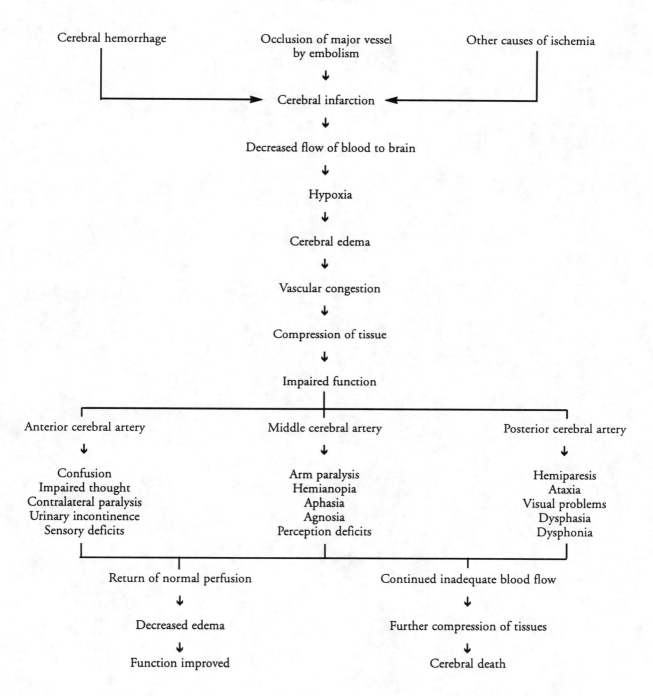

Cerebral hemorrhage   Occlusion of major vessel   Other causes of ischemia
by embolism

↓

Cerebral infarction

↓

Decreased flow of blood to brain

↓

Hypoxia

↓

Cerebral edema

↓

Vascular congestion

↓

Compression of tissue

↓

Impaired function

Anterior cerebral artery	Middle cerebral artery	Posterior cerebral artery
↓	↓	↓
Confusion	Arm paralysis	Hemiparesis
Impaired thought	Hemianopia	Ataxia
Contralateral paralysis	Aphasia	Visual problems
Urinary incontinence	Agnosia	Dysphasia
Sensory deficits	Perception deficits	Dysphonia

Return of normal perfusion   Continued inadequate blood flow

↓   ↓

Decreased edema   Further compression of tissues

↓   ↓

Function improved   Cerebral death

Head Injuries

Head injuries, both open and closed, are usually the result of some type of trauma, and include skull fractures, concussions, lacerations, contusions, and/or cerebral hemorrhages. The injury can be the result of a direct blow to the head, or may involve acceleration/deceleration injuries. Acceleration, or coup, injuries occur when the brain is forced against the cranium. Deceleration, or contrecoup, injuries occur after the initial impact when the brain is rotated or thrown in the opposite direction of the force.

Closed head injuries (CHI) result when a blunt trauma to the head causes a neurological deficit or loss of consciousness from bruising, hemorrhage, or laceration of brain tissues. This type of injury may be further categorized into mild concussion, classic concussion, diffuse injury with loss of consciousness greater than 24 hours, and diffuse shearing and disruption of brain structures.

A mild concussion occurs when forces on the brain stretch nerve fibers and result in impaired conduction of nerve responses. Neurological dysfunction is temporary with no residual effects. In a classic concussion, the loss of consciousness is usually less than 24 hours in length and the patient experiences disorientation and a degree of retrograde amnesia when consciousness is regained. Some patients may experience residual personality changes or impairment in memory recall. Patients may exhibit a focal deficit caused by an injury that occurs to a specific area.

With diffuse closed head injuries, the loss of consciousness is greater than 24 hours and the coma may last up to weeks. The patient can exhibit restlessness, withdrawal from painful or noxious stimuli, or purposeful movement. Disorientation and amnesia occur with the return of consciousness, and personality changes are permanent due to the widespread cerebrum disruption.

When injury to the axons and neurons in the hemispheres, brain stem, and diencephalon occur and result in diffuse shearing of white matter with concurrent cerebral edema, dysfunction results in coma. More than half of these patients die, and those who do survive, have severe residual dysfunction. Contusions of the brain stem result in coma, as well as cranial nerve dysfunction and cardiopulmonary instability.

Skull fractures are normally classified as linear, basilar, or depressed. If a linear skull fracture does not puncture the dura mater, the fracture will heal without treatment. If the dura is torn, there is an increased chance that the middle meningeal artery is also punctured, and this will cause an epidural hematoma.

A basilar skull fracture can occur in the anterior or posterior fossa, and classic symptoms include cerebrospinal fluid leakage from the nose or ears, or ecchymoses over the mastoid projection or around the eyes. With basilar fractures, there exists a high risk for cranial nerve injury and dysfunction, infection, and residual neurological impairment.

Depressed skull fractures that are not depressed more than the thickness of the skull are usually not treated. A depression more than 5 millimeters or more in depth will require surgery in order to relieve the compression on structures. If the dura mater is punctured, the possibility of bone fragments entering the brain tissue is increased, as well as the potential for infection.

Lacerations of the scalp may occur with head injury or skull fractures, and will potentiate the danger of infection.

Intracranial hematomas result after trauma to the head, and frequently occur in conjunction with scalp lacerations, skull fractures, contusions, or penetrating wounds to the head. Subdural hematomas (SDH) usually are caused by venous bleeding, most often from the superior sagittal sinus, and involves the area between the dura mater and the arachnoid space. It may be acute, happening within 24-48 hours of injury, subacute, within 3-20 days of injury, or chronic, greater than 20 days from injury, depending on the time elapsed from injury to the onset of symptoms. SDH may occur spontaneously if the patient has a blood dyscrasia or clotting problem.

Epidural hematomas (EDH) are usually caused by arterial bleeding, generally from the middle meningeal artery, and involve the area above the outer dura mater and below the skull. These occur frequently when skull fractures cross the middle meningeal artery, or transverse or superior sagittal sinus, and the bleeding causes the dura to be pulled away from the skull. A posterior fossa EDH is usually caused by a venous bleed and may result in delayed symptoms due to the slow oozing. With EDH, the patient may have a brief episode of unconsciousness, followed by a varying length of lucid behavior prior to neurological deterioration and increased intracranial pressure.

Intracerebral hemorrhage (ICH) into the brain may occur hours or days after a closed head injury, and many result after rupture of an aneurysm, AV malformation, tumor, or vessel that has been weakened from hypertension. If the hemorrhage occurs in the internal capsule of the brain, paralysis will ensue. Symptoms vary depending on site, size, cerebral edema, and blood accumulation rate.

Head injuries can result in varying severity from absence of neurological dysfunction to death, and each injury must be considered potentially critical. Cervical spine injury evaluation may be required depending on the mechanisms of the closed head injury.

MEDICAL CARE

CT scans: used to identify cerebral edema, lesions, hemorrhage, ventricle size, tissue shifts, or infarctions

X-rays: skull x-rays may be used to identify fractures or midline shifts, or presence of bone fragments, and to evaluate healing or resolution

MRI: used to reveal disruption of axonal pathways and white matter shearing

Angiography: cerebral angiograms may be used to identify circulatory anomalies, shifting of structures, hemorrhage, or edema

Lumbar puncture: may be used in diagnosis of subarachnoid hemorrhage; LP may be contraindicated in some cases

Laboratory: electrolyte imbalances may increase ICP or alter mental status; CBC to evaluate blood loss and hydration status; drug toxicology studies to identify drugs that may be responsible for consciousness level changes; anticonvulsant drug levels to monitor therapeutic maintenance levels

Arterial blood gases: used to evaluate hypoxemia and acid-base imbalances that can increase ICP; intracranial hematomas may result in respiratory alkalosis, or metabolic acidosis if patient is also in shock

Diuretics: may be used to draw water from brain cells in order to decrease cerebral edema and ICP

Steroids: may be used to decrease inflammation and edema

Anticonvulsants: may be required to treat and/or prevent seizure activity

NURSING CARE PLANS

Alteration in tissue perfusion: cerebral

Related to: hemorrhage, hematoma, lesions, cerebral edema, metabolic changes, hypoxia, hypovolemia, cardiac dysrhythmias

Defining characteristics: disorientation, confusion, changes in mental status, combativeness, inability to focus on topic, amnesia, memory loss, restlessness, inability to follow commands, increased intracranial pressure, vital sign changes, impaired motor function, impaired sensory function

Outcome Criteria

Patient will achieve and maintain consciousness, and will have normal cognition and motor function.

INTERVENTIONS	RATIONALES
Assess patient for cause of impairment, problem with perfusion, and potential for increased ICP.	Establishes plan of care and identifies appropriate choices for intervention. Depending on patient's condition/problem, surgical intervention may be required.
Evaluate neurological status every hour initially, then every 1-2 hours, and notify MD for pertinent changes. See Glasgow Coma Scale below.	Establishes a baseline from which to gauge changes or trends. Alterations in level of consciousness and behavior, as well as other symptoms may be helpful to determine area of damage.
Assess patient's arousal or lack of arousal to verbal and noxious stimuli.	Establishes level of consciousness which is the single most important measure of the patient's status. Extensive damage involving the cerebral cortex may result in delayed responses to commands, drowsiness and

INTERVENTIONS	RATIONALES
	inability to stay awake unless stimulated, or disorientation. Lack of response to stimuli may indicate that damage has occurred to the midbrain, pons, and/or medulla. If a minimal amount of damage has occurred in the cerebral cortex, the patient may be uncooperative or drowsy.
Assess patient's best verbal response to questions and whether words/sentences are appropriate.	Identifies speech ability and orientation levels.
Assess ability to follow simple commands, noting purposeful and non-purposeful movements bilaterally.	Identifies ability to respond to stimuli when patient is unable to open eyes or cannot speak. Purposeful movement, such as holding up two fingers or squeezing and releasing hands when instructed to do so, can help identify awareness and the ability to respond appropriately. Abnormal posturing may indicate diffuse cortical damage, and the absence of any movement to one side of the body usually indicates damage has been done to the motor tracts of the opposite side of the cerebral hemisphere.
Observe pupils bilaterally, noting equality, size, and reaction to light. Notify MD of significant changes.	Compression of the brain stem and impairment of the second and third cranial nerves will alter pupillary response.
Observe position of eyes, noting any deviation laterally or vertically. Observe for presence of doll's eyes.	Loss of doll's eyes, or the oculocephalic reflex, indicates impairment in the function of the brain stem. Positions and movement of the eyes may indicate which area of the brain has been involved. Problems with abduction of the eyes may be an early indication of increased intracranial pressure.
Observe for presence of blink reflex.	Loss of blinking reflex may indicate injury to the pons and medulla.

INTERVENTIONS	RATIONALES
Monitor intracranial pressure at least hourly, or use continuous monitoring per hospital policy.	Provides immediate information about changes in pressure of the cerebrospinal fluid and blood to facilitate detection of life-threatening increases that can lead to brain deterioration. ICP fluctuates continuously and maintained increases longer than 10-15 minutes should be reported.
Monitor ICP waves.	Plateau, or A waves, have rapid increases and decreases of pressure ranging from 15-50 mmHg, last from 2-15 minutes, and are usually noted in cerebral dysfunction caused by shifting of the brain. B waves last from 30 seconds to 2 minutes, and are usually less significant unless they occur in runs, which may precede changes to A waves. C waves are small and normally occur at the rate of 6/minute, and relate to variances in arterial blood pressure.
Obtain CSF sample as ordered and as per hospital protocol.	May be required for diagnostic testing or to relieve pressure.
Monitor vital signs; observe for widening pulse pressure, blood pressure changes, bradycardia, tachycardia, apnea, Cheyne-Stokes respiration, or fever.	Autoregulation may be impaired after cerebral vascular injury. Temperature elevation may increase cerebral blood flow and volume, which can increase ICP. Widening pulse pressure may indicate increasing intracranial pressure, especially when consciousness level is deteriorating concurrently. Hypotension from hypovolemia may occur when patient has associated multiple trauma. Cardiac dysrhythmias may result from brain stem pressure or injury, or may be seen in cardiac disease. Increasing ICP or compression of brain structures may result in loss of spontaneous respiration and may require mechanical ventilation. Damage to the hypothalamus may result in hyperthermia which can result in increased ICP.

INTERVENTIONS	RATIONALES
Monitor EKG for rhythm and rate changes and treat per hospital protocol.	Bradycardia is frequently seen with brain stem injury. Dysrhythmias may become life-threatening and require emergent intervention.
Assess for presence of cough and gag reflexes.	Injuries to the medulla will result in impairment of these reflexes and may cause further complications.
Observe for restlessness, moaning, or nonverbal changes in behavior.	May indicate presence of discomfort or pain and this may increase ICP.
Observe for presence of seizure activity and provide appropriate safety precautions.	Cerebral injury and irritation, hypoxemia, hypoxia, and increased ICP may result in seizures. Seizure activity increases metabolic demands which can also increase ICP.
Observe for nuchal rigidity.	May be present when meninges are irritated if dura mater has been punctured, or if infection develops.
Elevate head of bed 15–30 degrees as indicated.	Reduces intracranial pressure and cerebral congestion and edema.
Support head and neck in a neutral midline position utilizing pillows, sand bags, or towels.	Movement of the head to either side can compress jugular veins inhibiting venous drainage and can result in increased ICP.
Limit suctioning to only when needed.	Suctioning procedures can increase intrathoracic, intraabdominal, and intracranial pressures.
Administer oxygen as warranted.	Reduces hypoxemia which may result in increased ICP.
If patient requires mechanical ventilation, monitor hyperventilatory status.	Hyperventilation results in respiratory alkalosis, which results in cerebral vasoconstriction and decreases in ICP.
Administer sedation and neuromuscular paralyzing agents as ordered and warranted.	Paralyzing drugs may be ordered to prevent sudden rises in ICP caused by coughing, suctioning, or other muscular activity, but should never be given without sedation of patient.

INTERVENTIONS	RATIONALES
Monitor pulse oximetry and notify MD if levels remain below 90%.	Indicates respiratory insufficiency and impending/present hypoxia.
Monitor ABGs as warranted.	Identifies acid-base imbalances and presence of hypoxemia. Elevations in $PaCO_2$ will cause vasodilation in the cerebral vasculature with a resultant increase in ICP.
Monitor intake and output hourly.	Reflects amounts of total body water which influences tissue perfusion. Cerebral injury may result in inappropriate ADH or diabetes insipidus, and may lead to hypovolemia.
Provide calm, quiet environment without extraneous stimuli, and provide rest periods between care activities. Use restraints only when absolutely necessary.	Helps to reduce ICP. Use of restraints may be required to ensure the patient's safety, but may cause irritation and fighting against the restraints which can increase ICP.
Administer osmotic diuretics as ordered.	Drugs remove water from areas in the brain that maintain an intact blood-brain barrier, and helps to reduce ICP.

Information, Instruction Demonstration

INTERVENTIONS	RATIONALES
Instruct patient to avoid coughing, straining, or any valsalva-like maneuvers.	Activities increase ICP by increasing intrathoracic and intra-abdominal pressures.
Prepare patient/family for placement on mechanical ventilation as warranted.	Injury to certain areas of the brain may result in insufficient respiratory status and may require intubation and mechanical ventilation to maintain life support.
Prepare patient/family for surgical procedures.	Craniotomy or burr holes may be necessary to remove bone fragments, remove a hematoma, stop hemorrhage, remove necrotic tissue, or elevate a depressed skull fracture.

Discharge or Maintenance Evaluation

- Patient will be alert, oriented in all phases, with no speech or motor impairment.

- Patient will have no sensory impairment.

- Patient will have stable vital signs and no increase in ICP.

Risk for ineffective breathing pattern

Related to: respiratory center injury, obstruction, structural shifting, surgical intervention

Defining characteristics: dyspnea, Cheyne-Stokes respirations, bradypnea, apnea, hypoxia, hypoxemia, abnormal arterial blood gases

Outcome Criteria

Patient will maintain a patent airway with no evidence of respiratory insufficiency.

INTERVENTIONS	RATIONALES
Observe respiratory status for rate, depth, rhythm, irregularity, chest expansion and symmetry, and absence.	Changes from patient's baseline may indicate pulmonary complications or involvement of brain injured areas. Respiratory insufficiency may require mechanical ventilation.
Maintain patency of airway.	Depending on location of injury, patient may not be able to maintain his own airway or ventilation and may require artificial means of doing so.
Auscultate breath sounds for changes and presence of adventitious lung sounds.	May indicate hypoventilation, obstruction, atelectasis, or infection which may impair cerebral oxygenation.
Observe for presence of gag, cough, and swallow reflexes.	Lack of these reflexes may impair the patient's ability to handle his secretions and may require an artificial airway. Nasopharyngeal airways are preferred to avoid stimulation of the gag reflex which can increase ICP.

INTERVENTIONS	RATIONALES
Administer oxygen as warranted.	Provides supplemental oxygen to reduce hypoxia and prevent desaturation.
Elevate head of bed as warranted.	Promotes chest expansion and ventilation.
Avoid suctioning unless mandatory, and observe for changes in sputum color, consistency, or odor.	Suctioning may cause hypoxia and decreases cerebral perfusion, while increasing ICP. Changes in sputum characteristics may indicate impending or presence of infection.

Information, Instruction, Demonstration

INTERVENTIONS	RATIONALES
Instruct patient in deep breathing exercises.	Reduces potential for atelectasis and/or pneumonia.
Avoid chest physiotherapy during acute phases.	CPT is contraindicated with patients with increased ICP because this potentiates the increase.
Prepare patient/family for intubation/mechanical ventilation as warranted.	As time and condition permits, instruction may be given. Provides knowledge and decreases fear in patients who are awake.

Discharge or Maintenance Evaluation

- Patient will maintain his own airway and be able to sustain spontaneous respiration.

- Patient will be able to handle secretions and dispose of them adequately.

- Arterial blood gases will be within normal limits for the patient.

- Patient will be able to recall information accurately and be able to demonstrate appropriate deep breathing.

Alteration in thought processes

Related to: injury, psychological problems, medications

Defining characteristics: memory deficit, diminished attention span, inability to focus, disorientation to time, place, person, or situation, poor recall, distractibility, personality changes, inappropriate behavior, inability to problem-solve

Outcome Criteria

Patient will be oriented in all phases and will be able to recall data.

INTERVENTIONS	RATIONALES
Evaluate orientation status with regard to time, place, person, circumstance, and recent events.	Provides a baseline on which to begin and plan interventions.
Observe patient for ability to concentrate and attention span.	Ability to concentrate may be diminished due to injury and this further potentiates anxiety for the patient.
Assist family members to understand patient's aberrant behavior, personality changes, and other responses.	Head injury recovery includes agitation and hostility, anger, and disorganized thought sequences. Family members may have difficulty dealing with the patient's changed personality and behavior.
Encourage family to discuss news and family occurrences with patient.	Helps to maintain contact with normal events and assists with orientation.
Explain all procedures with clear concise explanations.	Patient may have lost the ability to reason or conceptualize, and may require repeated reinforcement. Retention of information may be decreased and result in further anxiety.
Reduce competing stimuli when conversing with the patient.	Brain injured patients may be overly excitable and become violent with excess stimulation.
Be consistent with staff assignments as much as possible.	Provides atmosphere of stability and allows patient some control in situation.

INTERVENTIONS	RATIONALES
Remain with patient during episodes of fright or agitation.	Offers support and helps to calm patient to reduce anxiety to prevent loss of control and panic.
Assist patient/family to set realistic goals and instruct in ways to control behavior.	Helps to maintain a sense of hope for improvement and to facilitate rehabilitation.

Information, Instruction, Demonstration

INTERVENTIONS	RATIONALES
Consult rehabilitation counselor for assistance with cognitive training as warranted.	Assists patient with methods to compensate for problems with concentration, memory, judgment, and problem-solving.
Make appropriate referrals to support groups or counseling as warranted.	Additional help may be needed to help with recovery.

Discharge or Maintenance Evaluation

- Patient will regain normal mental skills and be oriented in all phases.

- Patient will be able to recognize aberrant behavior and control negative reactions.

- Patient will participate in rehabilitation/counseling for retraining.

Risk for infection

Related to: trauma, lacerations, broken skin, open wounds, invasive procedures, surgery, use of steroids, cerebrospinal fluid leakage, nutritional deficiency

Defining characteristics: fever, tachycardia, elevated white blood cell count, shift to the left on differential, redness to wounds, purulent drainage or sputum, nuchal rigidity, bloody or purulent CSF

Outcome Criteria

Patient will be free of signs/symptoms of infection.

INTERVENTIONS	RATIONALES
Monitor temperature every 2-4 hours.	Elevation may indicate development of infection.
Observe wounds, incision lines, invasive line sites, or other skin breaks for drainage, redness, or edema.	Prompt identification of developing problems may result in prompt intervention to prevent systemic sepsis.
Observe for CSF leakage from ears and nose, and report to MD.	Indicates a serious complication from head injury and may result in meningitis.
Use aseptic or sterile technique when changing dressings or providing wound care.	Prevents spread of infection.
Utilize good handwashing practices.	Prevents nosocomial infections.
Monitor urine output for adequacy of amount, color, clarity, and presence of foul odor.	May identify presence of bacterial infection.
Obtain cultures of wound, urine, blood, stool, sputum, or other body fluids/surfaces as warranted, and as per hospital protocol.	Identifies the presence of infection and the causative agent, as well as identification of appropriate antimicrobial agent to treat infection.
Administer antibiotics as ordered.	May be given prophylactically when trauma, surgery, or CSF leakage occurs. Appropriate antibiotic may be ordered after results of culture and sensitivity are received.

Information, Instruction, Demonstration

INTERVENTIONS	RATIONALES
Instruct on isolation procedures as warranted. Instruct visitors on avoiding patient if they have upper respiratory or other type of infection.	Isolation may be required based on type of organism grown. Restriction of ill visitors may reduce exposure of an already susceptible patient.
Instruct on deep breathing and pulmonary exercises as warranted.	Promotes lung expansion and reduces potential for atelectasis and pneumonia. Postural drainage is contraindicated if patient has increased ICP.

Discharge or Maintenance Evaluation

- Patient will be normothermic with normal white blood cell count.

- Patient will exhibit no signs/symptoms of infection.

- Wounds will heal without complications.

Impaired physical mobility

Related to: trauma, immobilization, mental impairment, decreased strength, paralysis

Defining characteristics: inability to move at will, inability to transfer or ambulate, decreased range of motion, decreased muscle strength, muscle incoordination, footdrop, contractures, decreased reflexes

Outcome Criteria

Patient will achieve and maintain an optimal level of motor function.

INTERVENTIONS	RATIONALES
Evaluate patient's ability and function and injury.	Identifies impairments and allows for identification of appropriate interventions.
Assess patient for degree of immobility.	Provides a baseline on which to base interventions. Patient may only require minimal assistance or be completely dependent on caregivers for all body needs.
Observe skin for redness, warmth, or tenderness.	May indicate pressure is being concentrated in one area and may predispose patient to decubitus formation.
Provide kinetic bed or alternating pressure mattress for patient.	Helps to promote circulation and reduces venous stasis and tissue pressure to prevent formation of pressure sores.
Maintain good body alignment and use pillows/rolls to support body. Use high-top tennis shoes and remove/reapply every 4-8 hours.	Prevents further complications and contractures. Use of tennis shoes helps prevent footdrop.
Perform range of motion exercises every 4 hours.	Helps to maintain mobility and function of joints.
Provide skin care every 8 hours and prn. Change wet clothing and linens prn.	Helps to promote circulation and reduces potential for skin breakdown.
Instill artificial tears or lubrication ointment to eyes every 4 hours and prn as ordered.	Prevents eye tissues from drying out. If patient is unable to maintain closed eyes, eye patches or tape may be required.

Information, Instruction, Demonstration

INTERVENTIONS	RATIONALES
Instruct patient/family in range of motion exercises and mobility aids.	Helps patient to regain some control and allows family some involvement in reconditioning program.
Instruct patient/family in reasons for impairment and realistic goals for changes in patient's lifestyle as warranted.	Promotes understanding and compliance with treatment regimen.

INTERVENTIONS	RATIONALES
Consult physical and/or occupational therapy, as warranted.	Assists patient with identifying methods to compensate for impairments and provides for post-discharge care.

Discharge or Maintenance Evaluation

- Patient will be able to maintain skin integrity with no complications.

- Patient will be able to increase muscle strength and tone and achieve a functional level of muscle function.

- Patient will be able to demonstrate exercise program.

- Patient and family will become involved in recovery programs.

Risk for alteration in nutrition: less than body requirements

Related to: inability to take in sufficient nutrients, inability to chew or swallow, decreased level of consciousness, intubation, increased metabolism

Defining characteristics: weight loss, muscle wasting, catabolism

Outcome Criteria

Patient will be able to ingest sufficient nutrients to meet metabolic demands, and will experience no weight loss.

INTERVENTIONS	RATIONALES
Evaluate patient's ability to eat, swallow, chew, etc.	Identifies problems and establishes data for choices of interventions.
Weigh every day.	Establishes trends and helps to evaluate effectiveness of interventions.
Provide small, frequent meals.	Improves patient compliance and facilitates digestion.

INTERVENTIONS	RATIONALES
Encourage family to assist with feeding as warranted.	Involves family in patient's plan of care and provides opportunity for socialization that may improve intake.
Administer tube feedings as required.	Tube feedings may be required during the initial phase after injury until the patient is able to swallow without danger of aspiration.
Elevate the head of the bed at least 30 degrees while eating or giving tube feedings.	Helps to prevent aspiration.
Auscultate bowel sounds every 4 hours.	Quality of bowel sounds may indicate response to feedings or development of an ileus.
Consult dietitian as warranted.	Provides additional resources to establish nutrient needs based on many factors including metabolic demands.
Monitor serum albumin, prealbumin, transferrin, iron, renal profiles, and glucose levels.	Assists in identification of nutritional problems, body function, and response to nutritional support.

Information, Instruction, Demonstration

INTERVENTIONS	RATIONALES
Consult speech or occupational therapy for mechanical problems.	May be required to establish a functional method of eating for the patient.
Check gastric contents, vomitus, and stools for occult blood.	Bleeding may occur from stresses resulting from injury or from mechanical erosion.

Discharge or Maintenance Evaluation

- Patient will maintain optimal weight.

- Patient will be in a positive nitrogen balance, with laboratory values within normal limits.

- Patient will be able to ingest food in sufficient amounts to meet and maintain metabolic demands.

HEAD INJURIES

Brain trauma
↓
Bleeding
↓

Bruising of brain   Small petechial hemorrhages   Laceration of brain tissue
↓

Brain edema   Neuronal pathways disrupted
↓   ↓
Compression of blood vessels   Cranial nerve dysfunction

Blood flow decreased
↓
Brain ischemia
↓
Tissue hypoxia
↓
Arteriolar dilatation
Increased capillary pressure
Decreased venous return
↓
Celular metabolism impaired
↓
Cellular transport decreased
Sodium and water increased
↓
Increased cerebral edema
Increased ICP
↓
Shifting of brain structures
↓
Brain tissue destruction
Herniation/compression of brain and brainstem
↓
Cardiovascular and respiratory impairment
↓
Cardiopulmonary failure
↓
DEATH

HEAD INJURIES

CONCUSSION	DIFFUSE INJURY WITH LOC<24 HOURS	DIFFUSE WHITE MATTER SHEARING WITH DISRUPTION OF AXON/NEURON PATHS

MILD	CLASSIC		
↓	↓	↓	↓
Stretching of nerve fibers	Axonal disruption	Coma with purposful movement and restlessness	Coma with brainstem and autonomic dysfunction
↓	↓	↓	↓
Loss of nerve conduction	Cortical dysfuntion	Disorientation	Cardiovascular collapse
↓	↓	↓	↓
Temporary neurological dysfunction	Disorientation	Retrograde and post-traumatic amnesia	DEATH
↓	↓	↓	
Retrograde amnesia	Retrograde and post-traumatic amnesia	Increased cerebral edema	
↓	↓	↓	
Return to normalcy	Potential subtle personality and memory changes	Increased ICP	
		↓	
		Brain tissue destruction/compression	
		↓	
		Cardiovascular collapse	
		↓	
		DEATH	

Spinal Cord Injuries

Spinal cord injuries are traumatic injuries to the spinal cord caused by contusion, compression, or transection of the cord as a result of dislocation of bones, rupture of ligaments, vessels, or vertebral discs, stretching of neuron tissue, or impairment in blood supply. These lesions are classified as being complete or incomplete. Complete lesions involve the total loss of sensation as well as voluntary motor function, and incomplete lesions involve mixed losses of sensation and voluntary motor function.

The flexion, hyperextension and/or rotational types of injury that result in spinal cord injury are usually caused by trauma, motor vehicle accidents, falls, gun shot wounds, stab wounds, and diving injuries. The severity of the injury can vary depending on the amount of pathologic changes that are produced. Injury without intervention results in ischemia, edema, hemorrhage, and progressive destruction. After the initial cord compression, small hemorrhages occur in the central gray matter. The expansion and increase in number of hemorrhagic areas cause even more compression, edema, and finally, necrosis of the cord. The cervical area is the most vulnerable part of the spine because of the mobility of the head and poor support by the muscles, but cervical fractures do not necessarily cause neurological problems.

The level of the injury relates to how much functional ability is retained. At the C1 to C8 levels, the patient is a quadriplegic with variances in muscle function from complete paralysis of respiratory function to limited use of the fingers. At T1 to L1 levels, paraplegia is noted with intact arm movement. At L1 and below, there may be mixed dysfunction with bowel and bladder dysfunction.

In central cord syndrome, the central gray matter of the cord is contused, compressed, or hemorrhaged. This results in varying degrees of sensory loss and bowel/bladder dysfunction, and there is more motor loss in the arms than in the legs. In anterior cord syndrome, the injury has occurred to the anterior horn and spinothalamic areas resulting in a loss of motor function and pain/temperature below the lesion. Sensations of touch, position, pressure and vibration may be maintained. In Brown-Sequard syndrome, as a result of a transverse hemi-transection of the cord, motor loss, touch, vibration, pressure, and position are involved ipsilaterally, with a contralateral loss of pain/temperature sensation. Posterior cord syndrome is exceedingly rare and results in the loss of light touch below the level of injury, with motor function and sensation of pain and temperature maintained intact.

When spinal lesions at or above T6 level block sensory impulses from reaching the brain, an excessive and critical autonomic response to a stimulus occurs, and this is known as autonomic dysreflexia. It may be precipitated by bowel or bladder distention or by stimulation of the skin or pain receptors. Symptoms may include severe blood pressure increases, pounding headache, profuse sweating above the lesion, blurred vision, goosebumps, and bradycardia. Treatment is aimed at removing the stimulus that causes the problem, and treating the hypertensive episode.

Spinal shock occurs when there is an abrupt loss of continuity between the spinal cord and the higher nerve centers, with a complete loss of all reflexes and a flaccid paralysis below the level of injury. Normally, this spinal shock lasts 7-10 days and when it begins resolution, the flaccidity changes to a spastic type of paralysis.

MEDICAL CARE

Arterial blood gases: used to identify hypoxemia and acid-base imbalances

Radiography: chest x-rays used to identify diaphragmatic changes or respiratory complications; spinal x-rays used to identify fracture or dislocation and identifies level of injury

CT scans: used to identify structural aberrancies and localize injury site

Magnetic resonance imaging: used to identify cord lesions, compression, or edema

Surgery: may be required to align or stabilize fracture, or repair other traumatic injuries that may be concurrent

Traction: may be required to align and stabilize fracture or dislocation of the vertebral column

NURSING CARE PLANS

Risk for decreased cardiac output

Related to: neurogenic shock, sympathetic blockade, spinal shock

Defining characteristics: hypotension, bradycardia, vasovagal reflex, hypoxia, decreased venous return, decreased hemodynamic pressures

Outcome Criteria

Patient will be able to maintain systolic blood pressure above 90 mmHg and have stable vital signs and heart rhythm.

INTERVENTIONS	RATIONALES
Monitor vital signs, especially blood pressure and heart rate.	Transection of the spinal cord above the T5 levels may result in vasodilation, decreased venous return, and hypotension. Sympathetic blockade may cause bradycardia.

INTERVENTIONS	RATIONALES
Monitor EKG for changes in rhythm and conduction, and treat according to hospital protocol.	Sympathetic blockade may cause conduction problems such as escape rhythms, and vasovagal reflexes may provoke cardiac arrest.
Monitor hemodynamic parameters if feasible.	Fluid shifts, hypotension, and hemorrhage may be reflected in lowered pressures and lower cardiac output/index.
Administer oxygen as warranted, ensuring pre-oxygenation prior to suctioning or prolonged coughing exercises.	Assists in preventing hypoxia which can result in vasovagal reflex and cardiac arrest.
Administer vasopressors as warranted.	May be indicated if fluid resuscitation is not successful in maintaining systolic blood pressure above 90 mmHg.

Information, Instruction, Demonstration

INTERVENTIONS	RATIONALES
Instruct patient in avoidance of valsalva-type maneuvers.	May lower blood pressure and facilitate vasovagal response.

Discharge or Maintenance Evaluation

- Patient will exhibit no episodes of cardiac rhythm disturbances.

- Patient will have normotensive blood pressure with stable hemodynamic pressures.

- Patient will have optimal cardiac output and index.

- Patient will exhibit no hypoxic episodes and avoid desaturation with procedures.

Inneffective breathing pattern

Related to: trauma, spinal cord lesions at high levels, paralysis of respiratory musculature, ineffective coughing, pneumonia, pulmonary edema, pulmonary embolism

Defining characteristics: dyspnea, use of accessory muscles, diaphragmatic breathing, decreased tidal volumes, sputum, abdominal distention, abnormal arterial blood gases, apnea, oxygen desaturation

Outcome Criteria

Patient will maintain adequate oxygenation and ventilation without evidence of respiratory complications.

INTERVENTIONS	RATIONALES
Assess respiratory status for adequacy of airway and ventilation, rate, character, depth, increased work of breathing, or use of accessory muscles.	Spinal cord lesions below C4 level induces diaphragmatic breathing and hypoventilation.
Auscultate lung fields for presence of adventitious sounds and other changes.	May reflect the presence of infiltrates, pneumonia, atelectasis, or fluid overload.
Assist with/measure pulmonary parameters, such as spontaneous tidal volume, vital capacity, and negative inspiratory force. Obtain arterial blood gases as warranted.	Measurement of pulmonary parameters may facilitate prompt identification of deterioration in respiratory status. ABGs are drawn to identify acid/base disturbances and hypoxemia that may result from restriction of lung expansion and ineffective cough mechanisms.
Evaluate patient's ability to cough and assist with abdominal thrusting technique, or quad coughing, as warranted.	Paralysis of respiratory musculature may prevent sufficient pleural pressure to be produced to maintain effective cough. External technique can assist patient to cough effectively.
Monitor oxygen saturation continually and notify physician if levels stay below 90%.	Oximetry assists in identification of deterioration in ventilatory status, allowing for prompt intervention.
Suction patient only when required. Provide humidification of oxygen and utilize pulmonary toilette as warranted.	Suctioning may precipitate vasovagal reflexes, bradycardia, and cardiac arrest. Liquification of environmental air and secretions may prevent mucous plugs and thick mucoid secretions.

Information, Instruction, Demonstration

INTERVENTIONS	RATIONALES
Prepare patient/family for placement on mechanical ventilation as warranted.	Hypoxemia that cannot be corrected with addition of supplemental oxygen may require intubation and ventilation to maintain airway and oxygenation.
Prepare patient for bronchoscopy as warranted.	May be required to remove obstructive secretions.
Monitor for signs/symptoms of pulmonary embolism, pneumonia, or pulmonary edema.	Edema may result from fluid resuscitation efforts, and pneumonia may develop from immobility and ineffective cough ability. Pulmonary emboli may result from venous thrombosis as a complication of immobility or hemorrhagic causes.
Instruct family member in techniques to assist patient with coughing, repositioning frequently, and suctioning techniques as warranted.	Provides information that will be used when patient is discharged and facilitates feelings of control over situation and self-esteem.

Discharge or Maintenance Evaluation

- Patient will maintain adequate airway and ventilation.

- Patient will exhibit no signs/symptoms of respiratory complications.

- Patient/family will be able to verbalize understanding of instructions and give adequate return demonstration.

Alteration in temperature regulation

Related to: poikilothermism, injury to hypothalamic center or sensory pathways

Defining characteristics: elevated body temperature, decreased body temperature, change of temperature based on environmental temperature

Outcome Criteria

Patient will achieve and maintain body temperature above 95 degrees.

INTERVENTIONS	RATIONALES
Monitor temperature every 2 hours until stabilized, then every 4 hours and prn.	Interruption of the sympathetic nervous system pathways to the temperature control center in the hypothalamus causes body temperature swings in an effort to match environmental temperatures.
Maintain a slightly cool environmental temperature. If patient is hypothermic, apply warm blanket.	Hyperthermia may occur during periods of spinal shock because the sympathetic activity is blocked and the patient does not perspire on paralyzed areas of body.

Information, Instruction, Demonstration

INTERVENTIONS	RATIONALES
Instruct patient/family regarding variable body temperatures and methods to maintain comfort.	Provides knowledge and facilitates compliance.

Discharge or Maintenance Evaluation

- Patient will exhibit normal temperature and be able to maintain core body temperature using methods discussed.

Impaired physical mobility

Related to: spinal cord lesion, trauma, paralysis, spasticity, physical restraint, traction

Defining characteristics: contractures, inability to move as desired, spastic movements, muscle atrophy, muscle wasting, skin breakdown, redness, pressure areas

Outcome Criteria

Patient will be able to achieve maximum mobility within limitations of paralysis and will avoid skin breakdown and contractures.

INTERVENTIONS	RATIONALES
Assess motor strength and function at least every 4-8 hours, and prn. Identify level of tactile sensation, ability to move parts of body, spasticity, etc.	Identifies level of sensory-motor impairment and evaluates resolution of spinal shock. Specific injury level may have partially mixed or occult sensorimotor impairment.
Observe for muscle atrophy and wasting.	May be noted during flaccid paralysis stage of spinal shock.
Encourage independent activity as able.	C1-4 lesions result in quadriplegia with complete loss of respiratory function; C4-5 lesions result in quadriplegia with potential for phrenic nerve involvement that may result in loss of respiratory function; C5-6 lesions result in quadriplegia with some gross arm movement ability and some sparing of diaphragmatic muscle involvement; C6-7 lesions result in quadriplegia with intact biceps; C7-8 lesions result in quadriplegia with intact biceps and triceps but no intrinsic hand musculature intact; T1-L2 lesions result in paraplegia with variable amounts of involvement to intercostal and abdominal muscle groups; below L2 lesions result in mixed motor-sensory loss with bowel and bladder impairment.
Assist with/provide range of motion exercises to all joints.	Improves muscle tone and joint mobility, decreases risk for contractures, and prevents muscle atrophy.
Reposition every 2 hours and prn. Utilize kinetic bed therapy as warranted.	Decreases pressure on bony prominences and improves peripheral circulation. Kinetic beds can immobilize the unstable vertebral column and decrease potential for complications from immobility.

INTERVENTIONS	RATIONALES
Ensure proper alignment with each position.	Correct anatomic alignment prevents contractures and deformities.
Utilize footboards or high-top tennis shoes.	Prevents footdrop.
Observe for changes in skin status and provide frequent skin care.	Loss of sensation, paralysis, and decreased venous return predispose the patient for pressure wounds.
Assist with/consult physical therapists or occupational therapists to develop plan of care for patient.	Exercises help stimulation circulation and preserves joint mobility.
Maintain cervical traction apparatus as warranted.	Cervical traction provides for stabilization of vertebral column, reduction, and immobilization to maintain proper alignment. Halo brace/devices provide immobilization but can facilitate with active participation with rehabilitation processes.
Observe for redness and swelling to calf muscles. Measure circumference daily if problem is noted.	Thrombus formation may occur as a result of immobilization and flaccid paralysis.

Information, Instruction, Demonstration

INTERVENTIONS	RATIONALES
Instruct family in rehabilitative therapy, exercises, and repositioning, and involve them with patient's care.	Facilitates adaptation to patient's health status and allows for family members to contribute to patient's welfare.
Avoid improper placement of footrests, headrests, or padding when repositioning patient.	May create pressure resulting in pressure sores or necrotic injury.
Instruct in methods for shifting weight.	Improves circulation by reducing pressure to body surfaces.
Administer muscle relaxants as warranted.	May be required to reduce pain and spasticity.

Discharge or Maintenance Evaluation

- Patient will maintain appropriate body alignment and maximal function within limit of injury.

- Patient will avoid complications of immobility.

- Patient will be able to verbalize understanding and demonstrate effective therapeutic modalities.

- Patient will exhibit suppleness of joints and muscles.

Alteration in comfort
[See Guillain-Barré]

Related to: trauma, surgery, cervical traction

Defining characteristics: burning pain below lesion, muscle spasms, phantom pain, hyperesthesia above lesion level, headaches, communication of pain, facial grimacing, irritability, restlessness

Risk for impaired skin integrity
[See Fractures]

Related to: immobility, surgery, traction apparatus, changes in metabolism, decreased circulation, impaired sensation

Defining characteristics: wounds, drainage, redness, pressure sores, abrasions, lacerations

Sensory-perceptual alteration
[See CVA]

Related to: traumatic injury, sensory receptor and tract impairment, damaged sensory transmission

Defining characteristics: decreases sensory acuity, impairment of position relation, proprioception, motor incoordination, mood swings, disorientation, agitation, anxiety, abnormal emotional responses, changes in stimulation response

Bowel incontinence

Related to: trauma, impairment of bowel innervation, impairment of perception, modifications of dietary intake, immobility

Defining characteristics: inability to evacuate bowel voluntarily, ileus, gastric distention, hypoactive bowel sounds, absent bowel sounds, nausea, vomiting, abdominal pain, constipation

Outcome Criteria

Patient will be able to establish and maintain bowel elimination patterns.

INTERVENTIONS	RATIONALES
Observe for presence of abdominal distention.	Innervation may be impaired as a result of the injury with resultant decrease or loss of peristalsis, and potential for development of ileus. Bowel distention may precipitate autonomic dysreflexia after spinal shock recedes.
Auscultate for presence of bowel sounds, noting changes in character.	High-pitched tinkling bowel sounds may be heard when patient has an ileus, and bowel sounds may be absent during spinal shock phase.
Evaluate bowel habits, such as frequency, character, and amount of stools.	Establishes pattern and facilitates treatment options.
Establish bowel pattern by use of stool softeners, suppositories, or digital stimulation.	Effectively evacuates bowel.
Increase dietary bulk and fiber.	Promotes peristaltic movement through bowel and improves consistency of stool.
Provide frequent skin care.	Incontinence of stool increases potential for skin breakdown.

Information, Instruction, Demonstration

INTERVENTIONS	RATIONALES
Instruct patient/family regarding method for daily bowel program.	Promotes independence and self-esteem.

Discharge or Maintenance Evaluation

* Patient will establish and maintain daily bowel pattern.

* Patient will be able to verbalize understanding and demonstrate appropriate methods to accomplish bowel care.

* Patient will be able to avoid complications that may be caused by gastric distention or ileus.

Urinary retention

Related to: traumatic loss of bladder innervation, bladder atony

Defining characteristics: urinary retention, incontinence, bladder distention, urinary tract infections, kidney dysfunction, stone formation, overflow syndrome

Outcome Criteria

Patient will be able to achieve and maintain balanced intake and output with no signs/symptoms of complications.

INTERVENTIONS	RATIONALES
Monitor intake and output every shift, noting significant differences in amounts.	May identify urinary retention from an areflexic bladder.
Observe for ability to void and palpate for bladder distention. Insert Foley catheter as warranted.	Spinal shock is exhibited in the bladder when there is a loss of sensory perception and the bladder is unable to contract and empty itself. Bladder distention may precipitate autonomic dysreflexia.

INTERVENTIONS	RATIONALES
Monitor urinary output for changes in color or character.	Cloudiness, blood, concentration, or foul smell may indicate urinary tract infection.
Administer urinary antiseptic agents/acidifiers as ordered.	Vitamin C and mandelamine may be given to acidify the urine to hinder bacterial growth and prevent stone formation.

Information, Instruction, Demonstration

INTERVENTIONS	RATIONALES
Instruct patient/family in methods for intermittent catheterization when warranted.	Catheterization may be required for long-term due to injury and dysfunction to bladder. Intermittent catheterization is preferred and is performed at specific intervals to approximate physiological function and may decrease complications from indwelling catheter.
Increase fluid intake, when warranted, up to 3-4 L/day, including acidic juices, such as cranberry juice.	Decreases formation of kidney or bladder stones, helps prevent infection, and ensures hydration.
Ensure sterile technique for catheter insertions.	Decreases potential for urinary tract infection.

Discharge or Maintenance Evaluation

• Patient will have balanced intake and output without signs of urinary tract infection.

• Patient/family will be able to verbalize understanding of need for catheterization, and will be able to give return demonstration of procedure.

Risk for dysreflexia

Related to: spinal cord injury at T6 level and above, excessive autonomic reaction to stimulation

Defining characteristics: hypertension, blurred vision, throbbing headache, diaphoresis above the

level of the lesion, bradycardia, piloerection, pupil dilation, nasal congestion, nausea

Outcome Criteria

Patient/nurse will be able to recognize signs/symptoms and take appropriate action to prevent complications.

INTERVENTIONS	RATIONALES
Observe for hypertension, tachycardia, bradycardia, sweating above level of lesion, pallor below level of injury, headache, piloerection, nasal congestion, metallic taste, blurred vision, chest pain, or nausea.	Identification of potential life-threatening complication facilitates prompt and timely intervention.
Assess for bowel or bladder distention, bladder spasms, or changes in temperature.	May be indicative of precipitating factor for autonomic dysreflexia.
Monitor vital signs frequently, especially blood pressure every 5 minutes during acute phase.	Hypotensive crisis may occur once stimulus is removed, but dysreflexia may recur and should be monitored.
Palpate abdomen VERY gently for bladder distention, and irrigate catheter VERY slowly with tepid solution.	Palpation should be done gently, if at all, so as to not increase stimulating factor and worsen condition. Irrigation may identify and correct catheter obstruction which may have been predisposing factor.
Check for rectal impaction VERY gently, and only after anesthetic-type rectal ointment has been applied.	May increase rectal stimulation and worsen dysreflexia.
Position in high-Fowler's position in bed.	Promotes decrease in blood pressure to avert intracranial hemorrhage or seizure activity.
Administer medications as ordered.	Atropine may be required to increase heart rate if bradycardia is present; apresoline, hyperstat, or procardia may be required to decrease blood pressure.

Information, Instruction, Demonstration

INTERVENTIONS	RATIONALES
Instruct patient/family on signs/symptoms of syndrome, and methods for preventing occurrence.	Problem may be lifelong but can be prevented by avoiding pressure-causing sensation.
Administer antihypertensive drugs as ordered.	May be required for long-term use to alleviate chronic autonomic dysreflexia by relaxation of the bladder neck.
Prepare patient for nerve block as warranted.	May be required if dysreflexia is unresponsive to other treatment modalities.

Discharge or Maintenance Evaluation

- Patient/family will be able to verbalize understanding of condition and methods to reduce occurrence.

- Patient will exhibit no signs/symptoms of autonomic dysreflexia, and have no complications.

SPINAL CORD INJURIES

Disease processes
(Loss of function without trauma)
↓
Contusion
↓
Edema to cord
↓
Increased intradural
pressure
↓
Neurodysfunction
↓
Paralysis of muscles
↓
Hypoventilation
↓
Decreased VC, TV
ineffective cough

Compression
↓
Tumor or hemorrhage
↓
Muscle weakness
↓
Loss of autoregulation
↓
Poikilothermism
↓
Decreased spinal cord
blood flow

Trauma
(Flexion, hypertension, rotation)
↓
Transection of cord
↓
Incomplete   Complete
↓   ↓
Partial dysfunction   Total loss of
of spinal cord tracts   sensory and
                        motor function

Sympathetic   Release of
blockade   vaso-active
                        substances
↓   ↓
Bradycardia   Vasodilation
                        ↓
                        Decreased venous
                        return

Decreased oxygenation
↓
Hypoxia
↓
Spinal shock/vasovagal reflex
↓
Arrest
↓
DEATH

Guillain-Barré Syndrome

Guillain-Barré syndrome, also known as infectious polyneuritis, polyradiculoneuritis, and Landry-Guillain-Barré-Strohl syndrome, is an acute neuropathy in which inflammation and swelling of spinal nerve roots create demyelination and degeneration to the nerves beginning distally and ascending symmetrically.

Demyelination causes nerve impulse conduction to be delayed. Both dorsal and ventral nerve roots are involved, so both sensory and motor impairment is noted. The disease progress may cease at any point or continue to complete quadriplegia with cranial motor nerve involvement. Symmetrical muscle weakness occurs and moves upward, with associated paresthesias and pain. Dysphagia, facial weakness, and extraocular muscle paralysis occur. Blood pressure and heart rate can be affected with marked fluctuations in response to a dysfunctional autonomic nervous system. After demyelination stops, remyelination begins and frequently complete function is restored in approximately 70% of patients. The recovery phase may last from 4 months to 2 years.

The exact cause of the syndrome is not known but several factors have been known to be associated with Guillain-Barré, such as, viral infections occurring 2-3 weeks prior, vaccinations, surgery, pre-existing systemic disease, and autoimmune diseases.

Guillain-Barré syndrome may cause complications of hypertension, bradycardia, respiratory failure, and cardiovascular collapse. When sacral nerve roots are affected, incontinence becomes a problem.

MEDICAL CARE

Lumbar puncture: used in the diagnostic process; initially protein levels are normal for the first 48 hours but then increase as the disease progresses; cell count is usually normal; ICP may be elevated

Electromyography: helps to differentiate Guillain-Barré from myasthenia gravis; in Guillain-Barré, nerve impulse conduction speed is decreased

Nerve conduction studies: nerve conduction velocity is slowed

Plasmapheresis: may be used on an experimental basis to remove circulating antibodies that compromise nerve receptors

Laboratory: white blood cell count is elevated; sedimentation rate is elevated; electrolytes are done to identify hyponatremia that may occur due to problems with volume receptors

NURSING CARE PLANS

Risk for ineffective breathing pattern
[See Head Injuries]

Related to: muscle weakness, paralysis, inability to swallow

Defining characteristics: dyspnea, bradypnea, apnea, hypoxia, hypoxemia, abnormal arterial blood gases, inability to handle secretions

Impaired physical mobility
[See Head Injuries]

Related to: neuromuscular impairment, paralysis

Defining characteristics: inability to move at will, inability to turn, transfer, or ambulate, decreased range of motion, muscle weakness, muscle incoordination, decreased reflexes

Risk for alteration in nutrition: less than body requirements
[See Mechanical Ventilation]

Related to: neuromuscular impairment, intubation

Defining characteristics: weight loss, muscle wasting, catabolism, inability to take in sufficient nutrients, impaired cough/gag/swallow reflexes

Impaired verbal communication
[See CVA]

Related to: neuromuscular impairment, loss of muscle control, weakness

Defining characteristics: inability to speak, inability to write

Sensory-perceptual alterations: visual, kinesthetic, gustatory, tactile
[See CVA]

Related to: neuromuscular deficits, altered reception of stimuli, altered sensation, inability to communicate, hypoxia

Defining characteristics: paresthesias, hypersensitivity to stimuli, muscle incoordination, inability to communicate, anxiety, restlessness

Alteration in comfort

Related to: neuromuscular impairment

Defining characteristics: communication of pain or discomfort with minimal stimuli, muscle aches, tenderness, joint pain, flaccidity, spasticity

Outcome Criteria

Patient will have no complaints of pain, or pain will be controlled to patient's satisfaction.

INTERVENTIONS	RATIONALES
Monitor for complaints of pain/discomfort and for non-verbal indications that patient may be in discomfort.	Patient may be unable to verbalize complaints.
Administer medication as ordered.	Reduces or alleviates pain. Narcotics may cause respiratory depression.
Apply hot or cold packs as warranted.	Helps to alleviate discomfort and improves muscle and joint stiffness.
Use therapeutic touch, massage, imagery, visualization, or relaxation therapies as warranted.	Helps to refocus attention away from pain and provides for active participation in relieving pain.

Discharge or Maintenance Evaluation

- Patient will have no complaints of pain or paresthesias.

- Patient will be able to communication pain and requests for analgesics.

- Patient will have pain controlled effectively to his satisfaction.

Risk for alteration in tissue perfusion: cardiopulmonary, peripheral, renal

Related to: autonomic nervous system impairment, hypovolemia, electrolyte imbalance, hypoxemia, thrombosis

Defining characteristics: hypotension, hypertension, blood pressure lability, bradycardia, tachycardia, dysrhythmias, altered temperature regulation, decreased urine output, anuria, skin breakdown

Outcome Criteria

Patient will achieve and maintain normal perfusion of all body systems.

INTERVENTIONS	RATIONALES
Monitor vital signs at rest and with turning. Notify MD of significant changes.	Severe changes with blood pressure may occur as a result of autonomic dysfunction because of the loss of sympathetic outflow to maintain peripheral vascular tone. Postural hypotension may occur as a result of impaired reflexes which normally readjust pressure during changes in position.
Monitor EKG for changes, and treat dysrhythmias per protocol.	Rate changes may occur as a result of vagal stimulation and impairment of the sympathetic innervation of the heart. Hypoxemia or electrolyte imbalances may alter vascular tone and impair venous return.
Monitor temperature of skin and core body. Observe for inability to perspire.	Vasomotor tone changes can impair the ability to perspire and cause temperature regulation problems. The patient's impaired sensation may further promote difficulty with warming and cooling the body.
Measure hemodynamics if pulmonary artery catheter in place, and notify MD for significant changes.	Impairment in vascular tone and venous return can decrease cardiac output.
Observe skin surfaces for redness or breakdown. Place patient on kinetic bed, egg crate mattress, alternating pressure mattress, etc., if warranted	Decreases in sensation as well as circulatory changes may result in impaired perfusion and facilitate skin breakdown or ischemia. Special beds/mattresses help to reduce hazards of immobility.
Observe calves for redness, edema, or positive Homan's or Pratt's signs.	Venous stasis may increase potential for deep vein thrombosis formation, and patient may be unaware of discomfort due to paresthesias.
Provide anti-embolic hose or sequential compression devices to both legs and remove at least once every 8 hours.	Helps to decrease venous stasis and promotes venous return.
Monitor hourly intake and output. Notify MD if urine output is less than 30 cc/hr for 2	Circulating volume may be decreased by patient's inability to take in adequate hydration, fluid

INTERVENTIONS	RATIONALES
hours, or if significant imbalance in I&O occurs.	shifting, and decreases in vascular tone.
Administer IV fluids as ordered.	Fluids help to prevent or correct hypovolemia but impaired vascular tone may result in severe hemodynamic lability based on small increases in circulating volumes.
Administer heparin SQ/IV as ordered, if no contraindications.	May be given prophylactically due to immobilization.

Discharge or Maintenance Evaluation

• Patient will be able to maintain adequate perfusion.

• Patient will have stable vital signs and hemodynamic parameters.

• Patient will have regular cardiac rhythm with no dysrhythmias.

Risk for urinary retention

Related to: neuromuscular impairment, immobility

Defining characteristics: inability to void, inability to completely empty bladder

Outcome Criteria

Patient will be able to empty bladder with no signs/symptoms of infection or retention.

INTERVENTIONS	RATIONALES
Monitor for ability to void. Measure output carefully.	Provides information regarding neuromuscular progression. Progression of disease may predispose patient to retention which may lead to urinary tract infection or other complications.

INTERVENTIONS	RATIONALES
Observe and palpate for bladder distention.	Bladder may become distended as sphincter reflex is involved in neuromuscular progression.
Insert indwelling catheter as warranted.	May be required to facilitate urinary emptying until disease process has resolved and bladder control has been achieved.
Observe for concentrated urine, presence of blood or pus, changes in clarity or odor.	May indicate presence of urinary infection.

Information, Instruction, Demonstration

INTERVENTIONS	RATIONALES
Instruct on need and procedure for catheter placement.	Promotes understanding and facilitates patient compliance.

Discharge or Maintenance Evaluation

* Patient will be able to void sufficient amounts without presence of retention or infection.

* Patient will be able to accurately recall information regarding need and procedure for catheter placement.

* Patient will be able to achieve bladder control once disease process has resolved.

Risk for constipation

Related to: neuromuscular impairment, bedrest, immobility, changes in dietary habits, changes in environment, analgesics

Defining characteristics: inability to expel all or part of stool, passage of hard stool, frequency less than normal pattern, rectal fullness, abdominal pain/pressure, decreased bowel sounds, decreased peristalsis, weakness, fatigue, appetite impairment

Outcome Criteria

Patient will be able to eliminate soft formed stool on a normal basis.

INTERVENTIONS	RATIONALES
Evaluate elimination pattern, normal habits, ability to sense urge to defecate, presence of nausea/vomiting, presence of painful hemorrhoids, and history of constipation problems.	Provides baseline information to facilitate appropriate intervention for the patient's plan of care.
Observe for abdominal distention, tenderness, or guarding, nausea, vomiting, and absence of stool.	May indicate present or impending ileus or impaction.
Palpate rectum for presence of stool/impaction.	Manual removal of stool may be required, and should be performed gently to avoid vagal stimulation. Other interventions may be necessary to allow for bowel elimination.
Auscultate bowel sounds for presence, pitch, and changes.	Diminished or absent bowel sounds, or presence of high-pitched tinkling sounds may indicate that an ileus has developed.
Administer stool softeners, laxatives, suppositories, or enemas as warranted/ordered.	May be required to stimulate bowel evacuation and to establish a bowel regime until patient is able to regain normal musculature control.
Insert nasogastric tube as ordered. Connect with intermittent suction per hospital policy.	Decompresses abdominal distention that occurs with ileus formation, and helps prevent nausea and vomiting.
Increase fiber in diet/tube feedings as warranted.	Helps to promote elimination by adding bulk and helps to regulate fecal consistency.

Information, Instruction, Demonstration

INTERVENTIONS	RATIONALES
Instruct on increases in fluid intake, dietary requirements, use of fruits and juices to improve bowel elimination.	Promotes knowledge and can help facilitate improvement in bowel regime.
Instruct on need/procedure for nasogastric tube insertion.	Helps to promote understanding of complications that may occur with the loss of peristalsis due to the disease process.

Discharge or Maintenance Evaluation

- Patient will achieve normal bowel elimination.

- Patient will require no bowel aids to facilitate his normal routine.

- Patient will regain muscle control and be able to evacuate stool.

- Patient will be able to utilize dietary modification to maintain bowel regime.

- Patient will be able to recall information correctly.

Anxiety, fear

Related to: disease process, change in health status, paralysis, respiratory failure, change in environment, threat of death

Defining characteristics: restlessness, apprehension, tension, fearfulness, sympathetic stimulation, changes in vital signs, inability to concentrate or focus, poor attention span, uncertainty of treatment and outcome, insomnia

Outcome Criteria

Patient will be able to reduce and/or relieve anxiety with appropriate methods.

INTERVENTIONS	RATIONALES
Evaluate anxiety level frequently. Stay with patient during acute episodes.	Determination of severity of patient's anxiety/fear can help to determine appropriate intervention. Nurse's presence during acute anxiety may foster feelings of reassurance and concern for the patient's well-being.
Maintain consistency with nurse assignments.	Helps to decrease anxiety and builds trust in relationships.
Patient should be placed near nurse's station and within visual contact.	Reassures patient that assistance will be nearby should he be unable to use call bell.
Provide method for patient to summon assistance.	Reduces anxiety and fear of abandonment.
Involve patient and family in plan of care. Allow patient to make as many decisions as warranted.	Helps to foster understanding and facilitates feelings of control and improved self-esteem. Improves cooperation with procedures and care.
Provide time for patient/family to discuss fears and concerns. Offer realistic options and do not give false reassurance.	Discussion of fears provides opportunity for clarification of misperceptions and for realistic methods of dealing with problems.
Administer anti-anxiety medications or sedation as warranted/ordered.	Patient's anxiety may result in alterations in hemodynamic stability and may require medication to initially deal with situational crises. Patient may require medication to facilitate improved ventilation should mechanical ventilation be warranted.

Discharge or Maintenance Evaluation

- Patient will be able to deal with changes in health status effectively.

- Patient will be able to control anxiety and reduce fear to a manageable level.

- Patient will have decreased anxiety and fear.

GUILLAIN-BARRÉ SYNDROME

TRIGGERING EVENT
↓
Immunologic demyelination of perepheral nervous system
↓
Lymphocytes infiltrate into nerve roots, nerves, and CNS
↓
Schwann cells deposit myelin around axons
with interruption at intervals by the nodes of ranvier
↓
Nerve conduction slows as impulses are conducted from node to node
instead of along azonal pathway
↓
Anterior horn cells in spinal cord degenerate
↓
Loss of reflexes
(usually symmetrical and ascending)
↓

Paralysis of muscles   Decrease/loss of autonomic reflexes   Peripheral volume
↓   ↓   Receptors impaired

Vital capacity decreased   BP fluctuations   SIADH
NIF decreased   ↓
↓   Hyponatremia
Loss of respiratory muscles   ↓
↓   Hypovolemia
Apnea   ↓
↓   Dysrythmias
Hypoxia

                    DEATH   DEMYELINATION CEASES
                                              ↓
                                      Remyelination begins
                                              ↓
                              Return of nerve impulse transmission
                                              ↓
                                  Function restored proximally
                                  and proceeds in reverse from
                                    last area involved upward

          Complete recovery   Varying degrees of function restored

Status Epilepticus

Seizures occur when uncontrolled electrical impulses from the nerve cells in the cerebral cortex discharge and result in autonomic, sensory, and motor dysfunction. Status epilepticus is a series of repeated seizures, a prolonged seizure, or sequential seizures longer than 30 minutes in which the patient does not regain consciousness. This seizure activity has a high mortality rate of up to 30% as a result of neurological and brain damage.

There are three types of status epilepticus: convulsive, nonconvulsive, and partial status epilepticus. In the convulsive type, seizure activity may have a focal onset, but has tonic-clonic, grand mal type seizures without experiencing alertness between motor attacks. Nonconvulsive seizures are noted with a prolonged twilight state and are usually not motor activity. Partial status epilepticus occurs when continuous or repetitive focal seizures occur but consciousness is not altered.

Status epilepticus usually occurs in patients with pre-existing seizure disorders who have a precipitating factor occurance. These factors can include withdrawal from anticonvulsant medication, alcohol withdrawal, sedative or antidepressant withdrawal, sleep deprivation, meningitis, encephalitis, brain abscesses or tumors, pregnancy, hypoglycemia, uremia, cerebrovascular disease, cerebral edema, or cerebral trauma.

The initial stage causes sympathetic activity increases with a decrease in the cerebral vascular resistance. After 30 minutes, hypotension occurs with a decrease in cerebral blood flow because of loss of autoregulation. The continuing massive autonomic discharges can cause bronchial secretions and restriction, with increased capillary permeability and pulmonary edema. Dysrhythmias can occur and patients may develop rhabdomyolysis and renal failure. Other complications may occur as a result of the significantly elevated metabolic state.

MEDICAL CARE

Laboratory: glucose levels decreased; electrolytes to identify imbalances that may be precipitating factor or result from prolonged seizure activity; enzymes, especially creatine phosphokinase elevated after seizure activity; drug screen done to identify potential factor for drug withdrawal; CBC used to identify hemorrhage or infection with shift to the left on differential; drug levels for medications being given for seizures to evaluate therapeutic response and discern toxicity; renal profiles to evaluate renal function; urinalysis to identify hematuria or myoglobinuria

CT scans: may be done to identify lesions or precipitating factors

Electroencephalogram: used to identify presence of seizure activity

Arterial blood gases: used to identify hypoxia and acid-base imbalances; usually acidosis seen

NURSING CARE PLANS

Risk for impaired gas exchange
[See Mechanical Ventilation]

Related to: altered oxygen supply from repetitive seizures, cognitive impairment, neuromuscular impairment

Defining characteristics: restlessness, cyanosis, inability to move secretions, tachycardia, dysrhythmias, abnormal ABGs, decreased oxygen saturation

Risk for ineffective airway clearance
[See Mechanical Ventilation]

Related to: neuromuscular impairment, cognitive impairment, tracheobronchial obstruction

Defining characteristics: adventitious breath sounds, dyspnea, tachypnea, shallow respirations, cough with or without productivity, cyanosis, anxiety, restlessness

Hyperthermia
[See Pheochromocytoma]

Related to: continued seizure activity, increased metabolic state

Defining characteristics: fever, persistent tonic-clonic seizure activity, persistent focal seizures, persistent generalized seizures, tachycardia

Risk for fluid volume deficit
[See ARDS]

Related to: excessive loss of fluid, decreased intake

Defining characteristics: hypotension, tachycardia, fever, weight loss, oliguria, abnormal electrolytes, low filling pressures, decreased mental status, decreased specific gravity, increased serum osmolality

Risk for injury

Related to: seizure activity, increased metabolic demands

Defining characteristics: respiratory acidosis, metabolic acidosis, hypoxemia, hyperthermia, hypoglycemia, electrolyte imbalances, renal failure, rhabdomyolysis, exhaustion, death

Outcome Criteria

Patient will achieve and maintain seizure-free status with optimal oxygenation and ventilation without complications.

INTERVENTIONS	RATIONALES
Maintain patent airway and adequate ventilation.	Intubation and placement on mechanical ventilation may be required if seizures cannot be controlled.
Monitor oxygen saturation by oximeter.	Decreases in saturation that cannot be improved with supplemental oxygen may require mechanical ventilation. Seizure activity increases oxygen consumption and demand.
Provide supplemental oxygen as warranted.	May be required to maintain desired levels of oxygen.
Monitor ABGs for imbalances and treat per protocol.	Metabolic increases may lead to lactate formation and acidosis.
Administer medications as ordered.	Valium may be given IV at 5 mg/min rate to control seizure activity by enhancing neurotransmitter GABA. Ativan 2-4 mg IV may be given and repeated every 15 minutes as needed for seizure control. Caution should be exercised because respiratory and cardiovascular depression can occur. Phenobarbital IV at 60 mg/min may be given to depress excitation, decrease calcium uptake by nerves, and to strengthen repression of synapses. Dilantin IV at 50 mg/min rate may be given to decrease cellular influx of sodium and calcium and blocking neurotransmission release.
Maintain patient in seizure-free status.	Once seizures have stopped, anticonvulsant drugs must be given to prevent recurrence of seizure activity.
Monitor EKG for dysrhythmias and treat per hospital protocol.	Electrolyte imbalances, too-rapid administration of medications, and hypoxia may contribute to appearance of cardiac dysrhythmias that may require interventional care.
Monitor intake and output every 2 hours and prn.	Identifies imbalances with fluid status and fluid shifting.

INTERVENTIONS	RATIONALES
Monitor labwork for changes and trends.	Electrolytes may fluctuate because of cellular movement of ions. Myoglobin may be present in urine as a result of prolonged seizure activity and can lead to renal failure. Drug levels may rise to toxic levels and should be evaluated for therapeutic effectiveness.
Identify and treat underlying cause of seizures.	Identification may lead to timely intervention and treatment.

Information, Instruction, Demonstration

INTERVENTIONS	RATIONALES
Instruct patient/family in disease process and methods for reduction of seizures.	Promotes knowledge and facilitates compliance.
Instruct in drug regimen, effects, side effects, contraindications, and precautions.	Promotes knowledge and helps prevent lack of cooperation with medication regime with resultant seizure breakthrough activity. Presence of side effects may indicate the need for changes in doses or medication type. Interactions with other drugs may produce adverse reactions, such as potentiated anticoagulation effect when dilantin and coumadin are concurrently taken.
Instruct in oral care.	Prevents gingival hypertrophy that may occur while taking dilantin.
Instruct on use of medical alert bracelet.	May hasten emergency treatment in critical situations.
Instruct on methods to promote safety with activities, such as, driving, using mechanical equipment, swimming, or hobbies.	May facilitate prevention of injury to self or other if seizures occur without warning.
Instruct on contact people, community resource groups, counselors, as warranted.	May provide opportunities for long-term support and sharing ideas with others who have similar problems.

Discharge or Maintenance Evaluation

- Patient/family will be able to verbalize understanding of all instructions and comply with medical regimen.

- Patient will remain free of seizures and injury.

- Patient will be able to effectively access community resources for help and support.

- Patient will exhibit no signs of complications.

Disturbance in self-esteem

Related to: perception of loss of control, ashamed of medical condition

Defining characteristics: fear of rejection, concerns about changes in lifestyle, negative feelings about self, change in perception of role, changes in responsibilities, lack of participation in therapy or care, passiveness, inability to accept positive reinforcement, little eye contact, brief responses to questions

Outcome Criteria

Patient will be able to participate in own care and have positive perceptions of self.

INTERVENTIONS	RATIONALES
Encourage patient to initiate self-care or request assistance.	Participation in care facilitates feelings of normalcy.
Discuss patient's perceptions of illness and potential reactions of others to his disease.	Provides opportunities to establish patient's knowledge base, clear up any misconceptions, and opportunity to problem-solve responses to future seizures.
Discuss previous success episodes and patient's strengths.	Concentrating on the positive experiences may help to reduce self-consciousness and allow patient to begin to accept condition.

INTERVENTIONS	RATIONALES
Discuss concerns with family members, allowing ample time for members to discuss problems and attitudes.	Negative feelings from patient's family may affect his sense of self-esteem.
Consult with counselors, ministerial support, or resource groups.	Provides opportunity for patient to deal with stigma of disease and overcome feelings of inferiority.

Discharge or Maintenance Evaluation

• Patient will be able to identify ways to cope with negative feelings.

• Patient/family will be able to discuss concerns and effect realistic problem-solving plans.

• Patient will become more accepting of self, with increased self-esteem.

• Patient will be able to effectively access community resources to gain help and support.

Grieving
[See Amputation]

Related to: traumatic injury, loss of physical well-being

Defining characteristics: communications of distress, denial, guilt, fear, sadness, changes in affect, changes in ability and desire for communication, crying, insomnia, lethargy

STATUS EPILEPTICUS

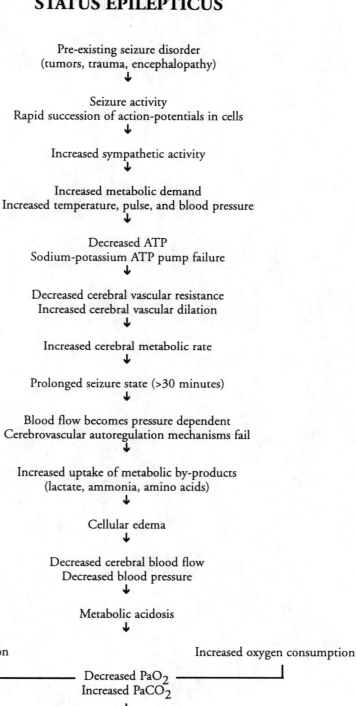

Pre-existing seizure disorder
(tumors, trauma, encephalopathy)
↓

Seizure activity
Rapid succession of action-potentials in cells
↓

Increased sympathetic activity
↓

Increased metabolic demand
Increased temperature, pulse, and blood pressure
↓

Decreased ATP
Sodium-potassium ATP pump failure
↓

Decreased cerebral vascular resistance
Increased cerebral vascular dilation
↓

Increased cerebral metabolic rate
↓

Prolonged seizure state (>30 minutes)
↓

Blood flow becomes pressure dependent
Cerebrovascular autoregulation mechanisms fail
↓

Increased uptake of metabolic by-products
(lactate, ammonia, amino acids)
↓

Cellular edema
↓

Decreased cerebral blood flow
Decreased blood pressure
↓

Metabolic acidosis
↓

Bronchial constriction   Increased oxygen consumption

Decreased PaO_2
Increased $PaCO_2$

Increased pulmonary ————————— Dysrhythmias
pressures

Meningitis

Meningitis is an acute infection of the pia and arachnoid membrane that surrounds the brain and the spinal cord caused by any type of microorganism. Bacterial meningitis is frequently caused by *Streptococcus pneumoniae, Haemophilus influenzae,* or *Neisseria meningitidis.*

Organisms are able to thrive because of opportune access during surgery, with invasive monitoring and lines, penetrating injuries, skull fractures, dura tears, otitis media, or with septic emboli. Once the organism begins multiplying, neutrophils infiltrate into the subarachnoid space and forms an exudate. The body's defenses attempts to control the invading pathogens by walling off the exudate and effectively creating two layers. If appropriate medical treatment is begun early, the outer and inner layers will disappear, but if the infection persists for several weeks, the inner layer forms a permanent fibrin structure over the meninges. This meningeal covering causes adhesions between the pia and the arachnoid membranes and results in congestion and increased ICP.

One of the major complications of meningitis is residual cranial nerve dysfunction, such as deafness, blindness, tinnitus, or vertigo. Sometimes these symptoms resolve, but cerebral edema may occur and cause seizures, nerve palsy, bradycardia, hypertension, coma, and even death.

The main goal of treatment is to eliminate the causative organism and prevent complications.

MEDICAL CARE

Laboratory: white blood cell count elevation to identify infection; cultures to identify the causative organism, CSF analysis to identify infection; urinalysis may show albumin and red and white blood cells; glucose levels elevated in meningitis, LDH elevated with bacterial meningitis, ESR elevated

Radiography: skull and spine x-rays used to identify sinus infections, fractures, or osteomyelitis; chest x-rays may be used to identify respiratory infections, abscesses, lesions, or granulomas

Lumbar puncture: treatment of choice to identify presence of meningitis, help identify type of meningitis, and identify causative organism

Electroencephalogram: may be performed to show slow wave activity

NURSING CARE PLANS

Alteration in tissue perfusion: cerebral
[See Ventriculostomy]

Related to: increased intracranial pressure

Defining characteristics: increased ICP, changes in vital signs, changes in level of consciousness, memory deficit, restlessness, lethargy, coma, stupor, pupillary changes, headache, pain in neck or back, nausea/vomiting, purposeless movements, papilledema

Risk for injury

Related to: infection, shock, seizures

Defining characteristics: presence of infection, elevated white blood cell count, differential shift to the left, positive cultures, hypotension, tachycardia, tremors, fasiculations, seizures, hypoxemia, acid-base disturbances

Outcome Criteria

Patient will be free of infection with stable vital signs.

INTERVENTIONS	RATIONALES
Assist with lumbar puncture.	Identifies presence of infection and can differentiate between types of meningitis. CSF with low white cell counts, less protein elevation, and glucose levels approximately half that of the blood glucose level may be indicative of viral meningitis. CSF that has an elevated initial pressure, high protein, low glucose, cloudy color, and high white cell count indicates bacterial meningitis.
Administer antimicrobials as ordered, as soon as possible.	Aqueous penicillin G is usually the drug of choice, but culture results may indicate a different agent needed to eradicate the organism. Antibiotics are usually given in larger doses at closer intervals in order to facilitate penetration across the blood-brain barrier.
Observe appropriate isolation techniques up to 48 hours after antibiotic regimen has begun.	Prevents spread of infection. After antimicrobial therapy has been instituted for 2 days, the patient is not considered infectious.
Administer anticonvulsants as ordered.	May be required for control of new seizure activity due to meningeal irritation.

Discharge or Maintenance Evaluation

- Patient will be free of infection with no complications from antimicrobial agents.

- Patient will be free of seizure activity.

- Patient will comply with isolation restrictions.

Alteration in comfort
[See Guillain-Barré]

Related to: infectious organisms, circulating toxins, invasive lines, bedrest

Defining characteristics: headache, muscle spasms, backache, photophobia, crying, moaning, restlessness, communication of pain, muscle tension, facial grimacing, pallor, changes in vital signs

Hyperthermia
[See Pheochromocytoma]

Related to: infection process

Defining characteristics: fever, tachycardia, tachypnea, warm, flushed skin, seizures

MENINGITIS

Infectious organisms gain access to meninges and subarachnoid spaces
(viral, bacterial, yeast)

Exudate forms
↓
Meningeal irritation/inflammation
↓
Cortical irritation
↓
Cerebral edema
↓
Increased ICP
↓

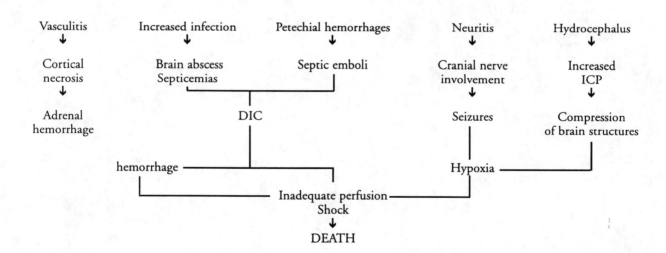

Vasculitis
↓
Cortical
necrosis
↓
Adrenal
hemorrhage

Increased infection
↓
Brain abscess
Septicemias

Petechial hemorrhages
↓
Septic emboli

DIC

Neuritis
↓
Cranial nerve
involvement
↓
Seizures

Hydrocephalus
↓
Increased
ICP
↓
Compression
of brain structures

hemorrhage

Hypoxia

Inadequate perfusion
Shock
↓
DEATH

Ventriculostomy/ICP Monitoring

The brain is housed in a nondistensible cavity that is filled to capacity with CSF, interstitial fluid, and intravascular blood, all of which possess very minimal ability for adjustment for increasing intracranial pressure. If the volume of any one of these constituents increases, there is a reciprocal decrease in the volume of one or more of the others, or else intracranial pressure becomes elevated. Intracranial pressure is normally between 2-15 mmHg or 50-200 cm H_2O, and fluctuates depending on positioning, vital signs changes, increased intra-abdominal pressure, and stimuli.

There are compensatory mechanisms that assist in decreasing intracranial hypertension. The most easily changed element is intravascular volume which results from compression of the venous system and decreases fluid level. The CSF is another element that can be used to compensate for increasing pressures. CSF can be displaced from the cranial vault to the spinal canal, which increases absorption of CSF by the arachnoid villi, slows production of CSF by the choroid plexus, and decreases ICP. Other compensatory mechanisms may be seen, such as skull expansion in infants whose sutures have not closed, as well as reduction of cerebral blood flow to a small extent, but these are not desirable.

Although auto-regulatory mechanisms can control small increases in ICP, rapid or sustained increases suppress these compensatory efforts, and decompensation occurs. As the ICP increases, the cerebral blood flow decreases because of pressure exerted on vessels. This causes brain ischemia and accumulation of lactic acid and carbon dioxide, resulting in hypoxemia and hypercapnia. Cerebral vasodilation ensues which increases blood volume and cerebral edema, which further increases ICP,

until a vicious cycle is established. When ischemia increases to a certain level, the medulla causes blood pressure to rise in an effort to compensate for the increasing ICP, but eventually the ICP will equal the MAP and precipitate curtailing of cerebral blood flow, resulting in vascular collapse and brain death.

ICP is increased when brain volume is enlarged by mass lesions, tumors, abscesses, hematomas or cerebral edema. Vasodilation and venous outflow obstructions cause changes in cerebrovascular status due to hypoventilation, hypercapnia, improper position of the head, or maneuvers that increase intrathoracic pressure. CSF volumes may increase from decreased reabsorption from an obstruction, such as with hydrocephalus.

Monitoring of ICP can be done from several sites. The lumbar or cervical subarachnoid area is simple to access, but potential for herniation exists. The lateral cerebral ventricles [per ventriculostomy] is highly accurate and allows for withdrawal of CSF and measurement of compliance, but infection to this area is catastrophic. Subdural sites are most easily inserted but carry serious infection risks, and an epidural site has less potential for infection, but lacks accuracy.

The three types of ICP monitoring are epidural sensor monitoring through a burr hole, subarachnoid screw or bolt monitoring through a twist drill burr hole, and ventricular catheter monitoring. Insertion of these may be performed in surgery or in the intensive care setting, but requires sterile field maintenance.

ICP monitoring may be performed on patients with head trauma, ruptured aneurysms, Reye's syndrome, intracranial bleeds, hydrocephalus, or tumors. A ventriculostomy is a cannula placed in the lateral ventricle and connected with a transducer for measurement of pressures of CSF directly, for periodic drainage of CSF, and for withdrawal of fluid for analysis.

Cerebral perfusion pressure (CPP) is the difference between the mean arterial pressure (MAP) and the mean ICP, and indicates the pressure in the cerebral vascular system and approximates the cerebral blood flow. A CPP of 60 mmHg is the minimum value for perfusion to occur, with normal ranges from 80-100 mmHg.

Increases in ICP can be manifested by signs such as systolic blood pressure elevations, widening pulse pressure, bradycardia, headache, nausea with projectile vomiting, papilledema, changes in level of consciousness, pupillary changes, respiratory changes, and cerebral posturing.

MEDICAL CARE

Surgery: may be required for traumatic injuries and/or placement of ICP monitoring device

Arterial blood gases: may be used to identify acid-base imbalances, hypoxemia, and hypercapnia; frequently patients are hyperventilated to keep $PaCO_2$ between 25-28

Osmotics: mannitol used to create osmotic diuresis in an attempt to decrease ICP

Barbiturate therapy: pentothal or nembutal used to place patient in coma to produce burst-suppression on the EEG and to reduce metabolic activity

Paralyzing drug therapy: pancuronium may be used to decrease metabolic requirements but must be used in conjunction with sedatives since drug only paralyzes muscles and does not change level of awareness

Adrenocorticosteroids: decadron has less sodium-retaining properties and is used to assist with decreasing edema

CT scans: used to identify lesions, hemorrhage, ventricular size, structural shifting, ischemic event (may be several days prior to visibility on scan)

Laboratory: electrolytes drawn to evaluate imbalances that may contribute to ICP increases; toxicology screens to identify other drugs that may be responsible for changes in mentation and level of consciousness; serum levels of drugs to assess therapeutic response versus toxicity

NURSING CARE PLANS

Alteration in tissue perfusion: cerebral

Related to: cerebral edema, space-occupying lesions, hemorrhage, substance overdose, hypoxia, hypovolemia, trauma

Defining characteristics: increased ICP, changes in vital signs, changes in level of consciousness, memory deficit, restlessness, lethargy, coma, stupor, pupillary changes, headache, nausea/vomiting, purposeless movements, papilledema

Outcome Criteria

Patient will have stable vital signs and mentation with no signs or symptoms of increased ICP.

INTERVENTIONS	RATIONALES
Monitor for changes in level of consciousness or mentation, speech, or response to commands/questions.	Alterations in levels of consciousness are among the earliest signs of increasing ICP and can facilitate prompt intervention. Progressive deterioration may require emergent care.
Monitor vital signs at least every hour, and prn.	As ICP increases, blood pressure elevates, pulse pressure widens, bradycardia may occur changing to tachycardia as ICP progressively worsens. Tachypnea is seen as an early sign but slows with increasingly longer periods of apnea. Fever may indicate hypothalamic damage or infection which can increase metabolic demands and further increase ICP.

INTERVENTIONS	RATIONALES
Perform pupillary checks, noting equality, position, response to light, and nystagmus every 1-2 hours and prn.	Increased ICP or expansion of a clot can cause shifting of the brain against the oculomotor or optic nerve which causes pupillary changes. Early increased ICP may be signified by impairment of abduction of the eyes as a result of injury to the fifth cranial nerve. Absence of the doll's eyes reflex may indicate brain stem dysfunction and poor prognosis. Uncal herniation produces ipsilateral pupillary changes.
Monitor neurological status utilizing the Glasgow Coma Scale (GCS).	GCS facilitates identification of arousability and level and appropriateness of responses. Motor response to simple commands or purposeful movement with stimuli assist with identification of problem. Abnormal posturing, decerebrate and decorticate, may indicate diffuse cortical damage. Inability to move one side of the body may indicate damage to the opposite side's cerebral hemisphere.
Monitor EKG for changes in heart rate and rhythm, and treat as per hospital protocol.	Brain stem pressure or injury may result in rate changes, normally bradycardia, or cardiac dysrhythmias.
Observe for presence of blink, gag, cough, and Babinski reflexes.	Reflex changes may be indicative of injury at the mid brain or brain stem level. Lack of blink reflex indicates damage to the pons and medulla. Cough and gag reflexes that are absent may indicate damage at medulla and presence of Babinski reflex indicates pyramidal pathway injury.
Observe for nuchal rigidity, tremors, fasiculations, twitching, seizures, irritability, or restlessness.	May indicate meningeal irritation from a break in the dura or the development of an infection. Seizures may occur from increased ICP, hypoxia, or cerebral irritation.

INTERVENTIONS	RATIONALES
Elevate head of bed 30-45 degrees as warranted.	Decreases cerebral edema and congestion, thereby decreasing ICP.
Maintain head placement in neutral, or midline, position using rolled towels or sandbags as warranted.	Moving head from side to side compresses jugular veins and increases ICP.
Avoid excess stimuli in room; allow visitation when warranted.	All stimulation increases ICP and should be limited to necessary tasks only in the presence of intracranial hypertension. Family members may have calming effect on patient and may facilitate decreased ICP.
Avoid suctioning unless mandatory, and when necessary, limit active suctioning to 15 seconds or less.	Minimizes hypoxia and acid-base disturbances. Hyperoxygenation prior to, during, and after procedure may also minimize complications.
Provide continuous monitoring of oximetry.	Provides for prompt recognition of deterioration in patient's ability to maintain saturation which allows for prompt intervention.
Apply oxygen at ordered concentrations; prepare for mechanical ventilation as warranted.	Supplemental oxygen decreases hypoxemia which results in increased ICP. Mechanical ventilation may be required if space-occupying lesions shift and destroy respiratory center enervation.
Administer medications as ordered.	Diuretics and/or mannitol may be used to draw water from cerebral cells to decrease edema and ICP. Steroids may be used to decrease tissue edema and inflammation. Anticonvulsants may be used prophylactically and for the treatment of seizures. Sedatives or analgesics may be used to control restlessness or agitation.

Information, Instruction, Demonstration

INTERVENTIONS	RATIONALES
Observe continuous intracranial pressure monitoring for fluctuations that are sustained, and for the presence of A, B, and C waves.	Increases above 25 mmHg that are sustained for at least 5 minutes may indicate severe intracranial hypertension. A waves, or plateau waves, have elevations from 60-100 mmHg and then drop sharply, and often coincide with headaches or deterioration. Cellular hypoxia is most likely to occur during A waves, and sustained A waves indicate irreversible brain damage. B waves have elevations up to 50 mmHg and occur every 1.5-2 minutes in a sawtooth-type pattern. B waves can precede A waves and/or appear in runs, and occur with decreases in compensation. C waves are rapid, rhythmic, and may fluctuate with changes in respiration or blood pressure, and are not of clinical significance.
Measure/obtain the mean ICP every hour and prn; set alarms for sustained elevations above ordered limits.	Provides direct measurement of changes in ICP and cerebral perfusion status.
Calculate CPP and do not allow CPP to fall below 50 mmHg.	CPP = MAP - MICP; normal CPP is 80-100 mmHg, and levels below 50 mmHg decrease cerebral blood flow and perfusion, which frequently precipitates death.
Recalibrate ICP monitoring device to level of foramen of Munro (eye canthus level approximately) every 4 hours and prn suspicious readings or position changes.	Ensures accuracy of readings.
Assist with removal of specified amounts of CSF through ventriculostomy utilizing sterile technique.	May be required to decrease severe ICP and prevent herniation from structural shifting.

INTERVENTIONS	RATIONALES
If ICP is increasing, ensure that airway is patent, and prepare for placement on mechanical ventilation.	Hyperventilation results in respiratory alkalosis that causes cerebral vasoconstriction, decreases cerebral blood volume, and can decrease ICP. Levels of $PaCO_2$ are usually kept from 25-35 to decrease ICP, but if allowed to go below 25, may adversely affect ICP.
Prepare patient/family for use of barbiturate therapy to produce coma.	Used as a last ditch effort, pentobarbital or other drugs are given to produce complete unresponsiveness, to reduce metabolic activity, and decrease ICP.

Discharge or Maintenance Evaluation

- Patient will exhibit no complications due to ICP monitoring.

- Patient will have ICP stabilized and controlled.

- Patient will have appropriate actions taken to control increasing ICP.

Risk for infection
[See Head Injuries]

Related to: invasive monitoring, lack of skin integrity, increased metabolic state, intubation, compromised defense mechanisms

Defining characteristics: increased temperature, chills, elevated white blood cell count, differential shift to the left, drainage, presence of wounds, positive cultures

Endarterectomy

Carotid endarterectomy is the removal of a thrombus or plaque from the carotid artery to reduce the risk of stroke in patients who have had a transient ischemic attack (TIA). Circulation is augmented by increasing blood flow from the internal carotid artery. The surgery is not without risk of its own due to the potential for shearing off pieces of plaque or material resulting in a stroke.

Initially, the major postoperative problem may be controlling labile blood pressures that occur because of impairment in carotid sinus reflexes. These blood pressure variances also predispose the patient to a stroke.

Respiratory insufficiency may occur if the trachea is compressed or shifted by a growing hematoma at the wound site, or by lack of responses to hypoxia with impairment of carotid body function.

MEDICAL CARE

Surgery: performed as described above

Vasoactive drugs: may be required to control blood pressures

Laboratory: CBC used to identify potential bleeding problems, occult bleeding into neck; electrolytes used to identify imbalances

Arterial blood gases: used to identify hypoxemia and acid-base imbalances

NURSING CARE PLANS

Alteration in tissue perfusion: cerebral
[See CVA]

Related to: occlusion, hemorrhage, vasospasms, cerebral edema, interruption of blood flow, surgery

Defining characteristics: changes in vital signs, mental status changes, restlessness, anxiety, sensory deficits, confusion, decreased level of consciousness

Risk for decreased cardiac output
[See Spinal Cord Injuries]

Related to: vasospasm, surgery, stroke

Defining characteristics: hypotension, hypertension, heart rate changes, decreased cardiac output/index, changes in systemic and peripheral vascular resistance, mental status changes, hypoxia

Risk for injury

Related to: surgery, predisposing health factors, injury to cranial nerves

Defining characteristics: muscle weakness, nerve injury, airway obstruction, hypoxia, dysphagia, facial weakness, asymmetry of face, facial drooping, vocal cord paralysis

Outcome Criteria

Patient will exhibit no complications from surgery and will have all cranial nerve function maintained.

INTERVENTIONS	RATIONALES
Observe for deviation of tongue toward side of operation, or weakness of tongue muscles.	May indicate hypoglossal nerve damage.
Observe for dysphagia, dysphasia, or impairment of upper airway.	May indicate bilateral hypoglossal palsy.
Observe for facial asymmetry, drooping at corner of mouth, and inability to manage salivary secretions.	May indicate facial nerve damage.
Monitor for changes in voice quality and sound.	May indicate vocal cord paralysis, injury to the vagus nerve, or recurrent laryngeal nerve.

Discharge or Maintenance Evaluation

- Patient will have facial symmetry and normal voice modulation.

- Patient will exhibit no signs/symptoms of cranial nerve injury.

- Patient will be free of any airway compromise and have stable vital signs.

Alteration in skin integrity
[See Cardiac Surgery]

Related to: surgical wounds, invasive lines, immobility

Defining characteristics: presence of wounds, drainage, redness, swelling, abrasions, pressure, lacerations, bruises, open skin

GASTROINTESTINAL/HEPATIC SYSTEM

Gastrointestinal Bleeding

Esophageal Varices

Hepatitis

Pancreatitis

Acute Abdomen/Abdominal Trauma

Liver Failure

Gastrointestinal Bleeding

Gastrointestinal bleeding may be massive and acute or occult and chronic in nature. GI bleeding results when irritation of the mucosal lining results in erosion through to the submucosal layer. Upper GI hemorrhage is considered to be a bleed from any site proximally to the cecum, and all ulcerative bleeding is arterial with the exception of a tear that cuts across all vessels, malignant tumors, and in patients with esophagitis.

When erosion into an artery occurs, it usually produces two bleeding sites because of arterio-arterial anastomoses. When the bleeding occurs at the ulcer base artery, it may be a life-threatening emergency.

Bleeding may occur from the lower gastrointestinal tract as well. Causes of lower GI bleeding include hemorrhoids, diverticulosis, inflammatory bowel disease, rectal perforation, or intussusception.

Acute upper GI bleeding may result from many causes, such as gastritis, peptic ulcer, stress, drugs, hormones, trauma, head injuries, burns, and esophageal varices.

Differential diagnosis between gastric and duodenal ulcers must be obtained. Duodenal ulcers usually account for approximately 80% of all ulcers noted and rarely become cancerous. Gastric ulcers, on the other hand, may become cancerous and are more likely to bleed.

Initial presenting symptoms of a GI bleed are either hematemesis, melena, or hematochezia. An acute bleed will have more than 60 cc/day of black tarry stool and usually greater than 500 cc, whereas occult bleeding is normally 15-30 cc/day. Stools can be positive for occult blood up to 12 days after an acute bleed. Of all GI hemorrhages, 80% usually stop spontaneously.

The goal of treatment is initially prevention and treatment of shock, with fluid volume replacement. Maintenance of circulating blood volume is imperative to prevent myocardial infarction, sepsis, and death. Endoscopic examination is the primary diagnostic procedure utilized. Once the lesion has been identified, treatment with Pitressin infusion may be used to control bleeding.

MEDICAL CARE

Laboratory: CBC to identify changes in blood volume and concentration, but may be normal during rapid loss because of the lapsed time required for equilibration of intravascular with extravascular spaces; MCV is useful to identify prolonged chronic loss with iron deficiency; B_{12} and folic acid levels used to identify anemia type; reticulocyte count may identify new RBC formation which occurs with an old bleed; platelet count, PT, PTT, and bleeding times to evaluate clotting status and platelet dysfunction; BUN and creatinine to evaluate effect on renal status; electrolytes to evaluate imbalances and treatment; ammonia levels may be used to identify liver dysfunction; gastric analysis to determine presence of blood and assess secretory activity of gastric mucosa; amylase elevated if duodenal ulcer has posterior penetration; pepsinogen level to help identify type of bleeding, with elevation seen in duodenal ulcer, and decreased levels seen in gastritis; stool specimens for guaiac

Arterial blood gases: may be used to show acid-base imbalances, compensation for decreased blood flow; initially respiratory alkalosis changing to metabolic acidosis as metabolic wastes accumulate

Esophagogastroduodenoscopy (EGD): primary diagnostic tool utilized for upper GI bleeding to visually identify lesion; can be performed as soon as lavage controls bleeding

Angiography: used when bleeding cannot be cleared for endoscopy; can identify bleeding site and allow for injection of vasopressin for active mucosal bleeding

Radiography: chest x-rays may be done to evaluate for free air/perforation; upper GI series may be done after endoscopy, but is never done before since the contrast media will adhere to mucosa and prevent further examination; may be done to identify other diagnosis; barium enema may be done once lower GI bleeding is stopped; radionuclide scanning, such as Red Cell Tags, identify source of bleeding, but may take an extended time for results to show

Electrocardiogram: used to identify changes in heart rate and rhythm and identify conduction problems or dysrhythmias that may occur with fluid shifting or electrolyte imbalances

Blood products: blood, plasma, and platelets may be required for replacement based on severity of bleed

Nasogastric tubes: large bore NG tube or Ewald tube is usually inserted to allow for iced/saline lavage, confirmation of bleeding, and for decompression of stomach

Levophed: may be used in solution with saline for lavage when plain saline is not effective in stopping bleeding due to its vasoconstrictor effects

Vasopressin: may be used for direct infusion into the gastric artery to control bleeding, or via intravenous route for specified length of time

Antacids: used to alter pH so that platelets can aggregate and stop bleeding, and to prevent digestion of raw mucosal surfaces

Histamine antagonists: used to inhibit gastric acid secretion; commonly used are cimetidine, ranitidine, pepcid, and axid

Sucralfate: used to help heal ulcer by forming protective barrier at site

Surgery: required in less than 10% of patients; may be necessary for control of hemorrhage

NURSING CARE PLANS

Fluid volume deficit

Related to: gastrointestinal bleeding

Defining characteristics: hypotension, tachycardia, decreased skin turgor, weakness, decreased urinary output, pallor, diaphoresis, decreased capillary refill, mental changes, restlessness, decreased filling pressures

Outcome Criteria

Patient will have no further bleeding and vital signs will be stable.

INTERVENTIONS	RATIONALES
Monitor vital signs, including orthostatic changes when feasible.	Patients with major GI blood losses will present with supine hypotension and resting tachycardia greater than 110/min, orthostatic DBP decreases of at least 10 mmHg, and orthostatic pulse increases of at least 15/min. Changes in vital signs may help approximate amount of blood loss and reflect decreasing circulating blood volume.
Monitor hemodynamic parameters when possible.	Facilitates early identification of fluid shifts. CVP values between 4-18 cm H_2O are considered adequate circulating volume.
Insert nasogastric tube for acute bleeding episodes, and monitor drainage for changes in bleeding character.	Facilitates removal of gastric contents, blood, and clots, relieves gastric distention, decreases nausea and vomiting, and provides for lavaging of stomach. Blood that is left in stomach can be metabolized into ammonia and can result in neurologic encephalopathy.

INTERVENTIONS	RATIONALES
Actively lavage stomach via NG tube per hospital protocol with cold or room temperature saline until return is light pink or clear.	Saline solution is utilized to reduce wash-out of electrolytes that may occur with use of water. Flushing facilitates removal of clots to assist with visualization of bleeding site, and may assist with control of bleeding through vasoconstrictive effect. The current consensus of opinion is that differences between using cold versus room temperature solutions is negligible, and in fact, iced solution may actually inhibit platelet function by lowering core body temperature.
Notify physician if bleeding clears and then becomes bright red again.	May indicate further bleeding or renewed bleeding.
Monitor intake and output, including amounts of lavage solution, bloody aspirate, blood products, and vomitus.	Helps facilitate estimation of fluid replacement required. Lavage amounts facilitate estimation of the magnitude of bleeding based on the volume of solution needed to clear the gastric return, and how long lavage is required before the aspirate clears.
Administer IV fluids through large bore catheters as ordered. Many facilities recommend at least two lines for active bleeding.	Facilitates rapid replacement of circulating volume prior to availability of blood products. Solutions of choice are normal saline or Lactated Ringer's, and should be run wide open until blood pressure is stabilized, and titrated to match volume requirements after that.
Administer blood transfusions, fresh frozen plasma, platelets, or whole blood as ordered.	Fresh whole blood may be ordered when bleeding is acute and patient is in shock so as to ensure that clotting factors are not deficient. Packed red blood cells are utilized most often for replacement, especially when fluid shifting may create overload. Frequently, fresh frozen plasma (FFP) will be concurrently administered to replace clotting factors and facilitate cessation of an acute bleed. For each unit of blood that is trans-

INTERVENTIONS	RATIONALES
	fused, a 3 point increase in the hematocrit may be noted. If this elevation is not noted, continued bleeding should be suspected.
Administer albumin as ordered.	May be used for volume expansion until blood products are available.
Administer vasopressin as ordered.	Intra-arterial infusion may be required for severe active bleeding and patient must be monitored closely for development of complications from the infusion. Rates are usually 0.1-0.5 Units/min into the artery supplying blood or peripherally at 0.3-1.5 Units/min.
Administer histamine blockers and/or omeprazole as ordered.	Histamine blockers decrease acid production, increase pH, and decrease gastric mucosal irritation. Omeprazole can completely inhibit acid secretion.
Administer sucralfate as ordered.	Decreases gastric acid secretion and provides a protective layer over the ulcer site. May decrease or inhibit absorption of other medications.
Administer antacids as ordered.	Facilitates maintenance of pH level to decrease chance of rebleeding.
Monitor labwork for changes and/or trends.	Hemoglobin and hematocrit help to identify blood replacement needs, but may not initially change as a result of loss of plasma and RBCs. BUN levels greater than 40 in the presence of normal creatinine may signify major bleeding, and BUN should normalize within 12 hours after bleeding has ceased.

Information, Instruction, Demonstration

INTERVENTIONS	RATIONALES
Administer antibiotics when ordered.	May be indicated when infection is thought to be the cause of the gastritis or ulcer.
Assist with and prepare patient for EGD/sclerotherapy.	EGD provides direct visualization of an upper GI bleeding site, and a sclerosing substance may be injected at site to stop bleeding or prevent a recurrence.
Prepare patient for surgery.	May be required to control gastric hemorrhage. Vagotomy, pyloroplasty, oversewing of the ulcer, and total or subtotal gastrectomy may be procedure of choice based on severity of bleeding.

Discharge or Maintenance Evaluation

• Patient will have stable fluid balance with normal vital signs and hemodynamic parameters.

• Patient will have adequate urine output.

• Patient will have no complications from fluid or blood replacement therapy.

• Patient will have labwork within normal limits.

• Patient will have no active bleeding or occult blood in stools.

Altered nutrition: less than body requirements
[See DKA]

Related to: nausea, vomiting, nasogastric tube

Defining characteristics: inability to ingest adequate amounts of food, weakness, fatigue, weight loss

Alteration in comfort
[See MI]

Related to: muscle spasms, ulceration, gastric mucosal irritation, presence of invasive lines

Defining characteristics: verbalization of pain, facial grimacing, changes in vital signs, abdominal guarding

Anxiety
[See MI]

Related to: change in environment, change in health status, fear of the unknown, life-threatening crisis

Defining characteristics: tension, irritability, restlessness, anxiousness, fearfulness, tremors, tachycardia, tachypnea, diaphoresis

Risk for altered tissue perfusion: gastrointestinal, cerebral, cardiopulmonary, renal, peripheral

Related to: hypovolemia, hypoxia, vasoconstrictive therapy

Defining characteristics: decreased blood pressure, tachycardia, decreased peripheral pulses, decreased hemodynamic pressures, abnormal ABGs, abdominal pain, decreased urine output, confusion, mental status changes, dyspnea, headache

Outcome Criteria

Patient will have adequate tissue perfusion to all body systems.

INTERVENTIONS	RATIONALES
Perform neurological checks every 4 hours and prn. Notify physician of changes in mentation or level of consciousness.	Decreases in blood pressure may result in decreased cerebral perfusion that may cause confusion. Increases in ammonia levels from

INTERVENTIONS	RATIONALES
	residual blood may result in cerebral encephalopathy.
Monitor for complaints of increasing severity of abdominal pain, as well as pain radiating to shoulders.	May indicate ischemia and necrosis from vasoconstrictive medication which may result when catheter is displaced, or may indicate peritonitis or further bleeding.
Monitor EKG for changes and treat according to hospital protocols.	Decreased blood pressure, electrolyte imbalances, hypoxemia, or response to cold injectate solution may cause cardiac dysrhythmias or changes with perfusion loss.
Palpate peripheral pulses for presence and character of pulses. Monitor for changes in color and temperature of extremities.	Decreased circulating blood volume may result in peripheral vasoconstriction and shunting to core.
Monitor urine output for decreases or changes in color or specific gravity. Notify physician for abnormalities.	Renal perfusion may be affected by hypovolemia.
Monitor for complaints of chest pain.	Myocardial ischemia and infarction may result if hypovolemic state decreases perfusion to crisis state.
Provide continuous pulse oximetry and notify physician for level below 90%.	Facilitates early identification of hypoxia and allows for timely intervention.

Discharge or Maintenance Evaluation

- Patient will have stable vital signs and hemodynamic parameters.

- Patient will have adequate and stable intake and output.

- Patient will have ABGs within normal limits, with no respiratory insufficiency or distress noted.

- Patient will have equally palpable pulses with equal color and temperature bilaterally to extremities.

Knowledge deficit
[See MI]

Related to: lack of information, lack of understanding of medical condition, lack of recall

Defining characteristics: verbalized questions regarding disease, care or instructions, inadequate follow-up on instructions given, misconceptions, development of preventable complications

GASTROINTESTINAL BLEEDING

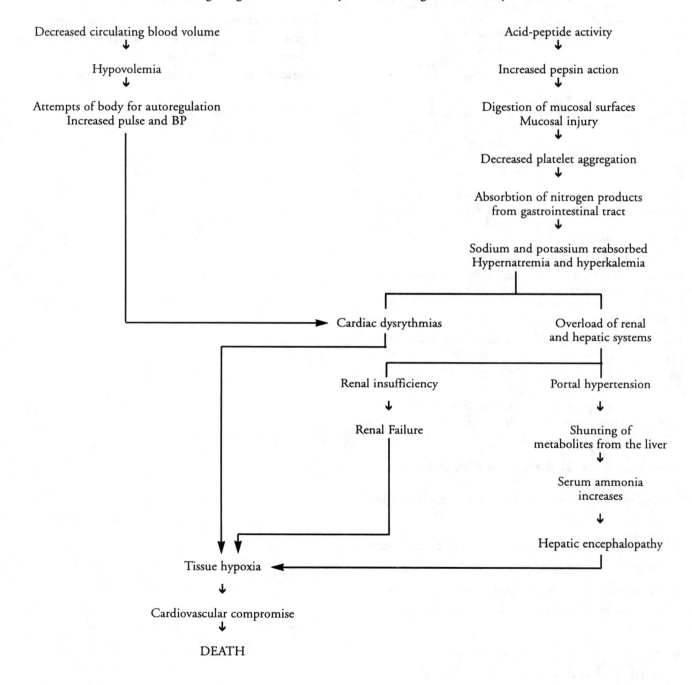

ACUTE BLOOD LOSS
(variceal bleeding, coagulation abnormality, cancer, ulcer, gastritis, Mallory-Weiss tears)

Decreased circulating blood volume
↓
Hypovolemia
↓
Attempts of body for autoregulation
Increased pulse and BP

Acid-peptide activity
↓
Increased pepsin action
↓
Digestion of mucosal surfaces
Mucosal injury
↓
Decreased platelet aggregation
↓
Absorbtion of nitrogen products
from gastrointestinal tract
↓
Sodium and potassium reabsorbed
Hypernatremia and hyperkalemia

Cardiac dysrythmias

Overload of renal
and hepatic systems

Renal insufficiency
↓
Renal Failure

Portal hypertension
↓
Shunting of
metabolites from the liver
↓
Serum ammonia
increases
↓
Hepatic encephalopathy

Tissue hypoxia
↓
Cardiovascular compromise
↓
DEATH

Esophageal Varices

Esophageal varices are twisting, dilated veins that are found in the gastrointestinal tract, but most frequently develop in the submucosal areas of the lower esophagus. Most esophageal varices occur as a result from liver disease and portal hypertension and the development of collateral esophageal veins. When these veins become eroded, the ensuing rupture causes extensive vigorous bleeding that is difficult to control.

Normally, the patient does not exhibit symptoms until coughing, vomiting, alcohol, or gastritis causes the varices to bleed. Mortality rates are high (above 60%) due to other complications of liver dysfunction, sepsis, or renal failure. Blood loss may be sudden, massive, and life-threatening, with shock and hypovolemia occurring.

Nearly all patients with esophageal varices have at least one of the precipitating factors of cirrhosis, portal vein thrombosis, hepatic fibrosis, schistosomiasis, hepatic venous outflow obstruction, or splenic vein or superior vena caval abnormalities.

The initial goal of treatment is to replace blood loss and prevent shock from hypovolemia. Balloon tamponade, utilizing the Sengstaken-Blakemore or Minnesota tube, may be required to produce hemostasis.

Complications that occur in conjunction with bleeding may become irreversible and lethal, such as hepatic coma, renal failure, myocardial infarction, or congestive heart failure.

MEDICAL CARE

Laboratory: hemoglobin and hematocrit decreased, BUN increased, liver function tests may be abnormal due to liver involvement and disease, sodium may be elevated, clotting studies may be abnormal due to liver involvement, ammonia may be elevated, stools for guaiac, bilirubin may be elevated if cirrhosis is a factor

Esophagogastroduodenoscopy (EGD): used to identify and sometimes treat variceal bleeding with sclerotherapy

Radiography: arteriogram used to identify tortuous portovenous vessels; chest x-ray used to identify other complicating problems with respiratory system

Arterial blood gases: may be used to identify acid-base imbalances; may show metabolic acidosis with bleeding

Nasogastric tube: used to keep stomach clear of blood and for lavage, but must be inserted cautiously so as to refrain from increasing bleeding

Balloon tamponade: Sengstaken-Blakemore (SB) or Minnesota tube is a multi-lumen tube that exerts pressure on part of the stomach and against bleeding varices to help control bleeding, and allows for removal of stomach contents; caution must be exercised since placement of this tube can create complications such as airway occlusion or esophageal rupture

Vasopressin: may be used as infusion through superior mesenteric artery or a peripheral vein to decrease splanchnic blood flow and promote hemostasis; may induce water intoxication or accentuate cardiac disease by increasing systemic vascular resistance

Nitroglycerin: may be used in conjunction with vasopressin to balance systemic vasoconstriction

Vitamin K: may be used to counteract increased prothrombin time

Cathartics: magnesium citrate or sorbitol may be used to decrease risk of ammonia-induced neuroencephalopathy

Surgery: may require distal splenorenal shunt, mesocaval and portocaval anastomoses, or devascularization of the varices all in the effort to lower pressure in the portal system

NURSING CARE PLANS

[Care plans in GI bleeding section also apply to this diagnosis]

Risk for alteration in tissue perfusion: cerebral, cardiopulmonary, gastrointestinal, renal, and peripheral
[See Infective Endocarditis]

Related to: variceal bleeding

Defining characteristics: decreased peripheral pulses, hypotension, tachycardia initially, bradycardia, cold and clammy skin, diaphoresis, mental status changes, lethargy, pallor, abnormal ABGs, decreased oxygen saturation, decreased urine output

Risk for decreased cardiac output
[See Cardiogenic Shock]

Related to: variceal bleeding, hemorrhage, exsanguination

Defining characteristics: decreased peripheral pulses, hypotension, tachycardia, cold and clammy skin, decreased urinary output, mental status changes, pallor

Risk for ineffective individual coping
[See Mechanical Ventilation]

Related to: bleeding disorder, alcohol abuse, hepatic disease

Defining characteristics: history of excessive alcohol usage, anxiety, fear, hostility, manipulative behavior, guilt, rationalization, blaming behavior

Risk for injury

Related to: utilization of balloon tamponade to control esophageal bleeding

Defining characteristics: increased bleeding, exsanguination, tube migration, air leakage, esophageal necrosis, encephalopathy, airway occlusion, asphyxia

Outcome Criteria

Patient will be free of complications and injury to self.

INTERVENTIONS	RATIONALES
Examine Sengstaken-Blakemore (or other type tube) balloons by testing inflation of balloons with air while tube is underwater.	Facilitates easier detection of leaks by escaping air bubbling, and ensures balloons are patent prior to insertion of tube into patient.
Refrigerate tube prior to insertion, and assist physician with insertion of tube into patient's nose/mouth by encouraging swallowing small sips of water.	Chilling firms the tube to facilitate easier placement.
Ensure that tube is patent in stomach by auscultating stomach for injected air bolus.	Proper positioning is crucial to ensure that the gastric tube is not inflated in the esophagus.
Obtain KUB x-ray after placement and securing of tube.	Verifies correct anatomical placement.
When placement is verified, inflate the gastric balloon with air and gently pull the tube back against the gastroesophageal junction. Secure tube, marking location at the nares, and clamp the gastric balloon.	Applies pressure against the cardia to attempt to control bleeding. Marking the tube facilitates prompt detection of accidental migration.
Balloon tubes should be adequately secured with some device [frequently used is a football helmet with face guard] with slight traction to the balloon tube.	Facilitates stable position of tube and prevents migration due to peristalsis or coughing, while exerting appropriate pull/pressure on anatomical sites.

INTERVENTIONS	RATIONALES
Attach a y-connector to the esophageal balloon opening, with a syringe on one side, and a manometer to the other. Fill balloon with air until manometer reading is between 25-35 mmHg and clamp balloon.	Maintains sufficient pressure to tamponade bleeding with pressure lower than level that may result in esophageal ischemia and necrosis.
Connect gastric port to intermittent suction and irrigate every hour.	Facilitates removal of old blood from stomach, allows observation of changes in bleeding, and relieves gastric distention.
Insert nasogastric tube above the level of the esophageal balloon and connect to intermittent suction. If tamponade tube has an esophageal suction port, attach it to intermittent suction.	Facilitates removal of salivary secretions and monitors for bleeding above the esophageal balloon, and reduces aspiration risk.
Clearly identify and label each port, checking connections frequently, and have scissors and resuscitative equipment at bedside.	Proper identification may prevent accidental deflation or improper irrigation. If the esophageal balloon migrates to the hypopharynx, the esophageal balloon must be cut immediately and removed to prevent airway obstruction.
Monitor for complaints of chest pain.	May indicate complication or esophageal rupture.
Monitor respiratory status for any changes, decrease in oxygen saturations, or changes in mental status.	May result from tube migration and asphyxia.
Keep head of bed elevated at least 30 degrees at all times.	Prevents regurgitation and decreases nausea.
Compare character and amounts of drainage coming from each lumen.	Facilitates identification of cessation of bleeding, as well as potentially identifying level of bleeding site.
Deflate esophageal balloon for 30 minutes every 12 hours, or as indicated per hospital protocol.	Decreases risk for esophageal mucosal ischemia and damage.

Information, Instruction, Demonstration

INTERVENTIONS	RATIONALES
Instruct patient/family regarding need for balloon tamponade, procedure of insertion, what to expect, etc.	Promotes knowledge and facilitates compliance. Decreases fear of the unknown.
Observation of patient should be constant.	Deterioration in patient's status can occur rapidly and continuous observation facilitates prompt intervention to prevent injury.

Discharge or Maintenance Evaluation

- Patient will have bleeding from varices controlled with no injury or complication from treatment modalities.

- Patient will be able to comply with treatment.

- Patient will have stable vital signs and oxygenation.

ESOPHAGEAL VARICES

Obstruction in portal system
↓
Increased pressure in portal vein
↓
Normal circulation disrupted
↓
Collateral channels form
Blood bypasses liver
↓
Portal hypertension increases
↓
Esophageal veins become varicosed and torturous
↓
Portal hypertension increases
Contributing factors cause inflammation/irritation
↓
Esophageal varicosities rupture
↓
Massive hemorrhage
↓
Hypovolemic shock
↓
DEATH

Hepatitis

Acute hepatitis is an infection of the liver that usually is viral in origin but may be induced by drugs or toxins. There are currently five types of hepatitis, denoted HAV, HBV, NANB or hepatitis C, HDV, and HEV, with HAV being the most common type. Hepatitis B, or HBV, is more severe and because it can be acquired from exposure to individuals who are asymptomatic, the potential for transmission is increased many-fold.

Hepatitis A, or HAV, is transmitted via fecal-oral route, with poor sanitation practices, with contamination of food, water, milk, and shellfish, or oral-anal sexual practices. HAV patients may exhibit no acute symptoms or have symptoms that are related to other causes.

Hepatitis B, or HBV, is transmitted via blood and blood products, breaks in the skin or mucous membranes, or from an asymptomatic carrier with Hepatitis B surface antigen (HBsAg).

Hepatitis C, or Non-A, Non-B hepatitis, is transmitted via intravenous drug use, sexual contact, blood or blood products, and from asymptomatic carriers.

Hepatitis D, or HDV, is transmitted through the same routes as HBV but must have hepatitis B surface antigen to replicate.

Hepatitis E, or HEV, is seen in developing countries and not encountered in the United States. It is transmitted through food or water contamination.

Once the disease has been contracted, treatment is symptomatic. Prophylactic therapy may assist in prevention of hepatitis from developing after being exposed to the virus. Immune globulin (IG) is generally given to provide temporary passive immunity. Hepatitis B vaccine provides active immunity and offers protection to people who are at high risk.

MEDICAL CARE

Laboratory: CBC shows decreased RBCs as a result of decreased lifespan from enzyme alterations or from hemorrhage; white blood cell count usually shows leukocytosis, atypical lymphocytes, and plasma cells; liver function studies are abnormal, up to 10 times normal values in some cases, albumin decreased, blood glucose may be decreased or elevated transiently due to liver dysfunction; Anti-HAV IgM presence shows either current infection or after 6 weeks may indicate immunity; hepatitis B surface antigen and hepatitis Be antigen show presence of HBV; Anti-HBc in serum indicates carrier status; Anti-HBsAg indicates HBV immunity; antidelta antibodies present without HBsAg indicates HDV; urine bilirubin elevated; prothrombin time may be elevated with liver dysfunction

Liver biopsy: may be used to delineate type of hepatitis and degree of liver necrosis

Liver scans: may be performed to identify level of parenchymal damage

NURSING CARE PLANS

Activity intolerance

Related to: infective process, decreased endurance

Defining characteristics: easy fatiguability, lethargy, malaise, decreased muscle strength, reluctance to perform activity

Outcome Criteria

Patient will achieve and maintain ability to perform normal activities without intolerance and fatigue.

INTERVENTIONS	RATIONALES
Maintain bed rest and quiet environment, allowing rest periods in between activities.	Decreases energy expenditure that is needed for healing. Activity can decrease hepatic blood flow and prevent circulation and healing to liver cells.
Reposition every 2 hours and provide good skin care.	Decreases potential for skin breakdown.
Increase activities as patient is able to tolerate.	Assists with return to optimal activity levels while enabling patient to have some measure of control over the situation.
Monitor labwork for liver function studies.	May assist with identification of appropriate levels of activity.
Administer medications as warranted.	Sedatives and antianxiety drugs may be required to effect needed rest. Caution should be taken to ensure drugs used are not hepatotoxic.

Information, Instruction, Demonstration

INTERVENTIONS	RATIONALES
Administer antidotes/therapeutic treatment modalities to remove causative agent with toxic hepatitis.	Removal of substance may restrict amounts of tissue damage.
Instruct patient/family on disease process and need for extended rest.	Promotes knowledge and facilitates compliance with treatment.

Discharge or Maintenance Evaluation

• Patient will be able to verbalize understanding of disease process and treatment program.

• Patient will be able to perform usual activities without fatigue.

• Patient will be able to gradually increase level of activities performed.

Social isolation
[See Transplants]

Related to: changes in health status, changes in physical status, imposed physical isolation, inadequate support system

Defining characteristics: feelings of loneliness, feelings of rejection, absence of family members/friends, sad, dull affect, inappropriate behaviors

Alteration in nutrition: less than body requirements
[See Liver Failure]

Related to: metabolism changes, anorexia

Defining characteristics: nausea, vomiting, anorexia, abdominal pressure, malabsorption of fats, altered metabolism of protein, carbohydrates, and fat, weight loss, fatigue, edema

Risk for infection
[See Transplants]

Related to: leukopenia, immunosuppression, malnutrition, exposure to causative organisms

Defining characteristics: increased white blood cells, differential with a shift to the left, fever, chills, hypotension, tachycardia, positive cultures

Risk for impaired skin integrity
[See Liver Failure]

Related to: bile salt accumulations on skin

Defining characteristics: jaundice, pruritus, itching, scratching

Knowledge deficit

Related to: lack of information, lack of recall, unfamiliarity of resources, misinterpretation of information received

Defining characteristics: questions, requests for information, statements of misperceptions, development of preventable complications

Outcome Criteria

Patient will be able to verbalize understanding of disease, treatment, and causative behaviors.

INTERVENTIONS	RATIONALES
Discuss patient's perceptions of disease process.	Identifies knowledge base and misconceptions to facilitate appropriate teaching plan.
Instruct on disease process, prevention and transmission of disease, and isolation requirements.	Types of isolation will vary according to type of hepatitis and personal situation. Family members may require treatment depending on type of hepatitis.
Instruct in appropriate home sanitation.	Dirty environment and poor sanitation methods may be responsible for transmission of the disease.
Instruct on activity limitations.	Complete resumption of normal activity may not take place until liver returns to its normal size and patient begins to feel better and this may take up to several months.
Instruct on all medications, side effects, effects, contraindications, and dangers of administration of over-the-counter drugs without physician approval.	Promotes knowledge and facilitates compliance. Some medications are hepatotoxic or are metabolized by the liver, increasing its workload.
Instruct to refrain from blood donation.	Most states do not allow anyone who has a history of any type of hepatitis to donate blood or blood products to prevent possible spread of the infection.

INTERVENTIONS	RATIONALES
Instruct on avoidance of recreational drugs or alcohol.	May jeopardize recovery from infection and increases liver dysfunction.
Consult with counselors, ministers, drug or alcohol treatment facilities as warranted.	May be required for assistance with substance withdrawal and for long-term support once discharged.

Discharge or Maintenance Evaluation

- Patient will be able to accurately verbalize understanding of all instructions given.

- Patient/family will be able to modify environment to control spread of disease.

- Patient will be able to effectively access community resources for treatment programs and discharge follow-up care.

- Patient will be able to effectively manage medical regimen with follow-up from physician.

HEPATITIS

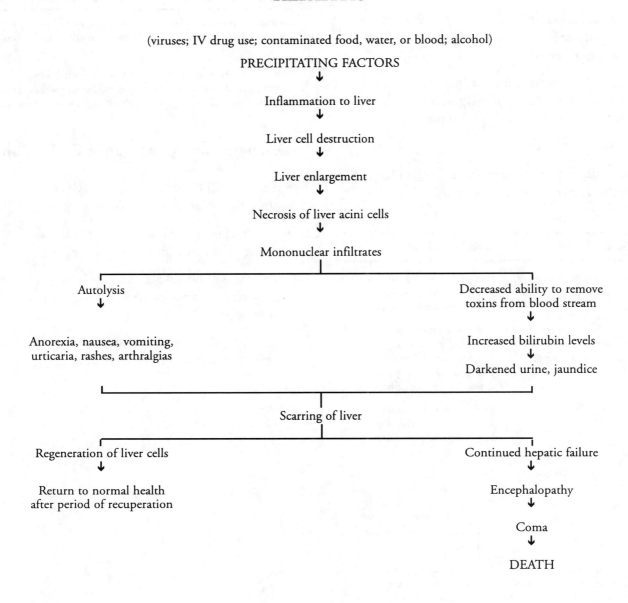

(viruses; IV drug use; contaminated food, water, or blood; alcohol)

PRECIPITATING FACTORS

↓

Inflammation to liver

↓

Liver cell destruction

↓

Liver enlargement

↓

Necrosis of liver acini cells

↓

Mononuclear infiltrates

Autolysis

↓

Anorexia, nausea, vomiting,
urticaria, rashes, arthralgias

Decreased ability to remove
toxins from blood stream

↓

Increased bilirubin levels

↓

Darkened urine, jaundice

Scarring of liver

Regeneration of liver cells

↓

Return to normal health
after period of recuperation

Continued hepatic failure

↓

Encephalopathy

↓

Coma

↓

DEATH

Pancreatitis

Acute pancreatitis is a life-threatening inflammatory response to an injury, in which pancreatic enzymes are abnormally activated and these enzymes destroy tissues in and surrounding the pancreas by autodigestion. Precipitating factors for the abnormal activation may be caused by effects of ethanol and its metabolite, acetaldehyde, diseases of the biliary tract, obstruction of the common bile duct, bile reflux into the pancreatic duct, ischemia, trauma, infections, surgical or invasive procedures, neoplasms, metabolic aberrations, use of oral contraceptives, corticosteroids, thiazide diuretics, or antihypertensives, or stimulation of vasoactive substances. Obstruction may result in widespread edema to the pancreas, which increases pressure in the pancreatic system. This increase in pressure results in the rupture of the ducts which allows the enzymes to spill into the cells, and begin the autodigestion process.

Trypsin activates the pancreatic enzymes, phospholipase A, elastase, and kallikrein. Trypsin may cause edema, necrosis, and hemorrhage in the pancreas. Elastase may attack the walls of smaller blood vessels and facilitate hemorrhage. Phospholipase A allows damage to the acinar cell membrane to occur, and may alter coagulation. Vasomotor changes and increases in vascular permeability may be caused by kallikrein, and this may also be the cause of the pain experienced with pancreatitis. If the disease is allowed to progress, the inflammation leads to massive hemorrhage, destruction of the pancreas, diabetes mellitus, acidosis, shock, coma, and death.

One of the predominant symptoms of this disease is the unrelenting abdominal pain located in the epigastric and/or periumbilical areas that may radiate to the chest and back. Nausea, continuous vomiting, low-grade fever, anorexia, diarrhea, weight loss, jaundice, diaphoresis, dehydration, and poorly defined abdominal mass may also be encountered.

Pseudocysts and abscesses in and around the pancreas may occur as a result of localized necrosis, and may exert pressure on the stomach or colon. They may develop slowly and may result in fistula formation.

The goal of therapy is to maintain adequate circulatory fluid volume with electrolyte replacement, pain relief, treatment of infection and treatment of hyperglycemia.

MEDICAL CARE

Laboratory: serum amylase is elevated up to 40 times the normal limit in the early stages and then decreases over 2-3 days; urine amylase elevated and lasts longer than serum amylase; elevated glucose, bilirubin, alkaline phosphatase, lactic dehydrogenase, aspartate transferase, potassium, triglycerides, cholesterol, and lipase; decreased albumin, calcium, sodium, and magnesium; white blood cell counts from 8,000-20,000 with increased polymorphonuclear cells; hematocrit may exceed 50%; prothrombin time may be increased; fat content in the stool increased; amylase-creatinine clearance ratio may indicate pancreatic disease; renal profiles used to evaluate renal function and hypovolemia

CT scans: used to identify size, shape, density, masses, or infiltrates in the pancreas

Ultrasonography: used to identify neoplasms, edema, inflammation, cysts, abscesses, or infiltrates in the pancreas, but cannot confirm the diagnosis of pancreatitis

Angiography: helps to visualize early pancreatic tumors or problems with vasculature

Endoscopic retrograde cholangiopancreatography (ERCP): used to directly visualize the pancreatic duct system by use of endoscopy and radiography; used to identify cysts, calculi, stenosis, pancreatic and biliary duct disease when other diagnostic tools are not conclusive

Surgery: may be necessary to drain abscesses or pseudocysts, or to anastomose the pseudocysts to an adjacent structure to provide internal drainage; chronic pancreatitis may require a pancreaticojejunostomy to relieve obstruction of the duct to relieve pain; experimental surgery for transplantation of the pancreas or islet cells may be performed

NURSING CARE PLANS

Alteration in comfort
[See MI]

Related to: pancreatic obstruction, autodigestion of pancreas, leakage of pancreatic enzymes, inflammation

Defining characteristics: unrelenting epigastric pain, patient curled up with both arms over abdomen, nausea, vomiting, tenderness, facial grimacing, groaning

INTERVENTIONS	RATIONALES
Administer Demerol IV as warranted/ordered.	Demerol is the drug of choice for pancreatitis. DO NOT GIVE Morphine because most opiate-type narcotics cause spasms of the Sphincter of Oddi, increasing patient's pain.

Alteration in nutrition: less than body requirements
[See DKA]

Related to: nausea, vomiting, anorexia, digestive enzyme leakage, increased metabolic needs, sepsis

Defining characteristics: increases in nausea and vomiting, retching, absent bowel sounds, decreased bowel sounds, anorexia, increased metabolism, lack of adequate food ingested

Fluid volume deficit
[See DKA]

Related to: nausea, vomiting, fever, diaphoresis, nasogastric drainage, fluid shifting, diarrhea

Defining characteristics: nausea, vomiting, ascites, nasogastric suctioning, hypotension, tachycardia, decreased urinary output

Risk for impaired gas exchange
[See Mechanical Ventilation]

Related to: complications from disease

Defining characteristics: altered arterial blood gases, dyspnea, use of accessory muscles, tachypnea, bradypnea, cough, sputum

Potential for injury

Related to: sepsis, pseudocysts, fistula formation, abscess formation, complications from disease

Defining characteristics: fever, abdominal pain, drainage, increased white blood cell count, shift to the left, systemic infection symptoms, DIC, electrolyte imbalances

Outcome Criteria

Patient will be afebrile and have no complications from disease.

INTERVENTIONS	RATIONALES
Monitor vital signs at least every 2 hours, and note changes.	Allows for prompt identification of early signs of infection to facilitate timely treatment. Third spacing, bleeding, and secretion of vasodilating substances may result in hypotension.

INTERVENTIONS	RATIONALES
Monitor hemodynamic pressures if possible.	Allows for actual measurement of cardiac output and other parameters to identify fluid shifts and hemodynamic alterations which may precede systemic complications.
Monitor EKG for cardiac rhythm, rate, and changes, and treat dysrhythmias per hospital policy.	Hypovolemia and electrolyte imbalances may precipitate cardiac dysrhythmias.
Auscultate heart sounds for changes, gallops, or murmurs.	JVD in conjunction with a new S_3 gallop may indicate heart failure or pulmonary edema.
Observe for changes in respiratory status, especially when occurring concurrently with fever and jaundice.	Gram negative sepsis may be seen symptomatically with cholestatic jaundice and decreases in pulmonary function.
Observe for increasing complaints of abdominal pain or tenderness, chills, fever, or hypotension.	May indicate formation of abscess, especially if symptoms occur while patient is receiving vigorous medical treatment. Abdominal rigidity or rebound tenderness may indicate peritonitis.
Observe for presence of petechiae, continued bleeding, or hematoma formation.	May indicate impending DIC as a result of circulating pancreatic enzymes.
Measure and monitor abdominal girth changes.	Identifies increases in fluid retention and ascites.
Monitor intake and output every 2 hours, noting hematuria, or significant imbalance.	Oliguria may occur as a result of renal involvement due to increases in vascular resistance or decreased renal blood flow. Hematuria may occur as a result from circulating pancreatic enzymes.

Information, Instruction, Demonstration

INTERVENTIONS	RATIONALES
Strict aseptic technique should be maintained when dealing with invasive lines or dressings.	Failure to maintain technique may result in sepsis, which is responsible for over 80% of deaths associated with pancreatitis.

INTERVENTIONS	RATIONALES
Prepare patient/family members for surgical procedures as warranted.	Surgical drainage of abscesses or pseudocysts may be required.
Instruct in usage of pancreatic enzyme supplements/bile salts.	Long-term replacement may be required for exocrine deficiencies from permanent pancreatic damage.

Discharge or Maintenance Evaluation

- Patient will be free of complications from pancreatitis, and will exhibit timely healing of all wounds.

- Patient will be able to accurately verbalize all instructed information.

PANCREATITIS

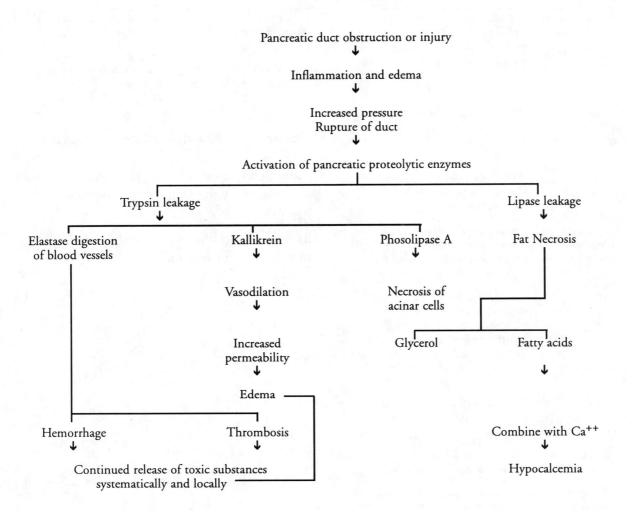

Pancreatic duct obstruction or injury
↓
Inflammation and edema
↓
Increased pressure
Rupture of duct
↓
Activation of pancreatic proteolytic enzymes

Trypsin leakage   Lipase leakage
↓   ↓
Elastase digestion   Kallikrein   Phosolipase A   Fat Necrosis
of blood vessels   ↓   ↓
                           Vasodilation   Necrosis of
                                ↓   acinar cells
                                               Glycerol   Fatty acids
                           Increased
                           permeability   ↓
                                ↓
                             Edema

Hemorrhage   Thrombosis   Combine with Ca^{++}
     ↓   ↓   ↓
   Continued release of toxic substances   Hypocalcemia
   systematically and locally

Acute Abdomen/ Abdominal Trauma

When someone is said to have an acute abdomen, it generally indicates that they have a sudden onset of severe abdominal pain that typically requires surgery to prevent peritonitis from contaminated materials spilling into the peritoneal cavity. There are numerous situations that could be responsible for this diagnosis, such as perforation of the appendix, peptic ulcer, bowel, gallbladder, diverticuli, or abdominal aortic aneurysm, ruptured ectopic pregnancy, or an abdominal injury.

Abdominal injuries may be caused from either blunt trauma or penetrating damage. Blunt trauma, with compression of abdominal structures against the vertebral column, can result from sports injuries, accidents, or falls, and can be caused as a result of a direct impact, rotary or shearing forces, or rapid deceleration. Any of these mechanisms can cause tearing of body structures that may involve substantial bleeding into the peritoneal cavity.

Penetrating injuries can cause perforation of the bowel or hemorrhage from lacerations to major vessels. These types of trauma can either be low-velocity, which damages tissues at the injury site, or high-velocity, in which tissues and organs surrounding the penetration path are damaged.

All of the types of injuries discussed have significant potential for critical emergencies, based on the severity of the wound, and how much damage it has caused. Mortality is approximately 10% from abdominal trauma due in part to the presence of structures involving many body systems being located in the abdomen. The goals of immediate treatment involve maintaining the hemodynamic status, control of hemorrhage, and preparation for surgical procedures.

MEDICAL CARE

Surgery: usually the treatment of choice due to potential or presence of peritonitis from injury; procedure is dependent on source of bleeding or contamination

Laboratory: urinalysis to identify bleeding or urinary tract injuries; CBC to identify sepsis and changes in hematological status; WBC is normally elevated in trauma; differential used to identify shifts to the left; amylase elevated with pancreatic injury or gastrointestinal perforations; renal and liver profiles to discern damage to the particular system; clotting profiles to monitor for coagulation status; myoglobin levels elevated with crush injuries, peritoneal fluid analysis for bleeding or infection

Radiography: chest and abdominal x-rays used to identify pneumothorax, free air below the diaphragm, foreign body that may have caused injury, or other complications; loss of psoas muscle outline indicates retroperitoneal bleeding

CT scans: may be used to identify abdominal and retroperitoneal injuries that may not be overt with regular x-rays; can identify cysts or abscesses that may require surgical intervention

Intravenous pyelogram: used to detect hematuria and trauma to renal structures

Retrograde urethrography/cystography: used to identify urethral or bladder injury

Ultrasound: use is limited; may be useful to distinguish between splenic hematoma from peritoneal blood or ascites

Paracentesis: may be used to identify presence of pus, blood, or other substance, and may be used for peritoneal lavage to identify effects of abdominal trauma and prevent unnecessary surgical intervention

NURSING CARE PLANS

Risk for infection

Related to: perforation of abdominal structures, laceration of vasculature, open wounds, peritoneal cavity contamination

Defining characteristics: fever, trauma, elevated white blood cell count, sepsis

Outcome Criteria

Patient will be free of infection, with stable vital signs and labwork within normal parameters.

INTERVENTIONS	RATIONALES
Monitor vital signs, especially temperature.	May indicate presence of or impending infection and sepsis. Decreasing pulse pressure, hypotension and tachycardia may signify impending septic shock from endotoxic vasodilation.
Observe skin color, temperature, and monitor for changes.	Patient may have warm, flushed, dry skin in shock's warm phase, changing to cold and clammy pale skin as shock progresses.
Obtain blood, urine, sputum, drainage, or other cultures as ordered.	Identifies causative organism and facilitates appropriate selection of antimicrobial agents.
Monitor intake and output every 2 hours.	Sepsis may impair renal perfusion and result in oliguria or anuria.
Administer antibiotics as ordered.	Cephalosporins and aminoglycosides are frequently used to fight these types of infections.
Ensure that universal precautions are utilized, and that sterile or aseptic technique is used when caring for wounds or inserting invasive lines or catheters.	Assists in preventing spread of infection by cross-contamination, as well as preventing other bacterial growth from invasion of skin/body.
Administer tetanus toxoid as ordered.	Decreases risk of development of tetanus.

Information, Instruction, Demonstration

INTERVENTIONS	RATIONALES
Prepare for surgery as warranted.	Surgical intervention may be the treatment of choice to drain abscesses or remove or repair perforated structures.
Assist with peritoneal aspiration as warranted.	May be performed to remove fluid and identify causative organism.
Change wound dressings as ordered.	Dressings protect wound and prevent spread of infection.
Monitor CBC, especially WBC count.	Facilitates assessment of effectiveness of antimicrobial therapy, as well as identifies blood loss or changes in infection.
Limit visitors as indicated, utilizing appropriate isolation precautions as warranted.	Decreases potential for cross-contamination.

Discharge or Maintenance Evaluation

- Patient will have stable vital signs and hemodynamic status.

- Patient will have white blood cell count within normal limits.

- Patient will have negative cultures.

- Patient will not exhibit further signs/symptoms of infection.

- Patient will not develop secondary infection.

- Family members will adhere to isolation regulations.

Risk for injury

Related to: trauma

Defining characteristics: hemorrhage, peritonitis, altered arterial blood gases, mental status changes, hypotension, tachycardia, bradycardia, arterial injuries, fractures, electrolyte imbalances

Outcome Criteria

Patient will be free of injury to self, and free of complications that may ensue from trauma.

INTERVENTIONS	RATIONALES
Monitor vital signs every 1-2 hours, and prn. Check blood pressure readings in both arms and legs.	Decreases in blood pressure or changes with orthostatic readings may indicate impending hypovolemia. Pulse pressures may increase during the latent effects of shock or with head injuries, and may decrease in early stages of shock. Differences between right and left sides greater than 20 mmHg may indicate aortic injury.
Monitor respiratory status, noting changes in breath sounds.	Injury to lungs or diaphragm may result in tachypnea and dyspnea. Breath sounds that are distant or absent may indicate pneumothorax or hemothorax.
Observe chest for symmetry, paradoxical movement, anatomical deformity, swelling, bruising, or crepitus.	Splinting by patient or obvious deformity or swelling may be seen if ribs are fractured. Paradoxical movement may indicate flail chest. Palpable crepitus may be present if lung or mediastinum has been punctured.
Auscultate heart sounds for changes or abnormalities.	Extra heart sounds or murmurs may indicate injury to valves or heart, and distant, muffled heart tones may signal cardiac tamponade.
Observe abdomen for wounds, masses, swelling, pulsations, hematomas, protrusion of organs or viscera, lacerations, and abrasions; auscultate for bowel sounds.	Bluish discolorations around the umbilicus may indicate retroperitoneal bleeding accumulating in abdomen. An odd number of bullet holes may indicate the remaining presence of a foreign object/bullet in the body. Decreased or absent bowel sounds may indicate ileus or peritonitis. Abdominal bruits may result when a vessel is partially occluded, venous hums auscultated over the upper

INTERVENTIONS	RATIONALES
	abdomen or liver may indicate hepatic or splenic vein thrombosis, and friction rubs heard over the spleen may indicate infarction or inflammation of spleen.
Percuss abdomen for changes, dullness or tympany.	Dullness that is decreased over liver may indicate presence of free air below the diaphragm. Upper abdominal distention and increased tympany over the stomach may indicate gastric dilation. Flank area dullness may indicate retroperitoneal hemorrhage.
Cover protruding abdominal viscera with saline-soaked sterile gauze or sterile towels, and position patient with knees flexed.	Protects viscera from drying, and positioning prevents additional protrusion/evisceration.
Palpate peripheral pulses for presence, quality, and character. Notify physician for significant changes.	Changes in pulse characteristics may indicate arterial or venous impairment which may require immediate treatment.
Observe for Grey Turner's and Coopernail's signs.	Grey Turner's sign is a bluish discoloration on flank that indicates retroperitoneal bleeding accumulation in abdomen. Coopernail's sign is ecchymoses on scrotum or labia and may indicate pelvic fracture.
Monitor for complaints of pain at the tip of the left shoulder or right shoulder.	May indicate rupture of spleen or irritation of the diaphragm from blood or other substance with left shoulder pain, and possible liver laceration with right shoulder pain.

Information, Instruction, Demonstration

INTERVENTIONS	RATIONALES
Assist with peritoneal tap and lavage.	Done to identify intraperitoneal bleeding which is diagnosed when fluid is analyzed.
Instruct on all procedures and testing; prepare for surgery as warranted.	Promotes knowledge and decreases anxiety which facilitates compliance with medical regimen.

INTERVENTIONS	RATIONALES
Instruct patient/family to notify physician for fever or abdominal pain.	Abdominal injury signs and symptoms may not appear for several hours to days.

Discharge or Maintenance Evaluation

* Patient will have no evidence of abdominal injury complication.

* Patient will have no intraperitoneal bleeding or structural damage to organs.

* Patient will be compliant with regimen.

* Patient will have successful surgical intervention with no postoperative complications.

Risk for fluid volume deficit
[See GI Bleeding]

Related to: fluid shifts, hemorrhage, nasogastric suctioning

Defining characteristics: hypotension, tachycardia, decreased urinary output, decreased hemoglobin and hematocrit, decreased filling pressures, electrolyte imbalances, presence of peritonitis

Alteration in comfort
[See MI]

Related to: trauma, surgery, edema

Defining characteristics: grimacing, complaints of pain, restlessness, splinting, shallow respirations, abdominal rigidity

Alteration in nutrition: less than body requirements
[See DKA]

Related to: trauma, surgery, nasogastric suctioning

Defining characteristics: abdominal pain, ordered nutritional status of NPO, increased metabolism, weight loss, nitrogen and electrolyte imbalance, decreased albumin and protein levels, vitamin deficiencies

ACUTE ABDOMEN/ABDOMINAL TRAUMA
(bowel obstruction, peritonitis, trauma, perforation)

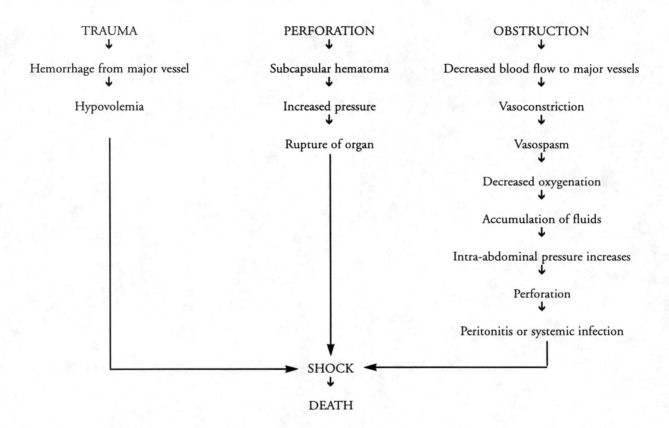

TRAUMA
↓
Hemorrhage from major vessel
↓
Hypovolemia

PERFORATION
↓
Subcapsular hematoma
↓
Increased pressure
↓
Rupture of organ

OBSTRUCTION
↓
Decreased blood flow to major vessels
↓
Vasoconstriction
↓
Vasospasm
↓
Decreased oxygenation
↓
Accumulation of fluids
↓
Intra-abdominal pressure increases
↓
Perforation
↓
Peritonitis or systemic infection

SHOCK
↓
DEATH

Liver Failure

The liver plays a vital role by providing multiple functions, such as, metabolism of carbohydrates, proteins, and fats, storing fat-soluble vitamins, vitamin B_{12}, copper, and iron, synthesis of blood clotting factors, amino acids, albumin, and globulins, detoxification of toxic substances, phagocytosis of microorganisms, and plays a role in glycolysis and gluconeogenesis. Liver functioning can be preserved until up to 75% of the hepatocytes become damaged or necrotic, at which time the liver can no longer perform its normal operation.

Early hepatic failure presents as a type of cirrhosis of the liver. Liver cells become inflamed and obstructed, which results in damage to the cells around the central portal vein. When the inflammation decreases, the lobule regenerates, and this cycle is repeated until the lobule is irreversibly damaged and fibrotic tissue replaces liver tissue.

Advanced hepatic failure develops when all compensatory mechanisms fail, causing the serum ammonia level to rise. The already-damaged liver is unable to synthesize normal products, so acidosis, hypoglycemia, or blood dyscrasias develop, and the patient becomes comatose.

Acute liver failure, also known as fulminant hepatic failure, may be precipitated by a stress factor that aggravates a preexisting chronic liver disease. Some stress factors include alcohol intake, ingestion of Amanita mushrooms, large amounts of dietary protein, gastrointestinal bleeding, and portacaval shunt surgery. An acute type of liver failure may occur as a result of viral or toxic hepatitis, biliary obstruction, cancer, acute infective processes, drugs, such as acetaminophen, isoniazid, and rifampin, severe dehydration, Reye's syndrome, or shock states.

Fulminant hepatic failure may begin as stage I hepatic encephalopathy, progressing to drowsiness and asterixis, stupor and incoherent communication, finally to stage IV with deep coma. The stages may progress over at little as two months. Distinguishing attributes between acute and chronic failure are the presence of cerebral edema and intracranial pressure increases.

The goal of treatment is to halt progression of the encephalopathy that occurs with increasing ammonia levels, and is accomplished with use of cathartics, decreasing dietary protein, and electrolyte replacement. Even with treatment, mortality rates are as high as 90%, depending on the age of the patient and severity of disease.

MEDICAL CARE

Laboratory: elevated ammonia levels, liver function studies elevated, elevated BUN; electrolytes tested to identify imbalances; serum bilirubin elevated; urine bilirubin may be present if direct serum bilirubin is elevated; albumin decreases and globulin increases in liver failure; cholesterol is elevated; PT prolonged; toxicology screens for ingestion of alcohol or other drugs that may have precipitated failure; magnesium level may be low with alcoholic cirrhosis and toxic if magnesium replacement is used

Medication: Neomycin or Kanamycin frequently used to prevent intestinal bacteria from converting protein/amino acids to ammonia; lactulose or sorbitol used to induce catharsis to empty intestines to decrease conversion to ammonia; thiazide diuretics may be given to decrease fluid retention

Hyperalimentation: may be used as diet of choice due to ability to control concentration of nutrients, electrolytes, and vitamins

Hemodialysis: may be used as a temporary measure for severe hepatic encephalopathy

Liver biopsy: may be done to establish diagnosis by study of biopsied tissue

Liver scans: may be used to detect degenerative cirrhosis changes or identify focal liver disease

NURSING CARE PLANS

Alteration in thought processes

Related to: serum ammonia levels, encephalopathy

Defining characteristics: increased ammonia, increased BUN, mental status changes, decreasing level of consciousness, changes in personality, handwriting changes, tremors, coma

Outcome Criteria

Patient will be conscious and stable, with ammonia levels within normal ranges.

INTERVENTIONS	RATIONALES
Monitor neurological status every 1-2 hours, and prn. Notify physician for abnormalities.	Identifies onset of problem and potential trend.
If possible, have patient write name each day and do simple mathematic calculation.	As hepatic failure progresses, the ability to write becomes more difficult, and writing becomes illegible at pre-coma stage. Inability to perform mental calculations may indicate worsening failure.
Administer cathartic agents as ordered.	Lactulose minimizes formation of ammonia and other nitrogenous by-products by altering intestinal pH. Neomycin or Kanamycin help prevent conversion of amino acids into ammonia. Sorbitol-type cathartics cause an osmotic diarrhea to empty the intestines to decrease ammonia production.

INTERVENTIONS	RATIONALES
Observe for asterixis or other tremors.	Rapid wrist flapping when arms are raised in front of body with hands dorsiflexed may indicate presence of encephalopathy.
Provide safe environment for patient.	Decreases risk of injury due to altered consciousness levels.
Provide low protein diet.	Decreased dietary protein may lessen serum ammonia levels.
Avoid sedatives and narcotics if at all possible.	May worsen decreasing level of consciousness and make identification of cause of decreased sensorium more difficult.

Information, Instruction, Demonstration

INTERVENTIONS	RATIONALES
Instruct patient/family in potential for altered sensorium and encephalopathy signs. Reorient patient as needed.	Provides knowledge and facilitates family involvement with maintaining optimal orientation level. Provides support with realistic expectations of disease process since outcome is poor.
Instruct in side effects of drugs used to facilitate decrease in ammonia levels.	Diarrhea will occur, and lactulose should be titrated to where patient has 3 stools per day.

Discharge or Maintenance Evaluation

• Patient will be awake, alert, and oriented.

• Patient will have serum ammonia levels within acceptable ranges.

• Patient and/or family will be able to verbalize understanding of instructions and be able to communicate concerns.

Alteration in nutrition: less than body requirements

Related to: metabolism changes, increased ammonia level

Defining characteristics: anorexia, nausea, vomiting, malabsorption of fats, malabsorption of vitamins, altered carbohydrate, fat, and protein metabolism, malnutrition, weight loss, fatigue, edema, ascites

Outcome Criteria

Patient will be able to achieve positive nitrogen balance and have stable weight.

INTERVENTIONS	RATIONALES
Provide diet that has protein in ordered amounts, with supplementation of vitamins and other nutrients.	Protein metabolism is altered with liver disease and results in increased ammonia levels. Vitamin/nutrient supplementation may be required due to malabsorption of element.
Ensure that patient is positioned in sitting position for meals.	Decreases abdominal tenderness and fullness, and prevents potential for aspiration.
Avoid sodium intake of amounts greater than ordered.	Sodium should be restricted to less than 500 mg per day to decrease edema and ascites.
If patient is unable to ingest adequate dietary intake, administer tube feedings or TPN as ordered.	Provides needed nutrients when patient is unable to eat.

Discharge or Maintenance Evaluation

* Patient will be able to ingest adequate amounts of prescribed diet to maintain weight and ammonia levels at acceptable levels.

* Patient will comply with dietary regimen and limitations.

* Patient will have no complications from enteral or parenteral therapies.

Fluid volume deficit
[See GI Bleeding]

Related to: osmotic changes, hydrostatic pressure changes

Defining characteristics: presence of ascites, oliguria, anuria, dry skin, decreased skin turgor, hypotension

Impaired skin integrity

Related to: poor nutrition, renal involvement, bile deposits on skin

Defining characteristics: edema, ascites, jaundice, pruritus

Outcome Criteria

Patient will maintain skin integrity.

INTERVENTIONS	RATIONALES
Observe skin for changes, abrasions, rashes, scaling, wounds, bleeding, redness, etc.	Facilitates identification of potential complications.
Turn at least every two hours and prn.	Prevents pressure area compromise of skin.
Apply lotions frequently when providing skin care; do not use soap when bathing; apply cornstarch or baking soda prn.	Soap may dry skin further and result in breach of integrity. Lotions and other agents may decrease itching.
Administer medications for pruritus as ordered.	Decreases itching which may cause wounds. Bile salts that are deposited on the skin of patients with hepatic or renal involvement cause chronic and severe pruritus.

Information, Instruction, Demonstration

INTERVENTIONS	RATIONALES
Instruct patient in methods to decrease itching: soothing massages, avoidance of extra covers, and use of clean white gloves at night.	Helps prevent patient from scratching during the night and reduces tendency to scratch.
Provide attention-diverting activity.	May refocus concentration to decrease scratching.

Discharge or Maintenance Evaluation

- Patient will exhibit no evidence of skin breakdown.

- Patient will be able to use discussed methods to avoid scratching.

- Patient will have no complications from lack of skin integrity.

Ineffective breathing pattern

Related to: increased pressure from ascites, elevated ammonia levels, decrease lung expansion, fatigue

Defining characteristics: presence of ascites, weakness, tachypnea, dyspnea, decreased lung expansion, altered arterial blood gases

Outcome Criteria

Patient will maintain effective respiration with normal ABGs and hemodynamics.

INTERVENTIONS	RATIONALES
Assist with paracentesis.	May be required to remove ascitic fluid if respiratory insufficiency cannot be corrected by other methods.
Prepare patient for placement of peritoneovenous shunt.	Surgical intervention may be required to provide method to return accumulations of fluid in abdominal cavity to the systemic circulation and provides long-term ascites relief.

Discharge or Maintenance Evaluation

- Patient will be free of shortness of breath and will have normal lung expansion with optimal arterial blood gases and oxygenation.

Risk for injury

Related to: hemorrhage, altered clotting factors, esophageal varices, portal hypertension

Defining characteristics: bleeding, exsanguination, decreased hemoglobin and hematocrit, decreased prothrombin, decreased fibrinogen, decreased clotting factors VIII, IX, and X, vitamin K malabsorption, thromboplastin release

Outcome Criteria

Patient will exhibit no evidence of bleeding.

INTERVENTIONS	RATIONALES
Monitor all bodily secretions for presence of blood; test stools and nasogastric drainage for guaiac.	GI bleeding may occur due to altered clotting factors and changes that occur with cirrhosis and liver disease.
Observe for bleeding from puncture sites, presence of hematomas or petechiae, or bruising.	May indicate a form of disseminated intravascular coagulation as a result of altered clotting factors.
Monitor vital signs and hemodynamic parameters. Avoid rectal temperatures.	Changes in vital signs may indicate loss of circulating blood volume. Vasculature in rectum may be susceptible to rupture.
Insert nasogastric tube gently and lavage as ordered.	Esophageal vasculature may be susceptible to rupture. Removal of blood from the stomach decreases synthesis to ammonia.
Administer vitamins as ordered.	Vitamin K facilitates synthesis of prothrombin and coagulation if liver is functional. Vitamin C may reduce potential for GI bleeding and facilitates healing process.
Administer stool softeners as needed.	Prevents straining to pass stool which may result in rupture of vasculature or increase in intra-abdominal pressures.

INTERVENTIONS	RATIONALES
Monitor labwork for CBC and clotting factors.	Helps to identify blood loss or impending DIC.

Discharge or Maintenance Evaluation

- Patient will have no active bleeding and labwork will be within normal limits.

- Patient will not exhibit any hemorrhagic complications from invasive line/tube placement.

Disturbance in body image

Related to: changes in physical appearance, ascites

Defining characteristics: presence of ascites, biophysical changes, negative feelings about body, fear of rejection, fear of reaction from others, fear of death, fear of the unknown

Outcome Criteria

Patient will be able to verbalize concerns and accept body/self perception within situational limits.

INTERVENTIONS	RATIONALES
Encourage patient to discuss concerns, fears, and questions regarding diagnosis being careful to recognize and accept his fears without minimizing them.	Validates patient's feelings and concerns regarding changes in body.
Discuss causes of alteration of appearance with patient and family members.	Validates realistic changes and allows for reinstruction on areas that may not have been understood. Jaundice, bruising, and ascites may be considered unattractive by patient and/or family, and may precipitate feelings of low self-esteem and body worth.
Encourage family to support patient without rejection or fear of his appearance.	Patient and family may experience guilt, especially if the cause is alcohol or drug-related. Emotional support from loved

INTERVENTIONS	RATIONALES
	ones may enhance patient's ability to accept changes.
Consult with social services, counseling, psychiatric services, minister, or other community resources.	Additional professional and community resources may be required to deal with alcohol or drug rehabilitation, or with perceptions of body image.

Discharge or Maintenance Evaluation

- Patient will be able to verbalize concerns over his appearance.

- Patient will be able to verbalize understanding of disease process and changes that may occur.

- Patient will be able to effectively utilize methods for coping with changes.

- Family will be supportive of patient's altered appearance and self-esteem.

- Patient will be able to effectively access community resources for continuing needs.

LIVER FAILURE

HEMATOLOGIC SYSTEM

Disseminated Intravascular Coagulation (DIC)

HELLP Syndrome

Anemia

Disseminated Intravascular Coagulation (DIC)

Disseminated intravascular coagulation, also known as consumptive coagulopathy, defibrinogenation syndrome, or DIC, is an acute disorder that accelerates the activation of the intrinsic and/or extrinsic cascade clotting mechanism and depletes both clotting factors and platelets. DIC is usually a complication of another disease process in which excessive thrombin is produced, converting fibrinogen to fibrin, and the fibrin creates damaging thrombi in the microcirculation. Fibrin blocks the capillary flow to the organs and results in ischemic tissue damage, and as the clotting factors, platelets, and fibrin split products (FSP) are consumed, hemorrhage and shock results. As the fibrin and FSP repolymerize, a secondary fibrin mesh forms in the microcirculation and when blood travels through this, the red blood cells become damaged and a hemolytic anemia can occur.

Some of the precipitating factors include sepsis, neoplasm necrosis, eclampsia, abruptio placentae, saline-induced abortions, retained dead fetus, amniotic fluid embolus, hemolysis, giant hemangiomas, systemic lupus erythematosus, transfusions, trauma, shock, burns, head injuries, transplant rejection, snake bite, fractures, anoxia, heat stroke, surgery utilizing cardiopulmonary bypass, and necrotizing enterocolitis.

Bleeding in a patient with no other previous history of bleeding or coagulopathy problems should raise questions as to the possibility of the presence of DIC. DIC may be acute or chronic (usually seen with neoplasms) and can vary in severity from mild oozing to exsanguination from all orifices. Treatment is aimed at correction of the underlying problem, correction of shock, acidosis, and sepsis, supportive care to restore circulatory volume and adequate oxygenation of tissues, and to replace blood loss due to hemorrhage.

MEDICAL CARE

Laboratory: prothrombin time (PT) to measure activity level and patency of the extrinsic and final pathways, increased in DIC; partial thromboplastin time (PTT) to measure activity level and patency of the intrinsic and final pathways, increased in DIC; thromboplastin time increased, platelet count decreased, fibrinogen usually decreased showing increased hypercoagability and decreased bleeding tendency, FSP elevated, usually > 10; clotting factor analysis used to identify factors being depleted; CBC used to evaluate anemia and RBC fragmentation; BUN and creatinine used to assess renal involvement from thrombosis; guaiacs on all body fluids to identify occult bleeding; cultures of sputum, blood, urine, CSF and other drainage used to identify causative organism of infection and to ascertain appropriate antimicrobial for therapy

Blood components: used as replacement therapy for significant blood loss; RBCs given to increase the oxygen-carrying capability; whole blood, plasma, plasmanate and albumin used to expand volume; fresh frozen plasma (FFP) and albumin used to replace proteins; FFP, cryoprecipitate, and fresh whole blood used to replace coagulation factors; platelet concentrate used to replace platelets

IV fluids: used to treat hypovolemia and shock

Antibiotics: used to treat infection that may cause DIC

Heparin: use is controversial; heparin inhibits micro thrombi formation by neutralizing free circulating thrombin; shouldn't be used unless bleeding is unmanageable by replacement therapy of FFP and platelets

NURSING CARE PLANS

Risk for impaired gas exchange
[See GI Bleeding]

Related to: bleeding, disease

Defining characteristics: decreased PaO_2 below 80 mmHg, dyspnea, tachypnea, increased work of breathing, restlessness, irritability, mental status changes, changes in blood pressure and pulse, decreased hemoglobin and hematocrit

Risk for fluid volume deficit
[See GI Bleeding]

Related to: blood loss, altered coagulability

Defining characteristics: weight loss, oliguria, abnormal electrolytes, hypotension, tachycardia, decreased central venous pressures, decreased filling pressures, altered coagulation studies, lethargy, mental status changes

Risk for injury

Related to: hemorrhage, blood loss, altered coagulability

Defining characteristics: bleeding, exsanguination, decreased hemoglobin and hematocrit levels, increased fibrin split products, increased prothrombin time, decreased platelet count, increased partial thromboplastin time, decreased fibrinogen

Outcome Criteria

Patient will be free of unexplained bleeding and will have stable vital signs and hemodynamic pressures.

INTERVENTIONS	RATIONALES
Identify and treat underlying disorder.	Treatment of cause and correction of coagulation problem is major goal of treatment. DIC is most often seen as the complication of an underlying infection, malignant disease, trauma, or shock state.
Administer IV fluids as ordered.	Large volumes may be required to maintain circulating volume due to bleeding, and to maintain hemodynamic status.
Administer blood and blood by-products, such as cryoprecipitate, fresh frozen plasma, etc. as ordered.	May be required to replace circulating blood volume and to help correct thrombocytopenia or hypofibrinogenemia.
Administer supplemental oxygen as warranted.	Decreased blood volume impairs oxygen carrying capability and supplemental oxygen may be required to maintain oxygenation.
Observe patient for petechiae, bruising, overt and occult bleeding.	May be present with impending DIC.
Monitor for dyspnea, hemoptysis, and decreased saturation; auscultate lung fields for adventitious breath sounds.	Crackles may be present and patient may exhibit these signs if microemboli in the pulmonary circulation are present.
Monitor intake and output.	Microemboli or deposits of fibrin within the renal system may present as renal insufficiency or failure.
Administer heparin therapy as ordered.	Controversial treatment may be given to disperse clumped clotting factors, but is rarely used today.
Monitor labwork for coagulation studies and CBC.	Provides identification of effectiveness of therapy or worsening of condition.

Discharge or Maintenance Evaluation

- Patient will have stable vital signs and hemodynamic pressures.

- Patient will exhibit no bleeding tendencies or active hemorrhage.

- Patient will exhibit no complications from other disease processes.

- Patient will achieve and maintain adequate blood volume.

- Patient will have underlying disease process corrected.

DISSEMINATED INTRAVASCULAR COAGULATION (DIC)

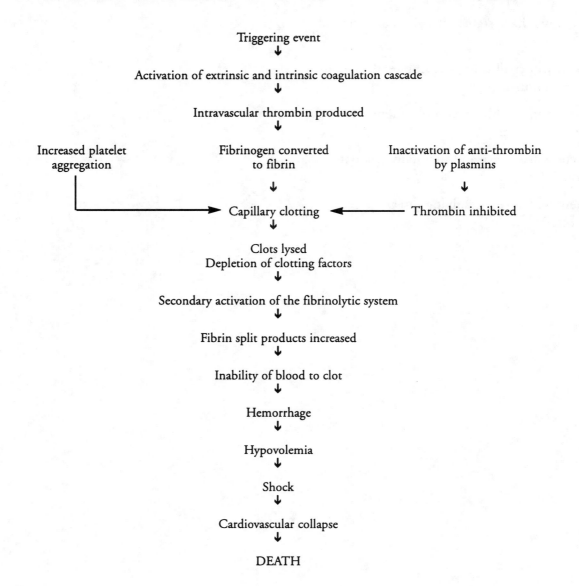

Triggering event
↓
Activation of extrinsic and intrinsic coagulation cascade
↓
Intravascular thrombin produced
↓

Increased platelet aggregation   Fibrinogen converted to fibrin   Inactivation of anti-thrombin by plasmins
↓   ↓
Capillary clotting   ←   Thrombin inhibited
↓
Clots lysed
Depletion of clotting factors
↓
Secondary activation of the fibrinolytic system
↓
Fibrin split products increased
↓
Inability of blood to clot
↓
Hemorrhage
↓
Hypovolemia
↓
Shock
↓
Cardiovascular collapse
↓
DEATH

H E L L P Syndrome

HELLP syndrome is an acute and severe complication that presents as a multi-organic disease process occurring concurrently with pregnancy-induced hypertension (PIH). The initials are compiled from the symptoms that comprise the syndrome: hemolysis, elevated liver enzymes and low platelets. These same findings may also be associated with DIC and frequently is diagnosed as such.

PIH usually occurs after the twentieth week of gestation in approximately 5% of all pregnancies, and most often in the primagravida patient. PIH results in increased edema, proteinuria, and hypertension. Although the cause is unknown, theories often involve immunologic, endocrine, and chorionic villi exposure.

HELLP may represent an acute autoimmune state in which the red blood cells lyse, liver enzymes are elevated as a result of fibrin thrombi blocking blood flow to the liver, and platelets decrease due to vasospasm and platelet aggregation. Vasospasm results in increases in systemic and peripheral vascular resistance, which increase blood pressure further. Sensitivity to angiotensin II is increased, and vasoconstriction may result in increases in vascular permeability and hemoconcentration.

The pathological changes in the liver may develop due to generalized activation of the intravascular coagulation process. Fibrin deposits and hemorrhagic necrosis develops in periportal areas and may lead to subcapsular hematomas or liver rupture. A decrease in antithrombin III and an increase in thrombin-antithrombin III complex (TAT) and the appearance of fibrin monomers and D-dimers is found in almost all cases of HELLP, but decompensated intravascular coagulation with increased PT and PTT and decreased fibrinogen levels is found only in severe forms. Decompensated coagulation occurs with other complications such as liver hematoma, abruptio placentae, renal failure, and pulmonary edema.

There is usually a low recurrence rate (5% or less), and the HELLP syndrome usually resolves with delivery of the baby. Treatment involves prophylaxis against postpartum worsening, curettage of the uterus, and treatment with calcium antagonists and decadron, as well as intense monitoring for a decline in liver function and for potential for bleeding.

MEDICAL CARE

Laboratory: hematocrit used to assess intravascular fluid status; protime and partial thromboplastin time used to evaluate clotting; magnesium levels used to evaluate therapeutic levels for treatment; urine collection for protein used to diagnose complications

Magnesium: used to prevent and treat convulsions by decreasing the neuromuscular irritability and depressing the central nervous system

Antihypertensives: apresoline is the drug of choice; used to relax arterioles and stimulate cardiac output and is utilized with diastolic blood pressures greater than 110 mmHg

Beta-blockers: occasionally used to control acute hypertensive crises

Valium: used to control seizure activity

NURSING CARE PLANS
Risk for impaired gas exchange
[See GI Bleeding]

Related to: bleeding, disease

Defining characteristics: decreased PaO$_2$ below 80 mmHg, dyspnea, tachypnea, increased work of breathing, restlessness, irritability, mental status changes, changes in blood pressure and pulse, decreased hemoglobin and hematocrit

Risk for fluid volume deficit
[See GI Bleeding]

Related to: blood loss, altered coagulability

Defining characteristics: weight loss, oliguria, abnormal electrolytes, hypotension, tachycardia, decreased central venous pressures, altered coagulation studies, lethargy, mental status changes

Risk for injury

Related to: administration of magnesium

Defining characteristics: CNS depression, venous irritation, dyspnea, shallow respirations, decreased oxygen saturation, oliguria, absence of deep tendon reflexes, changes in vital signs

Outcome Criteria

Patient will receive medication without experiencing side effects.

INTERVENTIONS	RATIONALES
Monitor for convulsions or tremors.	Identifies precipitation of problem.
Administer magnesium sulfate as ordered.	Magnesium is used to prevent and treat convulsions by decreasing the neuromuscular irritability and depression of the central nervous system. Normally, MgSO$_4$ is given IV, with a loading dose of 3-4 Grams, followed by an infusion of 1-4 Grams/hr. It may be given IM with dosage of 5 Grams in each hip every 4 hours using the Z-tract method. Some facilities add xylocaine to the medication to decrease the pain of IM injections.

INTERVENTIONS	RATIONALES
Monitor vital signs every 1-2 hours, and prn, especially respiratory status.	Depression of CNS can result in respiratory insufficiency or paralysis. Hypothermia may occur with toxicity of drug. MgSO$_4$ should be held for respirations less than 16 per minute.
Monitor EKG for changes and dysrhythmias, and treat per hospital protocol.	Dysrhythmias may occur with administration of magnesium or with its antidote, calcium.
Monitor intake and output every 2 hours.	Magnesium sulfate may cause toxicity with large doses and result in renal insufficiency and oliguria.
Monitor fetal heart tones every hour.	Fetal heart rate may decrease with use of magnesium sulfate.
Assess deep tendon reflexes.	Absence of DTRs may indicate hypermagnesemia and toxicity. Decreased DTRs may occur with therapeutic ranges.
Have calcium gluconate at bedside and give as warranted/ordered.	Calcium gluconate is the antidote for magnesium sulfate.
Monitor labwork for magnesium levels.	Normal levels are 4-7.5 mEq/L, with toxic levels above that.

Information, Instruction, Demonstration

INTERVENTIONS	RATIONALES
Instruct on signs and symptoms to report to nurse/physician.	Facilitates prompt identification of problem to allow for timely intervention.
Observe IM injection sites for redness, firm areas, warmth, and pain.	May indicate presence of sterile abscess from injections which have a variable rate of absorption given in this manner.

Discharge or Maintenance Evaluation

- Patient will have stable vital signs.

- Patient will be free of convulsions.

- Fetal heart rates will remain unaffected and activity will be within normal range.

- Patient will exhibit no signs of magnesium toxicity or complications from therapy.

HELLP SYNDROME

Pregnancy-induced hypertension
+
DIC
↓

Hemolysis	Fibrin thrombi mobilized	Platelet adhesion
↓	↓	↓
Abnormal morphology	Decreased blood flow to liver	Clumping of platelets
	↓	↓
	Liver congestion	Decrease in circulating platelets
	↓	
	Elevated liver enzymes	

Increased sensitivity to angiotension II
↓

Vasospasm

↓

Vasoconstriction
Increased vascular resistance
↓

Increased arterial blood pressure

↓

Increased vascular permeability
↓

Edema

↓

Proteinuria

Anemia

Anemia is a condition in which the red blood cell count, hemoglobin, and hematocrit are decreased. This decrease results in a decrease in the oxygen-carrying capability and causes tissue hypoxia. As the body tries to compensate, blood is shifted from areas that have a plentiful amount in tissues that have low oxygen requirements to those areas that require higher oxygen concentrations, such as the heart and brain.

There are several types of anemias; those that are due to decreased red blood cell production, those that are due to blood loss, and the hemolytic anemias caused from G6PD deficiency, autoimmunity, or physical causes. Microcytic, or iron deficiency anemia, develops when the transportation of iron by transferrin is insufficient to meet requirements of the erythropoietic cells. Macrocytic, or megaloblastic anemia, occurs because of a deficiency in vitamin B_{12} or folic acid. Pernicious anemia is a type of megaloblastic anemia in which the absence of vitamin B_{12} as well as lack of the intrinsic factor is noted. Normocytic, or aplastic anemia, is caused from the failure of the bone marrow or destruction of bone marrow by either chemical or physical means. Autoimmune anemia is an acquired condition that involves premature erythrocyte destruction from the person's own immune system. Hemolytic anemia results when erythrocyte destruction is increased and cells have a shortened life span. Sickle cell anemia is an inherited condition in which hemoglobin S is present in the blood resulting in sickling and abnormal hemolyzation that obstructs capillary flow. Thalassemia is a group of inherited anemias that result from faulty production of alpha or beta hemoglobin polypeptides.

Anemia can occur as the direct result of prosthetic heart valves or extracorporeal circulation and the destruction of red blood cells. Anemias can also be precipitated by toxic substance exposure or chronic disease processes, such as uremia or chronic liver disease.

MEDICAL CARE

Laboratory: CBC to help differentiate type of anemia—RBCs reduced; hemoglobin decreased with mild considered 10-14 G/dl, moderate 6-10 G/dl, and severe below 6 G/dl; hematocrit decreased; MCH, MCHC variable dependent on type of anemia; MCV 80-100 fl with normocytic, greater than 100 fl with macrocytic, and less than 80 fl with microcytic; platelet count usually decreased, but may be elevated after hemorrhage; RDW increased in iron depletion anemia; B_{12} level decreased, folate decreased; serum iron and TIBC may be decreased; stool guaiac may be positive if blood loss is from GI tract

Radiography: chest x-ray to discern pulmonary or cardiac complications; upper and lower gastrointestinal series may be done to identify active or current bleeding

Bone marrow aspiration: may be performed to determine type of anemia

Bone marrow transplants: may be required for severe aplastic anemia

Blood transfusions: may be required to replace blood volume with hemorrhage

NURSING CARE PLANS

Alteration in tissue perfusion: cardiopulmonary, renal, cerebral, gastrointestinal, peripheral

Related to: altered oxygen-carrying capability, blood loss

Defining characteristics: decreased hematocrit and hemoglobin, chest pain, palpitations, pallor, dry mucous membranes, cold intolerance, oliguria, nausea, vomiting, abdominal pain, abdominal distention, increased capillary refill time, confusion, lethargy, changes in pulse rate and blood pressure

Outcome Criteria

Patient will have adequate perfusion to all body systems with stable vital signs and hemodynamics

INTERVENTIONS	RATIONALES
Monitor vital signs every 1-2 hours and prn.	Facilitates identification of changes that may require intervention.
Monitor neurological status for mental confusion or level of consciousness changes.	May be indicative of impaired cerebral perfusion.
Auscultate lung fields for adventitious breath sounds. Auscultate for abnormal heart tones.	Crackles and/or new presence of cardiac gallops may indicate impending or present congestive failure that may have resulted from the body's compensatory mechanism of increasing cardiac output. Mild anemia can cause exertional dyspnea and palpitations; moderate anemia can cause increased palpitations and dyspnea at rest; severe anemia causes tachycardia, increased pulse pressure, systolic murmurs, intermittent claudication, angina, congestive heart failure, orthopnea, and tachypnea.
Administer supplemental oxygen as warranted.	Decreases in red blood cells decreases oxygen carrying capability since oxygen is bound to the hemoglobin for transport, and may require supplementation to maintain oxygenation.
Monitor EKG for changes in cardiac rhythm or conduction.	Changes may occur with imbalances of electrolytes, with fluid shifts, or with hypoxia.

INTERVENTIONS	RATIONALES
Monitor for complaints of chest pain, pressure, palpitations, or dyspnea.	May indicate decreased cardiac perfusion from hypoxia or ischemia.
Administer blood and/or blood products as warranted.	Blood replacement may facilitate improved oxygen-carrying ability due to increased number of red blood cells and correct volume deficiency.
Monitor labwork for changes.	May facilitate identification of deficiencies and allow for assessment of effectiveness of treatment.

Information, Instruction, Demonstration

INTERVENTIONS	RATIONALES
Maintain environment temperature within normal ranges.	Reduction of peripheral perfusion may result in cold intolerance to vasoconstriction. Excessive heat may cause vasodilation and further reduce organ perfusion.
Prepare patient/family for surgical procedures as warranted.	May require transplantation of bone marrow, or surgical repair for site of bleeding.

Discharge or Maintenance Evaluation

* Patient will achieve and maintain adequate perfusion to all body systems.

* Patient will have stable vital signs and hemodynamic pressures.

* Patient will exhibit no evidence of GI bleeding.

* Patient will exhibit no signs of complications of disease or therapy.

Risk for fluid volume deficit
[See GI Bleeding]

Related to: bleeding

Defining characteristics: hypotension, tachycardia, decreased skin turgor, weakness, decreased urinary output, pallor, diaphoresis, decreased capillary refill, mental changes, restlessness, decreased filling pressures

Activity intolerance
[See COPD]

Related to: decreased oxygen-carrying capability

Defining characteristics: weakness, lethargy, fatigue, dyspnea, activity intolerance, chest pain, palpitations, tachycardia, decreased oxygen saturation, increased respiratory rate with exertion, hypertension

Alteration in nutrition: less than body requirements
[See DKA]

Related to: inability to absorb required nutrients for red blood cell production

Defining characteristics: weight loss, activity intolerance, dyspnea, fatigue, weakness, loss of muscle tone, anorexia

Knowledge deficit

Related to: lack of information, unfamiliarity with information, lack of recall, misinterpretation of information

Defining characteristics: questions, communication of misconceptions, development of preventable complications, incorrect follow-up with instructions

Outcome Criteria

Patient will be able to verbalize understanding of disease process, treatment regimen, and procedures, and comply with therapy.

INTERVENTIONS	RATIONALES
Instruct on particular type of anemia that patient has developed.	Provides knowledge and facilitates compliance.
Instruct on labwork and other procedures.	Decreases anxiety and fear of the unknown.
Instruct on dietary requirements.	Increasing iron sources from red meat, egg yolks, dried fruits and green leafy vegetables may facilitate correction of anemia. Folic acid and vitamin C which augments iron absorption may be found in green vegetables, whole grains, citrus fruits, and liver.
Instruct on signs and symptoms of which to notify physician.	Decreased leukocyte count may potentiate the risk of infection and patient should seek medical assistance for timely intervention.
Instruct on medications, effects, side effects, contraindications, and avoidance of over-the-counter medications without physician approval.	Iron or vitamin B_{12} replacement may be necessary for life, and knowledge regarding therapeutic management will increase compliance with treatment and allow for prompt identification of complications that may require changes in dosages, types of medication, or schedule of administration.

Discharge or Maintenance Evaluation

• Patient will be able to verbalize and demonstrate understanding of all instructed information.

ANEMIA

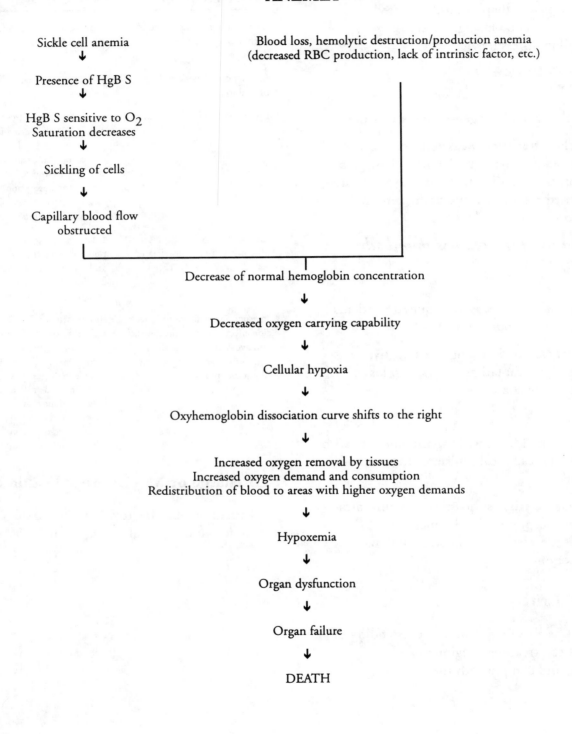

Sickle cell anemia
↓
Presence of HgB S
↓
HgB S sensitive to O_2
Saturation decreases
↓
Sickling of cells
↓
Capillary blood flow
obstructed

Blood loss, hemolytic destruction/production anemia
(decreased RBC production, lack of intrinsic factor, etc.)

Decrease of normal hemoglobin concentration
↓
Decreased oxygen carrying capability
↓
Cellular hypoxia
↓
Oxyhemoglobin dissociation curve shifts to the right
↓
Increased oxygen removal by tissues
Increased oxygen demand and consumption
Redistribution of blood to areas with higher oxygen demands
↓
Hypoxemia
↓
Organ dysfunction
↓
Organ failure
↓
DEATH

RENAL/ENDOCRINE SYSTEMS

Acute Renal Failure (ARF)

Diabetic Ketoacidosis (DKA)

Hyperglycemic Hyperosmolar Nonketotic Coma (HHNK)

Syndrome of Inappropriate ADH Secretion (SIADH)

Diabetes Insipidus (DI)

Pheochromocytoma

Thyrotoxicosis (Thyroid Storm)

Acute Renal Failure (ARF)

Acute renal failure (ARF) is noted when there is a sudden deterioration in function of the renal system that may be caused by renal circulation failure or glomerular or tubular dysfunction. The build-up of waste materials that accumulates affects multiple organ systems.

ARF can be subclassified according to the etiology of condition, such as prerenal, intrarenal, and postrenal. Prerenal conditions occur when blood perfusion is inadequate, such as with hypotension, hemorrhage, myocardial infarction, congestive heart failure, pulmonary embolism, burns, third spacing, septic shock, diuretic abuse, or volume depletion. This dysfunction causes glomerular filtration rates to decrease, and decreased reabsorption of sodium in the tubules.

Intrarenal renal failure occurs either from damage to the tubular epithelium, known as acute tubular necrosis (ATN), or from damage to glomeruli and the small vessels. This condition causes renal capillary swelling that decreases the glomerular filtration rate (GFR), or decreased GFR is secondary to the obstruction of the glomeruli by edema and cellular debris. ATN is the most common type of ARF and is the result of nephrotoxins or ischemia. Intrarenal failure may take many weeks to repair damage and is usually seen with trauma, sepsis, DIC, transfusion reactions, renal vasculature blockages, heavy metal poisoning, and with use of aminoglycosides, penicillins, tetracylines, dilantin, and amphotericin. Glomeruli damage is seen with acute glomerulonephritis, polyarteritis nodosa, lupus erythematosus, Goodpasture's syndrome, endocarditis, abruptio placentae, abortion, serum sickness, malignant hypertension, or hemolytic uremic syndromes.

Postrenal failure may occur as a result of an obstruction anywhere in the system from the kidney to the urethra. Some clinical conditions in which this type of failure is seen includes urethral obstruction, prostatic hypertrophy, bladder carcinoma, bladder infection, neurogenic bladder, renal calculi, and abdominal tumors.

There are three phases in ARF—an oliguric phase, a diuretic phase, and a recovery phase. Oliguria occurs when the tubule obstruction and damage makes absorption unstable, and BUN, creatinine, and potassium levels increase. During the diuretic phase, tubular function begins to return but the patient must be monitored for excessive diuresis with loss of electrolytes. When diuresis is no longer excessive, the recovery phase begins with gradual improvement in kidney function for up to one year. There may be a permanent decrease in renal function that, depending on severity, may require dialysis.

MEDICAL CARE

Laboratory: CBC— hemoglobin decreased with anemia, RBCs decreased due to fragility, white blood cell count elevated if sepsis or trauma is precipitating event; BUN and creatinine elevated with ratio of 10:1; serum osmolality increased above 285 mOsm/kg; electrolytes used to show imbalances, with elevated potassium due to retention, hemolysis, or acidosis; sodium usually increased, but may be normal; bicarbonate, pH, and calcium decreased; magnesium, phosphorus, and chloride increased; complement studies may be used to identify lupus nephritis; serum electrophoresis may be used to identify abnormal proteins that may damage kidneys permanently; ASO titer may be used to diagnose recent streptococcal infection that could cause poststreptococcal glomerulonephritis; UA: Urine color is dirty, tea-colored brown, volume is less than 400 cc/day, specific gravity less than 1.020 indicates renal disease and fixed at 1.010 indicates severe renal damage; pH greater than 7.0 seen with UTI, ATN, and chronic renal failure; osmolality less than 350 mOsm/kg indicates tubular damage; creatinine clearance decreased; sodium decreased but may be greater than 40 mEq/L if kidney does not reabsorb sodium; RBCs may be present if infection, renal stones, trauma, or tumor is cause; protein of 3 or 4+ indicates glomerular damage, 1+ or 2+ may indicate infection or interstitial nephritis; casts indicate renal disease or infection, brownish casts and numerous epithelial cells indicate ATN, and red casts indicate acute glomerular nephritis

Electrocardiogram: used to identify dysrhythmias and cardiac changes that may occur with acid-base imbalances or electrolyte imbalance

Radiography: KUB to identify size of structures, cysts, tumors, stones, or abnormal kidney location; chest x-ray to identify fluid overload that may occur with fluid shifts

Radionuclide imaging: may be used to identify hydronephrosis, calicectasis, or delayed filling or emptying, or other causes of ARF

Retrograde pyelogram: may be used to identify abnormalities of ureters or renal pelvis

Renal arteriogram: may be used to identify extravascular irregularities or masses, and provides visualization of renal circulation

Magnetic resonance imaging: may be used to evaluate soft tissue

CT scans: may be used to detect presence of renal disease

Dialysis: emergency and chronic dialysis may be required for ARF; ultrafiltration and CAVH may also be utilized

Surgery: may be required for renal calculi removal, resection of the prostate, or placement of fistula for long-term dialysis

NURSING CARE PLANS

Fluid volume excess

Related to: impairment of renal system regulation, retention of water

Defining characteristics: oliguria, anuria, changes in urine specific gravity, intake greater than output, weight gain, elevated blood pressure, edema, ascites, increased central venous pressure, neck vein distention, dyspnea, orthopnea, crackles, muffled heart tones, decreased hemoglobin and hematocrit, altered electrolytes, increased filling pressures, restlessness, anxiety, water intoxication

Outcome Criteria

Patient will have balanced intake and output, stable weight, stable vital signs and hemodynamic parameters, and have effective dialysis when required.

INTERVENTIONS	RATIONALES
Monitor vital signs and hemodynamic parameters every 1-2 hours.	Hypertension with increases in heart rate may occur when kidneys fail to excrete urine, changes occur within the renin-angiotensin cascade, or with fluid resuscitation. Hemodynamic pressures can facilitate identification of changes with intravascular volume.
Monitor intake and output every 2 hours and prn, noting balance or imbalance per 24 hour period. Estimate insensible losses through lungs, skin, and bowel.	Facilitates identification of fluid requirements based on renal function. Insensible losses can add up to 800-1000 cc/day and metabolism of carbohydrates can liberate up to 350 cc/day of fluid from ingested foods.
Weigh daily.	Changes in body weight help to identify fluid status. Gains over 1 pound/day indicate fluid reten-

INTERVENTIONS	RATIONALES
	tion. Fluid amounts of 500 cc are equivalent to 1 pound.
Auscultate lungs for adventitious breath sounds.	Adventitious breath sounds, such as crackles, will be heard with development of pulmonary edema or congestive heart failure.
Measure urine specific gravity, and note changes in character of urine output.	Specific gravity is less than 1.010 in intrarenal failure and signifies inability to appropriately concentrate the urine.
Administer fluids as warranted with restrictions per physician orders.	Prerenal failure is treated with fluid replacement, occasionally with use of vasopressors. Management of fluids is based on replacement of output from all sources.
Administer diuretics as ordered.	May be given to convert oliguric phase to nonoliguric phase, to flush debris from tubules, decreased hyperkalemia, or foster improved urine output.
Insert Foley catheter as warranted.	Catheterization eliminates potential lower GU tract obstruction and provides for accuracy of measurement of urine output, but may not be treatment of choice due to potential for infection.
Observe for presence and character of edema.	Dependent edema may be present, but pitting edema may not be discernable until the patient has more than 10 pounds of fluid in body. Periorbital edema may be the first clinical evidence of edema and indication of fluid shifting.
Monitor for mental status changes.	May indicate impending hypoxic state, electrolyte imbalances, acidosis, or sepsis.
Monitor arterial blood gases.	May indicate presence of acidosis and facilitate intervention for hypoxemia.
Monitor labwork for alterations.	Electrolyte imbalances may occur from impaired sodium reabsorption, fluid overload, or lack of excretion of potassium.

INTERVENTIONS	RATIONALES
	Hyperkalemia may occur as body attempts to correct acidosis, hypernatremia may indicate total body water deficit, and hyponatremia may result from fluid overloading or inability to conserve sodium. BUN/creatinine ratio, which is normally 10:1 is greater than 20:1 with prerenal failure.
Monitor urine specimen labwork for changes.	Urine sodium less than 20 mEq/L, osmolality above 450 mOsm/kg, and urine creatinine above 40 indicates prerenal failure. Urine sodium above 40 mEq/L, osmolality below 350 mOsm/kg, and urine creatinine below 20 indicates ATN.

Information, Instruction, Demonstration

INTERVENTIONS	RATIONALES
Identify and correct any reversible reason for ARF.	Improvement of perfusion, enhancing cardiac output and hemodynamics, or removal of obstruction may facilitate recovery from ARF and limit residual effects.
Obtain chest x-rays and compare with previous films.	May be used to identify increasing cardiac silhouette, effusions, infiltrates, pulmonary edema, or other complications that may occur with fluid overload.
Administer antihypertensives as warranted/ordered.	May be required to treat hypertension that occurs from decreased renal perfusion or fluid overload.
Instruct patient/family on necessity for fluid restriction.	Promotes understanding and facilitates compliance.
Prepare patient/family for dialysis treatment as warranted.	Dialysis may be required to remove toxic wastes and to correct electrolyte, acid-base, and fluid imbalances.

Discharge or Maintenance Evaluation

- Patient will achieve and maintain urinary output within normal limits for character and amount.

- Patient will have stable weight, vital signs, and hemodynamic parameters.

- Patient will exhibit no respiratory dysfunction and have normal arterial blood gases.

- Patient/family will be able to verbalize understanding of instructions and comply with treatment.

- Patient will have no signs of edema.

- Patient will tolerate dialysis procedure without complications.

Risk for fluid volume deficit

Related to: fluid loss, diuretic phase

Defining characteristics: weight loss, output greater than intake, hypotension, tachycardia, decreased central venous pressure, decreased hemodynamic pressures, increased temperature, dilute urine with low specific gravity, oliguria with high specific gravity, weakness, stupor, lethargy

Outcome Criteria

Patient will exhibit equivalent intake and output, have stable vital signs and weight, and will have urine output within acceptable levels.

INTERVENTIONS	RATIONALES
Monitor vital signs and hemodynamic pressures.	Hypovolemia may result in hypotension and tachycardia.
Observe for complaints of thirst, dry mucous membranes, poor skin turgor, or lethargy.	May indicate presence of dehydration. When extracellular fluid or sodium is depleted, the thirst center is activated. Continued

INTERVENTIONS	RATIONALES
	losses without adequate replacement may lead to hypovolemia and shock.
Measure intake and output every 1-2 hours, or prn, including insensible fluid losses. Compare for balance at least every 24 hours.	Facilitates identification of fluid loss and replacement requirements.
Supply allowed amounts of fluid throughout the day ensuring that all fluids are counted.	Lack of fluid intake maintenance may predispose nocturnal dehydration.
Administer IV fluids as ordered.	May require intermittent fluid boluses to challenge fluid shifting.

Discharge or Maintenance Evaluation

- Patient will have stable weight.

- Patient will have equivalent intake and output.

- Patient will have stable vital signs and hemodynamic parameters.

- Patient will have urine output within normal limits.

- Patient will have normal neurological status.

Alteration in tissue perfusion: renal, cardiopulmonary, cerebral, gastrointestinal, peripheral

Related to: fluid shifts, renal obstruction, impairment of renal function, septic shock, trauma, burns, uremia

Defining characteristics: oliguria, anuria, dehydration, hypotension, abnormal vital signs, abnormal blood gases, abnormal electrolytes, mental status changes, lethargy, nausea, vomiting, skin changes

Outcome Criteria

Patient will have adequate perfusion to all body systems.

INTERVENTIONS	RATIONALES	INTERVENTIONS	RATIONALES
Monitor vital signs and hemodynamic parameters.	Hypertension and fluid volume increases may increase cardiac workload, increase myocardial oxygen demand, and possibly lead to cardiac failure. Blood pressure below 70 mmHg interferes with autoregulatory mechanisms.	Monitor intake and output every 1-2 hours and prn. Measure specific gravity and note changes in character of urine.	Oliguria, with output less than 400 cc/day, and anuria, or no output, may be seen with fluid volume excess or decreased perfusion states. Decreases in urinary output that do not respond to fluid challenges cause renal vasoconstriction and decreased perfusion from increased renin secretion.
Monitor EKG for dysrhythmias or changes in cardiac rhythm, and treat appropriately.	Renal failure and electrolyte imbalances may predispose patient to dysrhythmias and conduction problems. Hypokalemia may be reflected with flat T wave, peaked P wave, and sometimes the presence of a U wave. Hyperkalemia may be reflected with peaked T wave, widened QRS complex, increased PR interval, and flattened P wave. Hypocalcemia may be manifested with QT prolongation. Treatment of potentially-lethal cardiac dysrhythmias may prevent death from complication of renal failure.	Monitor labwork for electrolyte changes.	May have hyperkalemia in oliguric phase changing to hypokalemia with diuretic phase. Potassium levels above 6.5 mEq/L should be treated as a medical emergency. Hypocalcemia produces adverse cardiac effects and potentiates potassium. Hypermagnesemia may occur with use of antacids and cause neuromuscular dysfunction, or cardiac or respiratory arrest.
Monitor neurological status for changes in mentation or level of consciousness.	Decreased perfusion may result in cerebral perfusion decreases resulting in lethargy, weakness, and stupor or from uremic syndrome.	Maintain oximetry of at least 90% by using supplemental oxygen.	Facilitates oxygenation of tissues in the presence of decreased perfusion and increased workload.
Monitor for peripheral pulse presence and character, skin color, appearance of mucous membranes, turgor, capillary refill time.	Pallor may be present with vasoconstriction or anemia, and skin may be cyanotic or mottled with pulmonary edema or cardiac failure.	Monitor arterial blood gases.	Facilitates measurement of actual oxygen levels and identifies acid-base disturbances that may require further intervention.
Auscultate for breath sounds and heart tones, and notify physician of abnormalities.	Fluid overload and decreased perfusion may result in development of S_3 or S_4 gallops, and pericardial friction rub may indicate the presence of uremic pericarditis.	Administer inotropic agents as ordered.	May be required to improve cardiac output, increase myocardial contractility, and improve perfusion.
		Administer glucose/insulin combination as ordered.	May be used as temporary emergent treatment to decrease serum potassium by shifting potassium into the cells.
		Administer polystyrene sulfonate as ordered.	May be used to lower serum potassium by exchanging sodium for potassium in the GI tract. Solutions that also contain sorbitol may also decrease potassium levels by osmotic diarrhea.
Monitor for complaints of numbness, paresthesias, muscle cramps, tremors, twitching, or hyperreflexia.	May indicate impairment of neuromuscular activity, hypocalcemia, and potential for decreased cardiac perfusion and function.	Administer mannitol as ordered.	May be used with muscle trauma for osmotic diuresis, but should

INTERVENTIONS	RATIONALES
	not be given repeatedly if response is not achieved due to accumulations of hyperosmolar compounds that may result in further renal damage and decreased perfusion.

Information, Instruction, Demonstration

INTERVENTIONS	RATIONALES
Prepare patient/family for dialysis as warranted.	Dialysis may be required to remove toxins and excess fluids from body and maintain life until kidney function is restored.
Instruct on specifics of peritoneal dialysis.	Peritoneal dialysis, or PD, may be intermittent, continuous ambulatory peritoneal dialysis (CAPD), or continuous cycling peritoneal dialysis for use overnight. With PD, the peritoneum becomes the dialyzing membrane with dialysate solution infused into the peritoneal cavity, allowed to remain there for 30 minutes and then siphoned out through a closed system. The duration of this dialysis depends on the severity of the renal condition and proportions of the patient. Peritonitis may occur and antibiotics may be added to the dialysate prophylactically.
Instruct on specifics of hemodialysis.	Hemodialysis, or HD, may be used for chronic renal failure patients as well as acute renal failure patients who require short-term dialysis. Blood passes through a semipermeable membrane or kidney, to the dialysate fluid where toxic substances move from the blood to the dialysate solution and are then discarded. Requires circulatory access, and takes 3-4 hours 3 times per week. Complications may include infection, bleeding, or obstruction of vascular access.

Discharge or Maintenance Evaluation

- Patient will achieve normalized perfusion of all body systems.

- Patient will have no long-term effects from perfusion impairment.

- Patient will have normal urine output with no symptoms or signs of ARF.

- Patient will have stable vital signs and hemodynamic pressures.

- Patient will have balanced intake and output with stable weight.

- Patient will have precipitating illness stabilized/resolved.

Alteration in nutrition: less than body requirements

Related to: dietary restrictions, hypercatabolic state

Defining characteristics: elevated BUN and creatinine levels, anorexia, nausea, vomiting, distorted taste perception, fatigue, weakness, loss of weight (dietary restriction), weight gain (non-compliance with fluid restriction), pain, depression, lethargy, oral mucosal lesions

Outcome Criteria

Patient will achieve and maintain nutritional requirements and stable weight.

INTERVENTIONS	RATIONALES
Determine patient's dietary habits and intake. Perform calorie count.	Identifies nutritional deficiencies, non-compliance with restrictions, and metabolic requirements.
Provide several small meals rather than 3 large ones.	Decreases nausea that may occur because of diminished peristalsis.

INTERVENTIONS	RATIONALES
	Smaller meals may not be as overwhelming and may facilitate compliance with restrictions.
Give patient high caloric, low protein, low potassium, low sodium diet as ordered.	Protein requirements for renal failure patients are much less than normal to compensate for their impaired renal function. Increased carbohydrates satisfy energy requirements while restricting catabolism and preventing acid formation from protein and fat metabolism. Restriction of potassium, sodium, and phosphorus may be required to prevent further renal damage.
Assist with/encourage frequent oral care.	Reduces distaste and freshens oral mucosa that may be inflamed.
Weigh daily.	Patient may lose up to 1 pound per day during NPO status.
Administer vitamins/minerals as ordered.	Patient may have iron deficiency secondary to protein restriction, anemia, or impaired GI function and need supplemental iron. Calcium may be given to replace levels and facilitate coagulation and metabolism of bone. Vitamin B complexes are required to maintain cell growth.

Information, Instruction, Demonstration

INTERVENTIONS	RATIONALES
Instruct patient/family member on renal diet.	Protein and electrolytes are adjusted to prevent uremia and electrolyte imbalances. Instruction provides knowledge and may facilitate compliance.
Consult dietician and/or other dietary resources.	May be helpful to discuss choices for meals, replacements for foods previously enjoyed but now restricted, and to allow patient some measure of control over his situation.

Discharge or Maintenance Evaluation

- Patient will achieve and maintain desired weight.
- Patient will be able to tolerate diet without nausea/vomiting.
- Patient will exhibit no evidence of mucosal lesions in mouth.
- Patient will adhere to dietary restrictions.
- Patient will comply with medical regimen and supplementation.

Risk for infection

Related to: renal failure, uremia, debilitation, septic shock, invasive procedures and lines, malnutrition, impaired immune system

Defining characteristics: increased white blood cell count, shift to the left, BUN greater than 100 mg/dl, history of repeated infections, fever, chills, cough with or without sputum production, wound drainage, hypotension, tachycardia, impaired skin integrity, wounds, positive blood, urine, or sputum cultures, cloudy concentrated urine

Outcome Criteria

Patient will exhibit no signs or symptoms of infection.

INTERVENTIONS	RATIONALES
Monitor vital signs and hemodynamic pressures.	Systemic vascular resistance decreases, cardiac output initially increases, blood pressure decreases, and patient has tachycardia, tachypnea, and hyperthermia with warm flushed skin in early stages of septic shock.

INTERVENTIONS	RATIONALES
Obtain urine culture.	Urinary tract infections may be asymptomatic initially.
Avoid insertion of invasive lines, catheters, and procedures whenever possible. Use aseptic/sterile technique for changing IV sites, dressing changes, or caring for catheters.	Decreases potential of bacteria gaining entrance to body and prevents risk of cross-contamination.
Observe wounds for drainage, noting changes in amount, color, and character. Change IV sites per hospital protocol.	Allows for identification of detrimental changes in wound status and facilitates timely intervention. Early detection of infection may preclude the development of septicemia.
Observe PD return fluid for cloudiness.	May indicate presence of peritonitis from perforation or loss of albumin.
Maintain adequate nutrition.	Facilitates healing and body metabolism.
Utilize appropriate isolation techniques when warranted.	Prevents cross-contamination and minimizes patient's risk of secondary infection.
Reposition patient every 2 hours, and encourage coughing and deep breathing.	Decreases potential for atelectasis and facilitates mobilizing secretions to avoid respiratory infection.
Obtain cultures as ordered.	Facilitates identification of causative organism and allows for appropriate antimicrobial treatment.
Administer antimicrobials as ordered.	May be required to combat infection.

Information, Instruction, Demonstration

INTERVENTIONS	RATIONALES
Instruct patient to avoid scratching and to maintain skin integrity.	May precipitate infection and worsen renal dysfunction.
Monitor labwork, especially BUN and creatinine, CBC, and	BUN should be maintained lower than 100 mg/dl to decrease

INTERVENTIONS	RATIONALES
differential.	potential for infection. CBC will identify presence of infection, and will be helpful to monitor therapeutic response to antimicrobials.

Discharge or Maintenance Evaluation

- Patient will be free of infection.

- Patient will be able to verbalize understanding of instructions to prevent infection complications.

- Patient will not develop septic shock.

Risk for impaired skin integrity

Related to: uremia, malnutrition, immobility

Defining characteristics: dry skin, edema, presence of wounds, presence of invasive lines/grafts/fistulas, uremic frost, bruising, erythema, pruritus, changes in skin texture and thickness

Outcome Criteria

Patient will maintain skin integrity or will have wound healing in a timely manner.

INTERVENTIONS	RATIONALES
Observe skin for wounds, pressure areas, abrasions, drainage, redness, rashes.	Prompt identification allows for timely intervention.
Bathe patient daily using oil in bath, and scant soap. Provide skin care with lotion or creams.	Removes waste products from skin while keeping skin supple and moist.
Administer antipruritic drugs as ordered.	Persistent itching may cause patient to scratch body to the point of bleeding and medication will help allay strong urge to

INTERVENTIONS	RATIONALES
	scratch. Open areas of skin are more susceptible to infection.
Reposition every 2 hours. Avoid constricting garments.	Decreases potential for skin breakdown.

Discharge or Maintenance Evaluation

- Patient will have clean, dry, intact skin.

- Patient will be free of itching.

- Patient will have no signs/symptoms of infection.

- Patient will have timely wound healing with no complications.

Risk for injury

Related to: altered metabolism and excretion of medications, kidney failure

Defining characteristics: decreased cardiac output states, acidosis, decreased protein binding, presence of uremia, competition for binding sites, decreased body stores of fat, decreased GI motility, changes in gastric pH, electrolyte imbalances, decreased protein binding, present renal failure

Outcome Criteria

Patient will be able to tolerate all pharmacological agents without adverse effects on renal or other body systems.

INTERVENTIONS	RATIONALES
Determine methods of action and excretion of all drugs being taken, as well as interactions among them.	Facilitates understanding of how uremia may affect drug effects. Conditions that reduce renal perfusion limits the amount of drug that the kidney is exposed to and decreases the amount of metabolism or excretion of the drug.

INTERVENTIONS	RATIONALES
Monitor for presence of acidosis.	Acidosis may interfere with absorption of some drugs.
Ensure that nephrotoxic drugs are utilized only when absolutely necessary.	Nephrotoxics will further impair renal failure.
Monitor patient for signs and symptoms of drug toxicity, and obtain serum drug levels for specific drugs in use.	Excretion of drugs may be hindered by renal failure and result in toxic levels with normally safe dosages.

Information, Instruction, Demonstration

INTERVENTIONS	RATIONALES
Instruct patient on all medications being taken, with symptoms to be reported.	Facilitates knowledge and increases compliance.
Give reduced drug dosages with longer time intervals between doses.	Decreases potential for toxic reaction to dosage with impaired excretion and metabolism.

Discharge or Maintenance Evaluation

- Patient will comply and tolerate therapeutic regimen with no adverse drug effects noted.

- Patient will have serum drug levels within therapeutic ranges.

- Patient will exhibit no signs of toxicity to drugs.

- Patient will have stable renal function.

- Patient will be able to verbalize understanding of all instructions and be able to identify medications being taken.

Altered oral mucous membrane

Related to: uremia, restriction on fluids, lesions, thrush

Defining characteristics: dry mouth, dry mucous membranes, taste distortion, presence of lesions, inflammation, white patches on mucosa, coated tongue, stomatitis, gingivitis

Outcome Criteria

Patient will have moist mucous membranes and be free of oral lesions and inflammation.

INTERVENTIONS	RATIONALES
Observe mouth and oral cavity at least every shift, noting lesions, redness, drainage, vesicles, lacerations, or ulcers.	Facilitates identification of problem to permit prompt treatment and resolution.
Differentiate inflammation of the mucosa from thrush, and administer nystatin suspension as ordered.	Thrush is initially identified as white patches on the tongue and mucosa, and occurs frequently in the presence of multiple antimicrobial agents as a fungal growth. Nystatin is the drug of choice for thrush.
Provide oral care at least every 2 hours, with peroxide rinses or normal saline as ordered.	Removes build-up of debris, moistens mouth, and decreases bad taste.
Use topical anesthetics as ordered.	Viscous xylocaine or Chloraseptic may be used to anesthetize mucosal pain receptors.

Discharge or Maintenance Evaluation

- Patient will be free of oral mucosal lesions and pain.

- Patient will exhibit no evidence of inflammation or infection to mouth.

- Patient will be able to swallow without discomfort.

- Patient will have no taste distortion and will be able to ingest adequate nutrition.

Fatigue
[See DKA]

Related to: anemia, restriction on diet, increased metabolic needs

Defining characteristics: lack of energy, inability to maintain normal activities, lethargy, disinterest

Anxiety
[See MI]

Related to: change in health status, fear of death, threat to role functioning, threat to body image

Defining characteristics: restlessness, insomnia, anorexia, increased respirations, heart rate, and/or blood pressure, dry mouth, poor eye contact, decreased energy, irritability, crying, feelings of helplessness

ACUTE RENAL FAILURE (ARF)

Diabetic Ketoacidosis (D K A)

Diabetic ketoacidosis, or DKA, is a critical emergency state that is caused by a deficiency of insulin in patients with insulin-dependent diabetes mellitus. This deficiency can be caused by physiological causes, or by failure to take an adequate amount of insulin, and results in hyperglycemia, ketonuria, metabolic acidosis, and dehydration. Precipitating causes include failure to take an adequate amount of insulin on a daily basis or failure to increase and compensate for acute infection processes, surgery, trauma, pregnancy, or other acute stress events. Early symptoms include polyuria, polydipsia, fatigue, drowsiness, headache, muscle cramps and nausea/vomiting. Later symptoms, such as Kussmaul breathing, sweet, fruity breath odor, hypotension, and weak and thready pulses will precede stupor and coma.

Treatment is aimed at correction of the acidotic state, hyperglycemia, hyperosmolality, hypovolemia, and potassium deficits, in conjunction with treatment of the underlying cause of the problem.

MEDICAL CARE

Laboratory: serum glucose level is increased above 300 mg/dl and may be greater than 1000 mg/dl; serum acetone positive; lipids and cholesterol levels elevated; osmolality increased but normally less than 330 mOsm/L; potassium initially normal or elevated due to cellular shifting, then later decreased; sodium may be decreased, normal, or elevated; phosphorus is often decreased; amylase can be elevated if pancreatitis is precipitating cause; serum insulin may be decreased in type I DM or normal to high in type II suggesting that there is improper utilization of insulin or that insulin resistance may have developed secondary to antibody formation; BUN may be elevated if dehydration is severe and renal perfusion is decreased; urinalysis will show positive for glucose and acetone, specific gravity and osmolality may be elevated; hemoglobin A_{1C} helps to differentiate whether episode is due to poor control of DM over previous few months or whether episode is incident-related; hematocrit may be elevated with dehydration; elevation of WBCs may occur in response to hemoconcentration or to stress; cultures may be helpful to discern potential cause of infection which may be precipitating factor

Arterial blood gases: pH will be less than 7.3, bicarbonate levels will be decreased, usually less than 15 mEq/L

Electrocardiogram: may show changes associated with electrolyte imbalances, especially hyperkalemia, with peaked T waves

NURSING CARE PLANS

Fluid volume deficit

Related to: hyperglycemic-induced osmotic diuresis, vomiting, inadequate oral intake

Defining characteristics: dry mucous membranes, decreased skin turgor, thirst, hypotension, orthostatic changes, tachycardia, weak and thready pulse, weight loss, intake less than output, increased urinary output, dilute urine

Outcome Criteria

Patient will have stable vital signs, adequate skin turgor, intake and output equivalent, and electrolyte levels within acceptable ranges.

INTERVENTIONS	RATIONALES
Monitor vital signs, especially noting respiratory status changes or alterations in blood pressure.	Tachycardia and hypotension are classic symptoms of hypovolemia. When systolic BP drops more than

INTERVENTIONS	RATIONALES
	10 mmHg when position is changed may indicate severity of hypovolemic state. Kussmaul's respirations may be present depending on degree of hyperglycemia, and respiratory changes may occur as the lungs attempt to remove acids by creating a compensatory respiratory alkalosis. Fever, in conjunction with flushed, dry skin, may indicate dehydration.
Monitor intake and output every 2-4 hours.	Facilitates measurement and effectiveness of volume replacement and adequate circulating fluid volume.
Administer IV fluids per hospital protocol, usually at least 2-3 L/day, and usually initially, 3+ L.	Amounts and solution types may vary based upon the degree of dehydration and patient status. Usual solutions of normal or half-normal saline with or without dextrose are used, as well as occasional use of plasma expanders depending on unsuccessful fluid rehydration.
Weigh every day.	Assesses fluid status.
Observe for complaints of nausea/vomiting, abdominal bloating, or distention.	Gastric motility may be affected by fluid deficits, and vomiting or other gastric losses may potentiate fluid and electrolyte imbalances.
Auscultate lungs for crackles, and assess patient for presence of edema, or bounding pulses.	Congestive heart failure or circulatory overload may occur with rapid rehydration.
Insert catheter per hospital policy.	Provides for more accurate assessment of output, especially if urinary retention or incontinence is present.
Monitor laboratory tests for BUN and creatinine, serum osmolality, hematocrit, and electrolytes.	Hematocrit may be elevated because of hemoconcentration following osmotic diuresis. Dehydration may result in cellular destruction and may result in renal insufficiency. Dehydration will result in elevated osmolality. Potassium levels are usually ele-

INTERVENTIONS	RATIONALES
	vated initially in response to the acidosis, but with diuresis, a hypokalemic state will ensue. Sodium may be decreased with shifting of fluids, and high sodium levels may indicate either a severe fluid loss or sodium reabsorption in response to aldosterone secretion.
Administer electrolyte replacements as per hospital policy/doctor's orders.	Phosphate replacement may help with plasma buffering capacity, but excessive replacement can cause hypocalcemia. Potassium supplementation is usually done as soon as urinary output is adequate to prevent hypokalemic states. As insulin replacement occurs and acidosis is corrected, hypokalemia usually occurs.
Assess patient's mental status and observe for significant changes in status.	Mental status changes can occur with exceedingly high or low glucose levels, electrolyte imbalances, acidotic states, hypoxia, or with decreases in cerebral perfusion pressure.

Information, Instruction, Demonstration

INTERVENTIONS	RATIONALES
Instruct patient/family members regarding signs/symptoms of hyperglycemia.	Provides information and promotes more timely identification of complications.
Instruct in seeking medical attention for infective processes or illness that may deplete circulating volume.	Infection may predispose the patient to fever and a hypermetabolic state which may increase volume depletion.

Discharge or Maintenance Evaluation

• Patient will have vital signs and hemodynamic parameters within acceptable ranges.

• Patient will have normal skin turgor with adequate output.

• Patient will have electrolytes and glucose levels within normal ranges.

Alteration in nutrition: less than body requirements

Related to: insulin deficiency, excessive amounts of epinephrine, growth hormone, and cortisol, increased protein-fat metabolism, decreased oral intake, nausea, vomiting, altered mental status, infection

Defining characteristics: weakness, fatigue, increased levels of glucose and ketones, weight loss in spite of polyphagia, lack of adequate food intake, glycosuria

Outcome Criteria

Patient will be able to have intake of appropriate amounts and types of calories and nutrients, and have glucose levels within acceptable range for patient.

INTERVENTIONS	RATIONALES
Obtain weight every day.	Facilitates assessment of nutritional utilization and fluid shifts.
Provide high-nutrient liquids as soon as patient is able to tolerate oral intake, with progression to solid food as tolerated.	Provides nutrition and helps restore bowel function.
Auscultate bowel sounds every 4–8 hours, and observe for abdominal distention or pain.	Elevated glucose levels can cause altered electrolyte levels and both may decrease gastric function. DKA may also mimic an acute surgical abdomen.
Monitor for changes in level of consciousness, cool or clammy skin, tachycardia, extreme hunger, anxiety, headache, light-headedness, tremors, or irritability.	When carbohydrate metabolism begins and blood glucose level decreases, hypoglycemia can occur. Comatose patients may not exhibit any noticeable change in mentation status and should be monitored closely. Long-standing diabetic patients

INTERVENTIONS	RATIONALES
	may not show normal signs of hypoglycemia due in part to their diminished response to low glucose levels.
Administer regular insulin, either by continuous infusion after an IV bolus dose has been given, by intramuscular injections every 1-2 hours, or by subcutaneous injection.	Subcutaneous route may be an option if the patient's peripheral perfusion is adequate but the response will not be as rapid as with IV administration. Regular insulin is rapid acting and will assist in movement of glucose into cells. The continuous IV method is normally preferred because it optimizes transition to carbohydrate metabolism, and helps to reduce hypoglycemia. Normally, the infusion rate is 5–10 Units/hr until glucose levels decrease within a stated parameter. Another goal of IV administration of insulin is to decrease the acidosis.
Monitor serum glucose every hour while on insulin IV infusion, and notify MD per parameters of when blood glucose has dropped to 250 mg/dl.	Blood glucose levels will decrease with insulin therapy usually in increments of 75 to 100 mg/dl/hr. Once the blood sugar has dropped to 250 mg/dl, and depending upon the degree of acidosis that is present, dextrose is added to the IV infusion, and the insulin infusion should be stopped to prevent hypoglycemic episodes.
Administer subcutaneous insulin 1-2 hours before stopping the continuous insulin infusion.	Prevents recurrence of ketosis and rebound hyperglycemia.
Administer IV solutions containing dextrose as ordered.	Dextrose solutions are usually added after the blood glucose levels have decreased to 250 mg/dl in order to avoid hypoglycemia.
Administer Reglan IV or PO as ordered by physician.	May be used to treat symptoms related to neuropathies that affect the GI tract, and facilitate oral intake and nutrient absorption.

Information, Instruction, Demonstration

INTERVENTIONS	RATIONALES
Instruct patient/family member in dietary management, with ideal amounts of 60% carbohydrates, 20% fats, and 20% proteins to be divided in designated number of meals and snacks.	Complex carbohydrates decrease the amounts of insulin needs, reduce serum cholesterol, and help to satiate patient. Food should be scheduled for peak effects with insulin as well as patient preference. Snacks are important to prevent Somogyi responses and hypoglycemia during sleep.
Obtain consult with dietician.	Assists in facilitating adjustments to diet for patient's special needs, and can facilitate development of workable meal plans.
Instruct in correct procedure for fingerstick glucose testing, with return demonstration as needed.	Monitoring blood glucose levels is more accurate than urine glucose testing, and can facilitate identification of alterations in levels of glucose to promote tighter control of varying glucose levels/insulin usage.
Ensure that at least 50 cc of solution is flushed through the tubing prior to connection to patient when intravenous insulin drips are utilized.	Promotes saturation of binding sites on plastic tubing to decrease incidence of insulin adhering to tubing rather than staying in solution.

Discharge or Maintenance Evaluation

- Patient will have normalized blood glucose levels within their own special parameters.

- Patient will be able to ingest oral food of sufficient amounts and nutrients to maintain and stabilize weight.

- Patient will be free of ketosis.

- Patient/family member will be able to verbalize understanding of instructions and able to provide acceptable return demonstration of procedure.

Impaired gas exchange

Related to: accumulation of ketones and acids secondary to insulin deficiencies and excessive production of stress hormones

Defining characteristics: acid-base imbalances, acetone breath, tachypnea, Kussmaul respirations, serum and urine ketones present, decreased pH, decreased bicarbonate levels, hyperkalemia, decreased level of consciousness, confusion

Outcome Criteria

Patient will have normalized acid-base balance with stable vital signs and mentation level.

INTERVENTIONS	RATIONALES
Monitor respiratory status for changes in rate, rhythm and depth, and for presence of acetone smell on breath.	Acetone breath is due to breakdown of acetoacetic acids. The lungs remove carbonic acid through respiration process, and may produce a compensatory respiratory alkalosis for ketoacidosis. Increased work of breathing may indicate that the patient is losing the ability to compensate for the severe acidosis or respiratory fatigue.
Monitor for changes in neurological status.	Acidosis, hypoxia, or decreased cerebral perfusion may cause changes in mentation. Impairment in consciousness may predispose the patient to aspiration and its complications.
Administer IV fluids and insulin as ordered.	Promote correction of acidosis with DKA.
Administer sodium bicarbonate, if ordered, for severe acidosis only.	Current recommendations are for use only where pH is 7.1 or below because excessive use of sodium bicarbonate may induce hypokalemia as well as alter the oxygen dissociation curve causing prolongation of the comatose state.

INTERVENTIONS	RATIONALES
Monitor labwork for hypokalemia.	May occur as acidosis and volume deficits are corrected.
Administer supplemental oxygen as necessary per hospital protocol.	Provides needed oxygen especially in patients that may not be able to obtain adequate oxygenation with room air, and helps to improve acidosis.

Discharge or Maintenance Evaluation

• Patient will have pH, bicarbonate, potassium, serum and urine ketones within normal limits.

• Patient will have stable vital signs with respiratory rate within normal limits.

• Patient will be free of acetone on breath.

Risk for infection

Related to: elevated glucose levels, alterations in circulation, pre-existing infection, especially URI or UTI, decreased leukocyte function

Defining characteristics: increased serum and urine glucose levels, temperature elevation, chills, fever, elevated white blood cell count, differential with shift to the left

Outcome Criteria

Patient will be free of infection and able to verbalize methods to prevent or reduce risk of infection.

INTERVENTIONS RATIONALES	
Monitor for fever, facial flushing, drainage from wounds, urine cloudiness, changes in sputum, tachycardia.	Patient may have been admitted with undiagnosed infection or have developed a nosocomial infection.
Auscultate for changes in breath sounds.	Accumulation of bronchial secretions may be heard as rhonchi and may indicate the presence of

INTERVENTIONS	RATIONALES
	bronchitis or pneumonia, either of which may be the precipitating cause of the DKA. Crackles may indicate fluid overload or congestive failure as a result from rapid fluid replacement.
Provide perineal or catheter care frequently.	Elderly female diabetics are prone to the development of urinary tract and vaginal infections.
Reposition patient and provide skin care every 2 hours.	Facilitates lung expansion, decreases risk of skin irritation and breakdown, and improves peripheral circulation.
Obtain culture specimens as ordered or as per hospital policy.	Assists with identification of causative organism and appropriate antimicrobial therapy.
Administer antibiotics as ordered.	Early intervention may reduce the risk of sepsis or multi-system involvement.

Information, Instruction, Demonstration

INTERVENTIONS	RATIONALES
Ensure proper handwashing techniques are used by staff and patient.	Prevents cross-contamination and decreases risk of spread of infection.
Maintain aseptic technique with administration of IV medications, insertion of catheters and invasive lines, and maintenance care. Restart IVs per hospital protocol.	Elevated glucose levels provide an excellent culture medium for bacterial growth.
Instruct patients in perineal care, disposal of secretions and infected materials.	Promotes compliance, minimizes risk of spread of infection, and cross-contamination.
Instruct in importance of oral care.	Reduces risk of oral or gum disease.

Discharge or Maintenance Evaluation

• Patient will be able to identify actions to reduce or prevent infection and cross-contamination.

- Patient will be free of infective process.

- Patient will be able to adequately demonstrate techniques to prevent or reduce infection risk.

Potential for injury: hypoglycemia

Related to: insulin therapy, decreased insulin-antagonist hormones circulating in body, rebound action

Defining characteristics: blood glucose levels below 70 mg/dl, altered mental state, decreased level of consciousness, cool and clammy skin, pallor, tremors, tachycardia, irritability, visual disturbances, paresthesias, dizziness, hunger, nausea, fatigue, diaphoresis

Outcome Criteria

Patient will have stable blood glucose levels and be able to identify methods of treatment and identification of hypoglycemic episodes.

INTERVENTIONS	RATIONALES
Monitor for signs/symptoms of hypoglycemia.	Prompt identification of problem will facilitate prompt treatment and help prevent further complications.
Change IV fluid to solution containing glucose when blood glucose level reached 250 mg/dl, as well as change infusion rate on insulin drip.	Prevents excessive drop in blood glucose level and allows time for blood chemistry to normalize.
If hypoglycemia occurs, give the patient oral (if able to tolerate fluids and awake) or parenteral glucose solutions, as per policy.	Glucagon, 10-50% solutions, may be given IV, or 15 grams of a rapid-acting carbohydrate will be effective in elevating the blood sugar level. Milk and crackers will assist in protecting patient from recurrences of hypoglycemic episode.

Information, Instruction, Demonstration

INTERVENTIONS	RATIONALES
Instruct patient/family in signs of hypoglycemia and treatment for this condition.	Promotes knowledge and facilitates compliance. Assists patient and family to feel in control.

Discharge or Maintenance Evaluation

- Patient will have stable blood glucose level above 80 mg/dl.

- Patient/family member will be able to identify signs and symptoms of hypoglycemia and interventions for treatment.

- Patient will have no hypoglycemic symptoms.

Fatigue

Related to: insufficient insulin, increased metabolic demands, decreased metabolic energy production, infection

Defining characteristics: lack of energy, inability to perform normal routine, decreased performance, accident prone, lethargy, tiredness, alterations in consciousness

Outcome Criteria

Patient will have increased energy and be able to participate adequately in normal activities.

INTERVENTIONS	RATIONALES
Observe patient for activity tolerance.	Provides baseline information so that identification of problem and interventions may be planned. Elevations in pulse, blood pressure and respiratory rate may indicate physiologic intolerance of activity.
Provide period of rest or sleep	Prevents excessive fatigue.

INTERVENTIONS	RATIONALES
alternated with periods of activity as patient can tolerate.	
Increase activity and patient participation gradually.	Provides time to build up tolerance, and increases self-esteem.

Information, Instruction, Demonstration

INTERVENTIONS	RATIONALES
Discuss with patient/family member the importance of activity, planning schedules with alternating rest and activity, and methods of conserving energy.	Information may facilitate motivation to increase activity level knowing that decreased energy will be expended and he will be able to accomplish more activity.

Discharge or Maintenance Evaluation

- Patient will be able to tolerate increased activity with stable vital signs.

- Patient/family will be able to verbalize and/or demonstrate techniques to conserve energy while performing activities.

Knowledge deficit

Related to: lack of information, lack of recall, misinterpreted information, unfamiliarity with resources

Defining characteristics: requests for information, questions, misrepresentation of facts, inaccurate follow-through of instructions, development of preventable complications

Outcome Criteria

Patient will be able to verbalize understanding of diabetes disease process, identify signs and symptoms of complications, correctly demonstrate all procedures, and access community resources adequately.

INTERVENTIONS	RATIONALES
Instruct patient/family member about disease process, normal ranges for blood glucose, glucometer use, relationship between insulin and glucose levels, type of diabetes the patient has, etc.	Provides knowledge base on which further instruction can be performed.
Instruct patient/family member in glucometer use and urine testing, with return demonstration by patient.	Promotes tighter control of diabetes with self-monitoring at least four times per day, and may help prevent or delay long-term complications.
Instruct in dietary plan, allowances, caloric intake, meals outside the home, etc.	Dietary control with assist with maintenance of decreased blood glucose levels. Fiber may slow glucose absorption and decrease fluctuations in serum levels.
Instruct in medication regime, with actions, side effects, and contraindications noted.	Promotes understanding of drug use and facilitates compliance with regimen. Proper techniques with administration of insulin assist with understanding and identification of potential problems so that interventions may be found.
Instruct in activity and other factors that determine diabetic control.	Promotes control of diabetes and may help reduce incidence of ketoacidosis. Aerobic exercises promote effective utilization of insulin and strengthens the cardiovascular system. Illness management and management of other stress-type factors facilitates equilibrium with disease process during these episodes.
Instruct in avoidance of smoking.	Nicotine causes constriction of blood vessels which restricts insulin absorption up to 30%.
Instruct in examination and care of feet.	Identifies potential complications that may occur because of peripheral neuropathy or circulatory impairment, and allows for early intervention.
Instruct in protocols for sick days—to take medications, to notify MD, to monitor blood sugar every 2-4 hours, to check	Provides plan for complications that occur, and gives the patient the knowledge to enable him to adequately care for himself

INTERVENTIONS	RATIONALES
urine ketones if blood sugar is >240 mg/dl, and to replace carbohydrates with liquids	during times of illness.
Instruct in maintaining medical maintenance, including vision checks, and follow-up care.	Vision changes may be gradual and may be more pronounced in poorly-controlled diabetics. Visual acuity may deteriorate to retinopathy and eventual blindness. Follow-up care can assist in preventing exacerbations of diabetic complications and delay development of systemic problems.
Discuss sexual function and questions patient/family member may ask.	Impotence may occur as an initial symptom of diabetes mellitus. Penile prosthesis and/or counseling may be of help.
Instruct in avoidance of use of over-the-counter medications without physician approval.	May contain increased sugar content and may interact with other medications being taken.
Instruct in available community resources, support groups like the American Diabetic Association, smoking and weight loss clinics, etc.	Provides continued support post discharge, and assists to support lifestyle changes.

Discharge or Maintenance Evaluation

• Patient/family member will be able to accurately verbalize knowledge base regarding diabetic disease process.

• Patient/family member will be able to accurately verbalize all information given.

• Patient/family member will be able to accurately return demonstration for all necessary procedures.

DIABETIC KETOACIDOSIS (DKA)

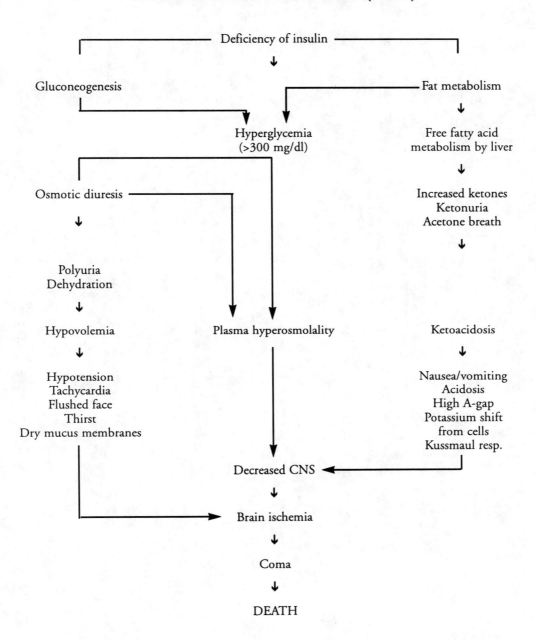

Deficiency of insulin

Gluconeogenesis

Fat metabolism

Hyperglycemia
(>300 mg/dl)

Free fatty acid
metabolism by liver

Osmotic diuresis

Increased ketones
Ketonuria
Acetone breath

Polyuria
Dehydration

Hypovolemia

Plasma hyperosmolality

Ketoacidosis

Hypotension
Tachycardia
Flushed face
Thirst
Dry mucus membranes

Nausea/vomiting
Acidosis
High A-gap
Potassium shift
from cells
Kussmaul resp.

Decreased CNS

Brain ischemia

Coma

DEATH

Hyperglycemic Hyperosmolar Nonketotic Coma (H H N K)

HHNK, or hyperglycemic hyperosmolar nonke-totic coma, may also be known as hyperglycemic nonacidotic diabetic coma, and presents a life-threatening emergency. Glucose transportation across the cell membrane is impaired by enough of an insulin deficiency that causes hyperglycemia without inhibiting lipolysis or ketogenesis in the liver. The hyperosmolality occurs from the hyper-natremia and hyperglycemia, and may further impair the secretion of insulin and prevent fatty acid release from adipose tissues. Extracellular fluid volume deficits occur as a result of osmotic diuresis in the body's attempt to offset increasing plasma osmolality. As fluid volume deficits increase, glomerular filtration rates decrease and reduces the ability of the kidneys to excrete the glucose.

HHNK occurs when insulin action or secretion is inadequate, and may occur in patients who have no previous history of diabetes mellitus. The elderly are especially prone to this because of the lower body water content and dehydration, and this may alter their buffering ability to respond to changes in osmolality. Illnesses, and other stress-provoking episodes, may either cause or hasten the development of HHNK by increasing glucose pro-duction in response to excessive stress hormone production.

HHNK has almost the same pathophysiologic pattern as DKA, but the difference is that with HHNK, a sufficient amount of insulin is being released to prevent the development of ketosis.

HHNK has also been associated with usage of thi-azide diuretics, glucocorticoids, phenytoin, sympathomimetics, diazoxide, chlorpromazine, sedatives, cimetidine, calcium channel blockers, and immunosuppressive agents because of their effects with glucogenesis and/or insulin.

Mortality is approximately 50% due in part to common complications that occur, such as shock, coma, acute tubular necrosis, and vascular throm-bosis. Correction of the problem is the main goal of treatment, with fluid balance the initial concern. The lack of insulin may be corrected by supplemental insulin administration and usually requires 100 Units or less in the first 24 hour period. Electrolyte imbalances are corrected and may require large amounts of potassium supple-mentation.

MEDICAL CARE

Laboratory: blood sugar level elevated, frequently over 1000 mg/dl; plasma osmolality elevated, fre-quently as high as 450 mOsm/kg; hematocrit elevated due to hemoconcentration; urine and serum acetone levels negative; BUN and creatinine elevated; marked leukocytosis; electrolytes to eval-uate deficiency; hypernatremia usually present

Arterial blood gases: used to identify acidosis; pH is usually greater than 7.30, bicarbonate is usually greater than 15 mEq/L; acidosis is mainly due to lactic acid or renal dysfunction

Electrocardiogram: used to identify dysrhythmias that may result as a consequence of electrolyte and fluid disturbances

NURSING CARE PLANS

Fluid volume deficit
[See DKA]

Alteration in nutrition: less than body requirements
[See DKA]

Potential for injury: hypoglycemia
[See DKA]

Potential for alteration in tissue perfusion: peripheral

Related to: dehydration, increased platelet aggregation, increased viscosity of blood

Defining characteristics: cool extremities, decreased peripheral pulses, extremity pallor or cyanosis, unequal extremity temperatures

Outcome Criteria

Patient will have bilaterally equal peripheral pulses, color and temperature to extremities, with no complications.

INTERVENTIONS	RATIONALES
Monitor and assess lower extremities for color, temperature, presence of pulses, and equality.	Identifies the status of circulation in the extremities and assists with prompt identification of complications.
Test for positive Homan's sign, redness, warmth, tenderness, or swelling to legs.	May indicate thrombus formation, but is not always present with thrombus formation.
Remove TED hose at least every 8 hours for 30 minutes to 1 hour.	Provides opportunity for thorough assessment and identification of changes, as well as for comfort of patient.
Assist with passive range of motion/encourage active range of motion exercises.	Prevents venous stasis.

Information, Instruction, Demonstration

INTERVENTIONS	RATIONALES
Instruct patient/family member to avoid constricting apparel, crossing legs or ankles, or any other activity that impedes circulation.	Prevents circulatory impairment and risk of complications.
Notify physician for any evidence of thrombus formation.	Prompt identification can lead to timely intervention.

Discharge or Maintenance Evaluation

• Patient will have equal pulses, color, and temperature to lower extremities bilaterally.

• Patient will have no evidence of thrombus formation.

• Patient/family will be compliant with methods to reduce risk of thrombus formation.

HYPERGLYCEMIC HYPEROSMOLAR NONKETOTIC COMA (HHNK)

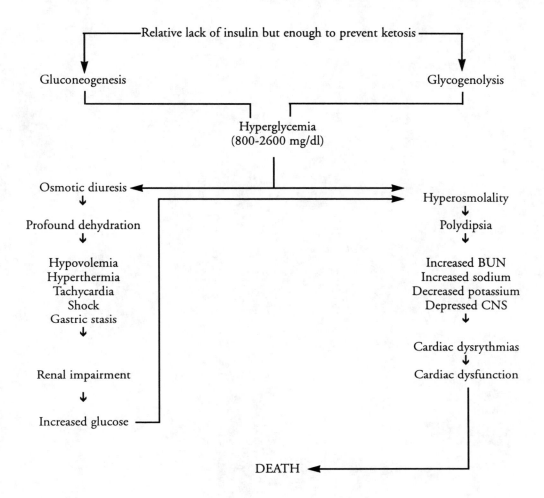

Relative lack of insulin but enough to prevent ketosis

Gluconeogenesis   Glycogenolysis

Hyperglycemia
(800-2600 mg/dl)

Osmotic diuresis   Hyperosmolality
↓   ↓
Profound dehydration   Polydipsia
↓   ↓

Hypovolemia   Increased BUN
Hyperthermia   Increased sodium
Tachycardia   Decreased potassium
Shock   Depressed CNS
Gastric stasis   ↓
↓   Cardiac dysrythmias
     ↓
Renal impairment   Cardiac dysfunction
↓

Increased glucose

DEATH

Syndrome of Inappropriate ADH Secretion (SIADH)

SIADH is another dysfunction of the antidiuretic hormone in which there is increased secretion or production of ADH. The increase is not related to osmolality, and therefore causes a slight increase in body water. Sodium concentration is decreased in the extracellular fluid and plasma. SIADH is usually caused by bronchogenic or pancreatic cancer, but can occasionally result from pituitary tumors. Other etiologies include central nervous system injuries, infections and tumors, pulmonary diseases, Addison's disease, hypopituitarism, aneurysms, AIDS, and use of tricyclic drugs, oral hypoglycemics, acetaminophen, chlorpropamide, thiazide diuretics, cytotoxic agents, and excessive vasopressin therapy.

Unlike diabetes insipidus, SIADH has a failure of the negative feedback system in which continued ADH secretion creates water intoxication because of low plasma osmolality and expanded volume. The primary initial goal is to restrict fluid intake and correct electrolyte imbalances. With severe cases, 3% hypertonic saline and IV lasix are used.

MEDICAL CARE

Laboratory: plasma sodium decreased, plasma osmolality decreased, urine sodium and osmolality increased, elevated plasma ADH levels; renal profiles used to assess renal status changes from imbalances and from nephrotoxic medications; thyroid profiles to assess thyroid function; electrolytes to evaluate concurrent imbalances

Electrocardiogram: used to identify cardiac dysrhythmias that may occur as a result of electrolyte or fluid imbalances

Nursing Care Plans

Fluid volume excess

Related to: inability to excrete water, inappropriate antidiuretic hormone secretion, failure of negative feedback system

Defining characteristics: hyponatremia, decreased plasma osmolality, increased urine osmolality, weight gain, neurologic disturbances, seizures

INTERVENTIONS	RATIONALES
Monitor for changes in level of consciousness, fatigue, weakness, headache or generalized pain.	May be early indication of impending water intoxication.
Monitor heart rhythm and hemodynamics as ordered.	Fluid shifts and electrolyte disturbances can precipitate cardiac dysrhythmias and changes in hemodynamic status.
Weigh patient every day, and maintain accurate I&O.	Assists with identification of fluid status/balance.
Administer IV and PO fluids as ordered, maintaining fluid restriction.	Restriction of fluid may be based partially on urine, nasogastric, or other fluid losses.
Administer hypertonic saline IV when ordered.	These types of infusions are generally reserved for severe hyponatremia or when accompanied by seizure activity. Fluid overload may worsen and deteriorate into heart failure. There are controversial theories that sudden increases in serum sodium can result in osmotic demyelination syndrome which may have adapted to the lower level of sodium.
Administer diuretics as ordered.	Assists with decreasing the action of ADH, but can also cause electrolyte losses.
Administer other drugs that help inhibit ADH action, as ordered.	Lithium and demeclocycline interfere with ADH at the renal tubular level, but can be nephrotoxic. Phenytoin inhibits ADH release.

INTERVENTIONS	RATIONALES
Administer supplemental electrolytes as ordered.	Facilitates replacement of required electrolytes to maintain function.

Information, Instruction, Demonstration

INTERVENTIONS	RATIONALES
Monitor lab studies, especially renal profiles for changes in renal perfusion.	Some medications are nephrotoxic and can worsen renal function.
Instruct patient/family regarding fluid balance, seizure precautions, drug therapy, procedures, lab studies, etc.	Promotes knowledge, and encourages compliance with medical regimen. Facilitates patient taking active part in his care.

Discharge or Maintenance Evaluation

- Patient will be neurologically stable with approximately equivalent intake and output, and vital signs will be stable.

- Patient will have normalized weight and be able to maintain weight.

- Patient will have laboratory values within normal parameters.

- Patient/family will be able to accurately verbalize understanding of all instructions.

Risk for injury
[See Status Epilepticus]

Related to: impairment of cognitive ability, physical inactivity, seizure activity

Defining characteristics: confusion, lethargy, memory impairment, irritability, personality changes, level of consciousness changes, restlessness, fatigue, weakness, seizures, imposed physical inactivity

Constipation

Related to: decreased gastric motility secondary to hyponatremia, fluid restriction, decreased activity

Defining characteristics: inability to pass stool, hard stools, painful, small stools

Outcome Criteria

Patient will be free of constipation.

INTERVENTIONS	RATIONALES
Assess bowel habits of patient; normal routines, frequency of stools, use of cathartics, etc.	Provides baseline from which to plan interventions.
Administer laxatives or stool softeners as ordered. Tap water enemas should be avoided.	Caution must be used in selection of pharmacological agent so as to not further add to fluid volume overload. Water in the enemas can be absorbed and increase overload.

Discharge or Maintenance Evaluation

- Patient will have normal bowel function with no complications to fluid status.

SYNDROME OF INAPPROPRIATE ADH SECRETION (SIADH)

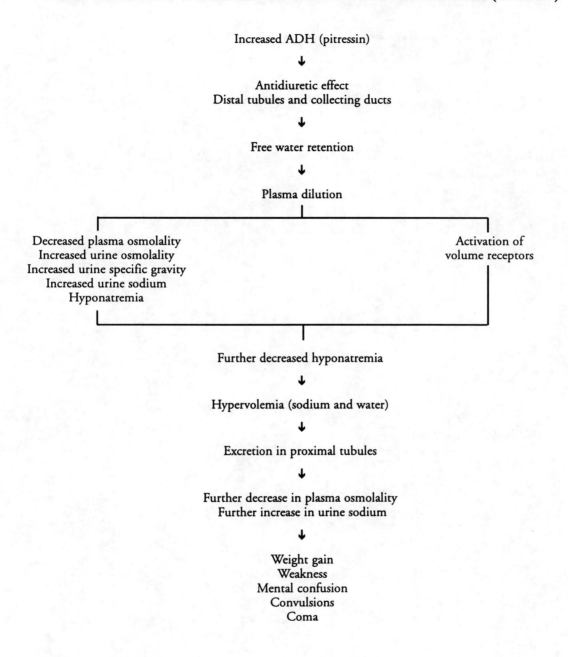

Increased ADH (pitressin)
↓
Antidiuretic effect
Distal tubules and collecting ducts
↓
Free water retention
↓
Plasma dilution

Decreased plasma osmolality
Increased urine osmolality
Increased urine specific gravity
Increased urine sodium
Hyponatremia

Activation of
volume receptors

Further decreased hyponatremia
↓
Hypervolemia (sodium and water)
↓
Excretion in proximal tubules
↓
Further decrease in plasma osmolality
Further increase in urine sodium
↓
Weight gain
Weakness
Mental confusion
Convulsions
Coma

Diabetes Insipidus (DI)

Diabetes insipidus, or DI, is a condition that results when damage or destruction of the neurons of the hypothalamus causes decreased levels of antidiuretic hormone (ADH) and severe diuresis and dehydration occur. The deficiency results in the inability to conserve water, and if the patient's thirst mechanism is not adequate, or if fluids are not accessible, the fluid balance will be altered.

The two main etiologies of DI are tumors of the hypothalamus or pituitary and closed head injuries that may have damage to the supraoptic nuclei or hypothalamus. Head injuries, neurosurgery, or hypophysectomy may lead to a loss of osmoreceptor function and/or damage to the areas that produce antidiuretic hormone. Sometimes, a transient type of DI occurs after surgical procedures, histiocyctosis, sarcoidosis, aneurysms, meningitis, encephalititis, or neoplastic conditions. All of the above respond to vasopressin.

DI that is nephrogenic is usually vasopressin-insensitive, and is seen in polycystic kidney disease, pyelonephritis, multiple myeloma, sarcoidosis, sickle cell disease, or any disorder that affects the kidneys. Usage of ethanol and phenytoin inhibit ADH secretion, and drugs such as lithium and demeclocycline inhibit ADH action in the kidney.

The main goal for treatment is to prevent dehydration and electrolyte imbalances, while determination and treatment of the underlying cause is underway. Vasopressin administration will control diabetes insipidus; D-amino-D-arginine vasopressin (DDAVP) is a nasal spray that has prolonged antidiuretic effects with minimal side effects.

MEDICAL CARE

Laboratory: serum osmolality elevated, usually greater than 295 mOsm/kg; urine osmolality decreased, generally less than 500 mOsm/kg and can be as low as 30 mOsm/kg; urine specific gravity low, generally 1.001 to 1.005; plasma ADH levels decreased in central diabetes insipidus; serum sodium elevated

Water deprivation test: used to demonstrate that in the presence of simple dehydration, kidneys cannot concentrate urine; used to differentiate psychogenic polydipsia from diabetes insipidus

Vasopressin test: used in conjunction with water deprivation test to identify that the kidneys can concentrate urine with exogenous ADH and differentiates nephrogenic from central diabetes insipidus

NURSING CARE PLANS

Fluid volume deficit

Related to: inability to conserve water, dehydration, decreased levels of ADH

Defining characteristics: extreme thirst, decreased skin turgor, dry mucous membranes, hypotension, tachycardia, weight loss, dilute urine output, increased urine output, hemoconcentration, hyperosmolality, increased serum sodium

Outcome Criteria

Patient will have fluid volume balance restored and be able to maintain adequate fluid volume.

INTERVENTIONS	RATIONALES
Assess and monitor vital signs.	Tachycardia and hypotension may result from hypovolemia.
Measure intake and output every 1-2 hours, and notify physician for changes. Record specific gravity measurements per hospital protocol.	Provides information to identify fluid imbalances and volume depletion. I&O should be continued in postoperative patients, especially neurosurgical patients,

INTERVENTIONS	RATIONALES
	to ensure that DI has not transiently resolved and then reappear only to become permanent. Urinary output may be as much as 15 L/day, and specific gravity is usually between 1.001 and 1.005.
Administer IV fluids as ordered. If able to take oral fluids, encourage patient to take in PO.	Helps to restore circulating fluid volume.
Weigh patient daily.	Provides identification of fluid balances and water losses.
Administer replacement therapy for central diabetes insipidus.	Aqueous pitressin (IV or SQ) is a short-acting ADH useful in transient DI. Nasal spray vasopressin is also short-acting and may be erratic in patients with respiratory infections or nasal problems. DDAVP (nasal or SQ) is a synthetic ADH that has a longer duration and can be given q12-24 hours. Vasopressin tannate in oil can last 24-72 hours and is not utilized as initial treatment due to inability to titrate dose.
Administer medication therapy for nephrogenic diabetes insipidus.	Chlorpropamide is used to stimulate ADH release and can augment the renal tubular response to ADH. Thiazide diuretics in conjunction with sodium restriction will reduce solute load and enhance water reabsorption.

Information, Instruction, Demonstration

INTERVENTIONS	RATIONALES
Ensure that vasopressin tannate in oil is warmed and vigorously agitated prior to injection.	Reduces pain from injection and ensures complete mixture.
Observe for water intoxication with pharmacologic replacement therapies.	May occur with shifting fluid balances.
Assist with diagnostic procedures such as water deprivation and	Ensures that correct sequence will be maintained for specimens

INTERVENTIONS	RATIONALES
vasopressin tests by obtaining accurate weights, vital signs, I&O, lab specimens at proper intervals, and maintaining deprivation for required amount of time.	and that procedure data will be accurate. The water deprivation test is usually terminated if the patient has a 3% weight loss.
Instruct patient/family member in methods to prevent dehydration when on long-term ADH therapy, as well as when hospitalized.	Promotes knowledge and facilitates compliance with medical regimen.

Discharge or Maintenance Evaluation

- Patient will have stable vital signs and balanced intake and output.

- Patient will be able to maintain normal hemodynamic parameters.

- Patient will have weight restored and be able to maintain weight.

- Patient/family will be able to verbalize accurately any information related to them.

Knowledge deficit

Related to: potential self-care management for permanent diabetes insipidus

Defining characteristics: newly diagnosed DI, requests for information, questions, inaccurate follow-through with instructions or medications, development of preventable complications, inability to recall information vital to disease process

Outcome Criteria

Patient/family member will be able to accurately verbalize medical regimen to manage diabetes insipidus.

INTERVENTIONS	RATIONALES
Assess for patient/family member comprehension of disease and medications.	Provides baseline of knowledge and facilitates plan for interventions.
Instruct in all medications, action, side effects, adverse reactions, schedule to be taken, method of administration, and importance of adherence to medical regime.	Promotes knowledge and facilitates compliance.
Instruct to notify physician for excessive water retention or urinary frequency and increased amount.	Prompt identification may facilitate timely intervention and treatment.
Discuss reasons for non-adherence to medication, if patient has previously been diagnosed with DI.	Explores patient's rationale and identifies any misconceptions he might have regarding his medical regimen.
Discuss obtaining medical alert bracelet identifying patient as having DI.	Promotes fast recognition of medical condition in cases where patient is not able to identify problems.

Discharge or Maintenance Evaluation

- Patient will be able to accurately verbalize purpose, side effects, and schedule of medications.

- Patient will adhere to medical therapeutics and take medication as prescribed.

- Patient/family will be able to accurately recall all information related to them.

- Patient/family will be able to identify fluid balance alterations that should be reported to physician.

- Patient will be compliant in obtaining medical identification bracelet.

DIABETES INSIPIDUS (DI)

Decreased ADH (Pitressin) or
low plasma ADH levels

↓

Renal tubular unresponsiveness

↓

Decreased permeability to waters

↓

Excess water excreted in urine

↓

Decreased urine osmolality
Decreased urine specific gravity

↓

Plasma volume loss
Increased plasma osmolality
Increased serum sodium

↓

Dehydration

Hypovolemic shock   Polydipsia
                                                     Weakness
                                                     Fever
                                                     Confusion

Pheochromocytoma

Pheochromocytoma is a vascular tumor, composed of chromaffin cells that secrete catecholamines or their precursors (epinephrine, norephinephrine, or dopamine). This, in turn, causes severe persistent or intermittent hypertension due to the severe vasoconstriction in response to the catecholamine excess.

Usually the tumor is encapsulated and located within the medulla of the adrenal glands, but can occur in the sympathetic paraganglionic areas of the abdomen, chest, brain, or cervical areas. These tumors are usually benign, but can be malignant in up to ten percent of patients. Frequently occurring between the ages of 30 and 50, attacks may occur paroxysmally if the tumor releases catecholamines on an intermittent basis. These episodes may range from once per year to several times per day. Attacks may be spontaneous, or be caused by palpation of the tumor, emotional stress or trauma, exposure to cold, beta-blockers, postural changes, abdominal compression, anesthesia induction, urination, defecation, or heavy lifting.

The tumor's hallmark symptom is high blood pressure with fluctuations up to 220/150 or higher. The catecholamine secretion causes symptoms of "flight or fight" reactions, typically beginning with palpitations, headache, pallor, cool, moist hands and feet, flushing, profuse sweating, and extreme anxiety.

Pheochromocytoma is also a part of the Multiple Endocrine Neoplasia (MEN) Syndromes and may be found in conjunction with neurofibromatoses, hemangiomas, and medullary thyroid cancers. Other diagnoses, such as angina, essential hypertension, hyperthyroidism, acute anxiety reactions, transient ischemic attacks, and menopause, must

be ruled out. Pheochromocytoma always leads to death if untreated.

MEDICAL CARE

Medications: use of alpha- and beta-blockers (phenoxybenzamine and propranolol, or phenoxylbenzamine and metyrosine) to control catecholamine excess symptoms; IV infusions of trimethaphan camsylate or sodium nitroprusside to control vasopressor effects

Laboratory: fasting serum glucose elevated, increased hematocrit; 24-hour urine for catecholamines, vanillymandelic acid and metanephrines to identify elevated levels

Electrocardiogram: used to identify tachycardia, bradycardia, LV enlargement and strain from elevated blood pressure, cardiac dysrhythmias

Radiography: chest and abdominal x-rays used to localize and identify tumor; CT scans, IVP, radionuclide imaging and selective venographic angiography also used to localize tumors; caution must be used due to potential for test to exacerbate hypertensive crisis

Surgery: surgical removal of the pheochromocytoma may be required

NURSING CARE PLANS

Altered tissue perfusion: cardiopulmonary, cerebral, gastrointestinal, peripheral, and renal

Related to: excessive catecholamine secretion

Defining characteristics: pulse and blood pressure changes, changes in cardiac output, changes in peripheral resistance, impaired myocardial oxygenation, chest pain, cardiac dysrhythmias, EKG changes, dyspnea, tachypnea, palpitations, nausea, vomiting, epigastric pain, constipation, slow digestion, weight loss, headaches, visual disturbances, paresthesias, oliguria, anuria, electrolyte imbalances, cold and clammy skin, decreased peripheral pulses, flushing, diaphoresis

Outcome Criteria

Patient will maintain adequate perfusion to all vital organs and will have adequate peripheral and systemic circulation.

INTERVENTIONS	RATIONALES
Monitor vital signs, including lying, sitting, and standing BP.	Provides information about heart rate and perfusion pressure which will affect blood flow and tissue perfusion. Chronic excessive secretion of catecholamines will affect the reflexes that are responsible for maintaining upright blood pressure and may result in orthostatic hypotension.
Monitor functional abilities in relation to the affected system.	Interrelationships of the body systems can cause overlapping signs and symptoms associated with tissue perfusion and can cause changes in oxygenation, cardiac output, metabolic demands, neurologic function, renal function, and nutrition.
Assess for presence and character of pulses, capillary refill time, skin color and temperature, urine output, mentation, gastric distention, presence of bowel sounds, and appetite.	May indicate decreased perfusion related to the particular body system.
Position patient in Fowler's position.	Helps to decrease the blood volume returning to the heart by pooling blood in dependent parts of the body. Decreases BP by use of orthostatic changes associated with the chronic catecholamine secretion.
Avoid any non-essential activities, especially pressure-causing movement. Avoid straining with bowel movements or urination.	Ambulation, exercise, and valsalva-type efforts may provoke an attack, increasing blood pressure and decreasing tissue perfusion.

INTERVENTIONS	RATIONALES
Administer medications as ordered.	Alpha- and beta-blockers may stabilize the condition prior to surgical intervention. Metyrosine interrupts the catecholamine synthesis, decreases levels of norepinephrine production, decreases levels of VMA, and decreases BP.
Titrate IV meds as needed to keep systolic blood pressure less than 170 mmHg, and diastolic pressure less than 100 mmHg.	Reduces risk of complications from severely elevated pressure.
Weigh every day.	Weight loss may occur due to increased metabolism, decreased appetite, nausea, or vomiting.
Monitor intake and output, and notify physician for urine output less than 30 cc/hr.	Decreased renal perfusion may lead to decreased urinary output, renal impairment, and failure.
Avoid palpation of abdomen; post sign near bed to refrain from palpation during assessments.	Prevents possible palpation of tumor and triggering of acute crisis.
Monitor labwork, especially FBS, hematocrit and renal function levels.	Catecholamine release can increase glycolysis and inhibit insulin release. Excess catecholamines can also increase erythropoietin stimulation and can elevate hematocrit, as well as decrease blood flow to the kidney resulting in renal impairment.

Information, Instruction, Demonstration

INTERVENTIONS	RATIONALES
Assist with obtaining 24-hour urine specimen for diagnosis.	Elevated levels may be diagnostic for pheochromocytoma, but coma and increased stress states must be ruled out. Normal values for VMA are < 10 mg/24 hrs, metanephrines < 1.3 mg/24 hrs, free epinephrine and norepinephrine < 100 mcg/24 hrs.
Avoid use of rauwolfia alkaloids, tetracycline, quinine, methyl-	These substances may interfere with the results and hamper

INTERVENTIONS	RATIONALES
dopa, catecholamines, large quantities of vanilla, coffee, chocolate, nuts, bananas, guaifenesin, and salicylates for at least 2 days prior to 24-hour test, if possible.	determination of diagnosis.
Instruct patient/family in causes of exacerbations or attacks, and methods to reduce frequency of occurrence.	Promotes understanding of the condition and risk of decreased perfusion to vital organs.
Instruct to avoid exposure to cold temperatures.	Cold may cause vasoconstriction, decreases circulation, and perfusion, as well as precipitate an attack.
Instruct in medications, effects, side effects, adverse reactions, complications, and symptoms to report to physician.	Promotes knowledge and facilitates compliance with medical regimen.
Instruct in methods to decrease emotional stress, such as relaxation techniques.	Reduces stress and lessens precipitating factors with intermittent attacks by facilitating vasodilation.
Instruct in having frequent blood pressure checks, keeping log of trends, ranges to report to physician, etc.	Primary indicator of the tumor activity is blood pressure increases, which cause decreased perfusion to tissues and organs. Increased knowledge will decrease fear and increase compliance with treatment, and provide opportunity for prompt treatment to prevent serious complications.
Instruct in avoiding rapid changes in position.	Facilitates body's attempt to cope with orthostatic hypotension by allowing time for body and circulatory system to adjust to changes.
Instruct to avoid wearing any clothing that may be tight or constrictive.	May result in an attack by compression of abdomen or tumor region.

Discharge or Maintenance Evaluation

- Patient will have normalized vital signs.

- Organ function will be within patient's normal parameters.

- Extremities will be warm, with normal color and sensation, and have equally palpable pulses.

- Patient will have adequate urinary output with equivalent intake and output.

- Patient will be free of abdominal or epigastric pain, and able to ingest adequate nutritional intake to maintain weight.

Anxiety

Related to: excessive catecholamine release, threat to health status, changes in health status, life-threatening crisis, possibility of surgical intervention

Defining characteristics: apprehension, sense of impending doom, fear of death, restlessness, fear, fear of death, fear of surgery, fear of the unknown, feelings of helplessness, anxiousness, worry, communication of uncertainty, voiced concern over changes in life events

Outcome Criteria

Patient will have less anxiety or anxiety will be within an acceptable and manageable level.

INTERVENTIONS	RATIONALES
Assess anxiety level, noting verbalizations of fear or sense of doom.	Catecholamine increases can produce marked anxiety which then increases oxygen demand on tissues.
Provide calm environment for patient to express fears, concerns, and feelings. Allow time for patient to ask questions.	Provides an opportunity to vent feelings and to obtain information. Decreases anxiety and promotes a caring and trusting atmosphere.
Encourage visits from family and friends who do not increase or	Provides emotional support and relieves anxiety when familiar

INTERVENTIONS	RATIONALES
provide patient with emotional stress.	people are available.
Decrease stimuli in environment.	Prevents further stressors.
Administer medications as ordered.	Assists to allay fear and anxiety.

Information, Instruction, Demonstration

INTERVENTIONS	RATIONALES
Instruct patient/family members about disease process, what to expect with procedures, pre- and postoperative care.	Decreases anxiety caused by fear of the unknown, and promotes knowledge and understanding.
Instruct on emotional stress and other precipitating triggers for attacks, and methods to reduce stress and anxiety.	Reduces anxiety and provides patient with some measure of control over the situation.
Instruct on medications, effects, side effects, contraindications, and symptoms to report to physician.	Promotes knowledge and understanding which facilitates compliance with medical regimen.

Discharge or Maintenance Evaluation

- Patient will have reduced anxiety and be able to vent feelings and concerns.

- Patient/family will be able to verbalize understanding of disease process, medications, and treatments, and will be compliant with regimen.

- Patient will be able to avoid stressful visitors, situations, or other provoking events, and will be able to perform relaxation exercises when stressed.

Hyperthermia

Related to: increased metabolic rate in response to catecholamines, decreased heat loss due to vasoconstriction

Defining characteristics: increase in body temperature greater than normal range, flushed warm skin, increased heart rate, increased respiratory rate, diaphoresis, delirium

Outcome Criteria

Patient will have temperature within normal range.

INTERVENTIONS	RATIONALES
Monitor temperature every 1-2 hours or use continuous monitoring.	Fluctuations in temperature can occur rapidly and temperature elevations can increase metabolism needs.
Adjust room temperature for patient comfort and maintain at or below 72 degrees.	Assists patient with comfort and decreases temperature.
Administer antipyretics as ordered.	Decreases fever.
Provide frequent tepid sponge baths and change linens if patient is diaphoretic.	Promotes patient comfort and reduces temperature by evaporation.
Avoid chilling or shivering of patient.	Shivering may increase metabolic requirements and actually increase temperature.
Place covered ice packs to groin, axillae, and/or behind neck, if warranted.	Decreases temperature by means of conduction.
Use cooling blanket for temperatures greater than 103 degrees if warranted. Cool body slowly— no faster than 1 degree/15 minutes. Blanket should be covered and continuous monitoring of temperature should be performed.	Assists in lowering temperatures by conduction. Blankets should be covered to prevent burns and tissue injury. Cooling that is done too rapidly can produce ventricular ectopy.
Administer thorazine IM/IV as ordered.	Thorazine is an alpha-adrenergic blocking agent that causes peripheral vasodilation which helps heat to dissipate and also can assist in decreasing shivering.

Information, Instruction, Demonstration

INTERVENTIONS	RATIONALES
Instruct patient/family in procedures, what to expect with cooling blanket application, etc.	Promotes knowledge and reduces anxiety.

Discharge or Maintenance Evaluation

• Patient will achieve and maintain normal body temperature.

• Patient will be compliant with medical regimen.

Sensory-perception alteration (visual, thought processes, kinesthetic)
[See CVA]

Related to: altered sensory reception, chemical alterations due to hypoxia, chemical alterations due to glucose/insulin and electrolyte imbalances, restrict environment, psychologic stress, vasoconstriction

Defining characteristics: confusion, anxiety, fear, disorientation, change in behavior patterns, hyperesthesia, restlessness, irritability, impaired decision-making

Alteration in nutrition: less than body requirements
[See Mechanical Ventilation]

Related to: hypermetabolic state, nausea, vomiting, anorexia, malabsorption

Defining characteristics: inadequate food intake, weight loss, muscle weakness, fatigue

Impaired gas exchange
[See Mechanical Ventilation]

Related to: increased respiratory workload, impaired oxygen to heart, hypoventilation, altered oxygen supply, altered blood flow, change in vascular resistance, altered oxygen-carrying capacity of blood, shift of the oxyhemoglobin dissociation curve, hypermetabolic state

Defining characteristics: confusion, restlessness, hypercapnia, hypoxia, cyanosis, dyspnea, tachypnea, changes in ABG values, changes in A-a gradient, changes in vital signs, activity intolerance, changes in mental status

Constipation

Related to: inadequate dietary/fluid intake, GI distress, changes in level of activity, decreased blood flow slowing digestion, malabsorption

Defining characteristics: nausea, vomiting, decreased appetite, epigastric pain, hard-formed stool, absence of stool, abdominal pain

Outcome Criteria

Patient will have normal elimination pattern reestablished and maintained.

INTERVENTIONS	RATIONALES
Determine patient's bowel habits, lifestyle, ability to sense urge to defecate, painful hemorrhoids, and history of constipation.	Assists with identification of an effective bowel regime and/or impairment and need for assistance. GI function may be decreased as a result of decreased digestion.
Auscultate bowel sounds for presence and quality.	Presence of abnormal sounds, such as high-pitched tinkles, suggest complications like ileus.
Monitor diet and fluid intake.	Adequate amounts of fiber and roughage provides bulk and adequate fluid intake (greater than 2 L/day) is important in determining stool consistency.
Monitor for abdominal pain and distention.	Gas, abdominal distention, or ileus could be a factor. Lack of peristalsis from impaired digestion can create bowel distention and worsen to the point of ileus.

INTERVENTIONS	RATIONALES
Provide bulk, stool softeners, laxatives, or suppositories as warranted.	May be required to stimulate evacuation of stool.
Provide high-fiber, whole grain cereals, breads and fresh fruits.	Improves stool consistency and promotes elimination.

Information, Instruction, Demonstration

INTERVENTIONS	RATIONALES
Determine pre-existing habits of laxative/enema usage.	Laxative dependence can predispose patient to constipation.
Instruct patient to avoid frequent use of enemas.	Promotes enema dependence and causes fluid loss which results in more difficult elimination.
Provide activity or exercise within limits of disease process.	Promotes peristalsis.

Discharge or Maintenance Evaluation

- Patient will have improved dietary and fluid intake.

- Patient will achieve bowel elimination pattern establishment and be able to maintain elimination of soft-formed stool without cramping or straining.

- Daily exercise will be maintained within level of confinement in ICU.

Decreased cardiac output

Related to: altered preload, altered afterload, inotropic changes in the heart from increased blood pressure and TPR, left ventricular enlargement and strain, and from accumulation of extra fluid in the lungs or systemic venous system, myocardial compromise due to vasoconstriction, decreased coronary blood flow, increased myocardial oxygen demands, hyperthermia, increased catecholamine receptor sensitivity

Defining characteristics: increased blood pressure and pulse, cold and clammy skin, jugular vein distention, dyspnea, crackles, edema, cough, frothy blood-tinged sputum, confusion, restlessness, nocturia, decreased urinary output, increased mean arterial pressure, increased systemic vascular resistance, decreased cardiac output and cardiac index

Outcome Criteria

Patient will have adequate cardiac output to maintain hemodynamic stability and perfusion to all organs.

INTERVENTIONS	RATIONALES
Identify other pre-existing conditions and assess cardiac function.	Other factors and disease states may further stress an already compromised heart and place an extra burden of myocardial oxygen supply.
Monitor blood pressure, heart rate and rhythm, apical and peripheral pulses, pulse deficits, respiratory status, presence of cough or adventitious breath sounds, presence and character of any sputum, and oxygenation.	Cardiac output and blood volume is decreased with elevated blood pressure. Afterload increases, pulse increases, and changes in contractility and conduction occur. Respiratory changes may result in decreased oxygen intake and hypoxia.
Measure cardiac output/cardiac index and other hemodynamic parameters as indicated.	Cardiac output < 5 L/min or cardiac index < 2.5 L/min/m² indicates severe vasoconstriction and decrease in myocardial oxygenation, leading to myocardial ischemia, cardiac failure, and death.
Monitor EKG for presence of dysrhythmias, and treat according to hospital protocol.	Dysrhythmias decrease the heart's pumping efficiency which affects the cardiac output. Dysrhythmias may indicate inadequate myocardial perfusion. Tachydysrhythmias decrease ventricular filling time and coronary blood flow; bradydysrhythmias decrease cardiac output and result in left ventricular failure.

INTERVENTIONS	RATIONALES
Auscultate heart sounds for presence of gallops and/or murmurs.	Accumulations of extra fluid can be heard as these abnormal heart sounds.
Monitor for edema to extremities, sacral region, or other dependent areas; assess for jugular vein distention, cold peripheral extremities, decreased urinary output, and sluggish capillary refill.	May indicate decreased venous return to the heart and a decrease in cardiac output. Fluid retention may result in a decrease in urinary output as a result of decreased venous return and perfusion.
Weigh every day.	Weight gain may indicate fluid retention.
Monitor intake and output every 2 hrs and prn.	Intake and output should approximate each other. A fluid deficit between output and intake indicates fluid retention and a weight gain (500 cc approximately = 1 lb).
Position in semi-Fowler's or high-Fowler's position.	Semi-Fowler's positioning prevents blood pooling and facilitates breathing and improved air exchange. High-Fowler's positioning reduces preload quickly by pooling blood but does not decrease stroke volume significantly. Afterload decreases by dilating peripheral arteries and decreasing LVEDP.
Balance rest with short, planned periods of activity; provide atmosphere that is conducive to rest.	Prevents increased demand on heart and myocardial oxygen supply.
Monitor for mental status changes, decreases in orientation, restlessness, agitation, or dizziness.	Central nervous system disturbances can occur with decreased cardiac output due to decreases in perfusion to these areas.
Administer vasoactive drugs as ordered, with titration based on ordered parameters.	These agents promote optimum cardiac output by changing blood pressure, and can reduce afterload and preload.
Administer anti-dysrhythmic drugs as ordered.	These agents decrease pacemaker activity, modify areas of impaired conduction, and blocks sympathetic effects of the heart; myocardial contractility is

INTERVENTIONS	RATIONALES
	decreased, heart rate is slowed, and oxygen consumption is preserved. Blood pressure decreases and coronary perfusion and myocardial oxygen supply is increased due to the decrease in the heart rate.

Information, Instruction, Demonstration

INTERVENTIONS	RATIONALES
Instruct to elevate legs when sitting or lying down.	Promotes venous return.
Instruct in signs to report: edema, weight gain, chest pain, headache, blood pressure or pulse rate changes.	May indicate complications as a result of decreased cardiac output and facilitate prompt intervention.

Discharge or Maintenance Evaluation

- Patient will have stable vital signs and hemodynamics will be within patient's acceptable parameters.

- Patient will have stable cardiac rhythm with no dysrhythmias, and perfusion to organs will be maintained.

- Patient will have clear lung fields with no adventitious breath sounds.

- Patient will have palpable peripheral pulses with warm, dry extremities.

- Patient will have adequate urinary output, with no edema or extra weight gain.

PHEOCHROMOCYTOMA

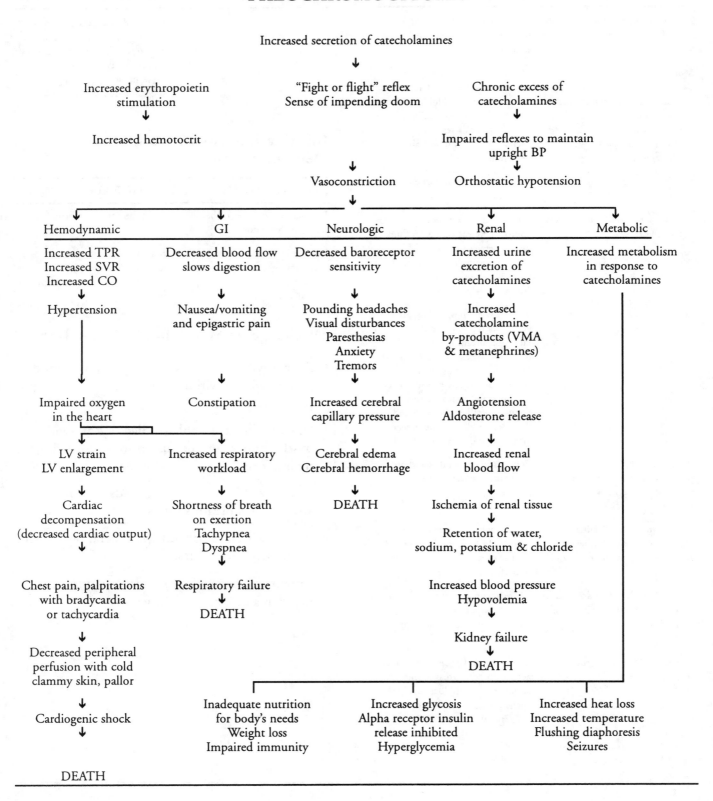

Thyrotoxicosis (Thyroid Storm)

Hyperthyroid crisis, also known as thyroid storm and thyrotoxicosis, is a life-threatening emergency characterized by greatly exaggerated signs of hyperthyroidism. Mortality is high, and symptoms appear rapidly when triggered by infection, trauma, surgery, diabetes, or abrupt withdrawal of thyroid medication. Thyroid storm may be difficult to diagnose because the precipitating illness may mask its detection.

Hyperthyroid patients are more susceptible to catecholamines because of the increased number of catecholamine receptors they possess. A triggering illness creates an outpouring of catecholamines, and so the elevated levels of thyroid and increased number of receptors create the crisis. A hypermetabolic state then ensues causing increased oxygen and nutrient consumption, fluid and electrolyte imbalances, and a catabolic state.

Patients in crisis typically have hyperthermia, tachydysrhythmias, dehydration, nausea, vomiting, weight loss, and neurologic changes. Treatment is usually begun without waiting for confirmation of lab tests and is aimed at supporting vital functions. Reversal of excessive thyroid hormone decreases the hypermetabolic state, and reduction of the circulating thyroid hormones further decreases the crisis. Once vital functions are preserved, treatment of the precipitating cause is begun. If the crisis is untreated, heart failure, exhaustion, and death will ensue.

MEDICAL CARE

Laboratory: serum and serum free T_4 and T_3 are increased; TSH levels are decreased; thyroglobulin is increased; electrolytes are used to identify imbalances; thyroid antibodies positive in Graves' disease; glucose levels elevated from insulin resistance, increased glycogenolysis, or impaired insulin secretion; serum cortisol decreased due to lower adrenal reserve; alkaline phosphatase increased; serum calcium increased; liver function abnormal, decreased serum catecholamines; urine creatinine increased

TRH test: used in some cases to identify TSH suppression with administration of TRH hormones

Electrocardiogram: used to identify elevated thyroid levels or electrolyte imbalances; atrial fibrillation may be present; cardiomegaly in elderly with masked hyperthyroidism

Oxygen: used to provide supplemental oxygen due to increased oxygen consumption and increased metabolic demands

Radiography: chest x-rays used to identify cardiac enlargement that may occur in response to increased circulatory demands, to identify presence of cardiac overload and congestion, respiratory infiltrates or other precipitating causes

Radioactive iodine uptake test: used to differentiate types of thyroid problems; usually high in Graves' disease and toxic goiter, but low in thyroiditis

Thyroid scan: may be used to aid diagnosis when thyrotoxicosis is caused from cancer or a multinodular goiter

Iodine solutions: used to slow the release of thyroid hormones; common solutions are Lugol's solution and sodium iodide

Beta-adrenergic blockers: used to reverse peripheral effects of excessive thyroid hormones and to decrease the hypermetabolic state; commonly used is propranolol; reserpine IM also helps to reduce peripheral effects and may help decrease the tachycardias

Corticosteriods: high doses of hydrocortisone help support body functions during hypermetabolic state

Digoxin: may be required for congestive heart failure patients prior to initiating beta-blockade

Diuretics: may be required if congestive heart failure occurs, and may also help decrease calcium level if neuromuscular function is compromised

Nutrients: high doses of vitamin B complex are used to provide necessary nutrient support for the catabolism state, as well as to facilitate increased glucose, protein, and carbohydrate absorption

Thyroid hormone antagonists: used to block the thyroid hormone production and effects; usually propylthiouracil (PTU) or methimazole (Tapazole) are used; lithium carbonate can also inhibit thyroid hormone synthesis and may be used in patients who cannot tolerate the other drugs

Sedatives: may be required to help patient rest and reduce myocardial oxygen consumption and cardiac workload, as well as control of shivering that may increase metabolic rate

Surgery: thyroidectomy or subthyroidectomy may be required

NURSING CARE PLANS

Hyperthermia

Related to: accelerated metabolic rate secondary to excessive thyroid hormone secretion, increased beta-adrenergic responses, increased sodium-potassium exchange in cells

Defining characteristics: increase in body temperature over 100 degrees, flushed warm skin, diaphoresis, tachypnea, tachycardia, delirium, lethargy

Outcome Criteria

Patient will have normal body temperature restored and be able to maintain temperature within acceptable range.

INTERVENTIONS	RATIONALES
Monitor temperature for elevation and/or pattern of elevation, chilling, shaking, or diaphoresis.	Hyperthermia up to 106 degrees may result from the acceleration of the metabolic rate caused from excessive thyroid hormone secretion. Chills may precede temperature elevation.
Monitor other vital signs and heart rhythm for alterations.	Elevated temperatures may result in elevations of blood pressure, respiration, and pulse. Cardiac dysrhythmias as a result of heart failure, electrolyte imbalance, or fluid overload may be noted promptly to allow timely intervention.
If required, use cooling methods such as cooling blankets, ice packs, etc., being careful to not cause shivering.	Assists in reducing temperature, but may cause shivering which increases metabolic rate and may worsen condition.
Administer antipyretic medications as ordered by physician, but avoid the use of aspirin.	Assists with reduction of temperature. Aspirin should be avoided because it increases free thyroid hormone levels and may worsen condition.
Administer antithyroid medications as ordered.	PTU or methimazole inhibits thyroid hormone synthesis, and PTU inhibits conversion of T_4 to T_3 in peripheral tissues. Iodine-containing agents inhibit the release of stored thyroid hormones and help to inhibit synthesis. Glucocorticosteroids block conversion of T_4 to T_3.
Administer beta-adrenergic blockers as ordered.	Propranolol and nadolol block the peripheral effects from excessive thyroid hormone and may block conversion of T_4 to T_3.
Administer IV fluids and electrolytes as ordered.	Replaces fluid losses from fever and diaphoresis.

INTERVENTIONS	RATIONALES
Administer antibiotics if ordered.	Assist in fighting infection when that is believed to be a precipitating factor in the crisis.
Ensure comfort of patient by frequent repositioning, changing of linens and clothing, cool cloths, lowering room temperature, etc.	Assists in reducing and maintaining temperature.

Information, Instruction, Demonstration

INTERVENTIONS	RATIONALES
Instruct patient/family in all medications being utilized.	Promotes knowledge and facilitates compliance with regimen.
Observe for depression, tremors, nausea, vomiting, or increased urine output.	Symptoms may indicate adverse effects from lithium carbonate.
Instruct in watching for fever, sore throat, or rashes, and to notify physician if he develops these symptoms.	May be indicative of an agranulocytosis caused from medication.

Discharge or Maintenance Evaluation

- Patient will have stable vital signs and be able to maintain values within normal ranges.

- Patient will have no adverse reactions to medications or treatment.

- Patient will be able to accurately recall all instructed information.

Risk for decreased cardiac output

Related to: excessive demands on cardiovascular system due to hypermetabolic state, increased cardiac workload, hyperthermia, increased sensitivity of catecholamine receptors, changes in venous return, changes in peripheral and systemic vascular resistance, changes in heart rhythm or conduction.

Defining characteristics: elevated blood pressure, elevated mean arterial pressure, elevated systemic vascular resistance, elevated peripheral vascular resistance, decreased cardiac output or cardiac index, tachycardia, decreased or absent peripheral pulses, EKG changes, hypotension, gallops, decreased urinary output, diaphoresis, deterioration in mental status, impending cardiovascular collapse.

Outcome Criteria

Patient will be able to maintain cardiac output at an acceptable level for tissue perfusion.

INTERVENTIONS	RATIONALES
Monitor vital signs, especially blood pressure for widening pulse pressures.	Peripheral vasodilatation and decreased fluid volume may result from excessive catecholamine secretion. Widening of pulse pressure may indicate compensatory changes in stroke volume and decreasing systemic vascular resistance.
Observe heart rate and respiratory rate while patient is sleeping.	Provides accurate assessment of tachycardia without increase demand of activity.
Auscultate heart tones for extra sounds, gallops, and murmurs.	Hypermetabolic states create prominent S_1 sounds and murmurs due to the forcefulness of the cardiac output, and S_3 gallop development may indicate impending cardiac failure.
Monitor cardiac rhythm for changes, and treat accordingly per hospital protocol.	Excessive thyroid hormone secretion creates excessive catecholamine stimulation to myocardium which can result in tachycardia and dysrhythmias, and may worsen condition by decreasing cardiac output.
Assess for weak or thready pulses, decreased capillary refill, decreased urinary output, and decreased blood pressure.	May indicate dehydration and reduction in circulating volume which compromises cardiac output.
Auscultate lung fields for changes in breath sounds.	Adventitious breath sounds may indicate early signs of pulmonary congestion or impending cardiac failure.

INTERVENTIONS	RATIONALES
Administer IV fluids as ordered.	Fluid replacement may be indicated to increase circulating volume, but may result in cardiac failure or overload.
Administer atropine if indicated.	Beta-blockers that are given to control tachycardia and tremors during the crisis may decrease heart rate, and may result in symptomatic bradycardia requiring treatment.
Administer digoxin if indicated.	CHF patients may require digitalization prior to initiating beta-blockers.
Administer sedatives and/or muscle relaxants as ordered.	Reduces metabolic demands by promoting rest, and may be helpful to reduce shivering that occurs with fever.
Administer supplemental oxygen as ordered.	Assists to support increased metabolic needs and with increased oxygen consumption.
Assist patients by restricting activity or assisting with activity when required.	Reduces energy expenditure which increases oxygen consumption and contributes to increase metabolic needs.

Information, Instruction, Demonstration

INTERVENTIONS	RATIONALES
Identify patients who may be at most risk from complications of disease, such as elderly, preexisting coronary disease or cardiac risk, pregnancy, asthma, or bronchoconstrictive diseases.	Allows for closer assessment and monitoring of patients who may develop cardiovascular compromise from therapeutic measures designed to relieve thyroid crisis, and enable appropriate choices of beta-blockers or other agents.
Once PTU therapy has begun, avoid abrupt withdrawal of drug.	May result in further thyroid crisis. PTU may not have rapid effect on thyroid crisis.
If oral iodine solution is utilized, it should be started 1-3 hours after beginning anti-thyroid medication.	Minimizes hormone formation from the iodine. Iodine may interfere with radioactive iodine treatment and has been known to exacerbate the crisis in some individuals.

INTERVENTIONS	RATIONALES
Monitor lab studies, i.e., potassium, calcium, etc.	Hypokalemia may cause cardiac dysrhythmias and hypercalcemia may interfere with contractility, both of which decrease cardiac output and function.
Monitor cultures for infection.	Identifies causative organism that may be responsible for thyroid crisis. The most frequent factor of thyrotoxicosis is respiratory infection.
Assist with hemofiltration, hemodialysis, or plasmapheresis procedures.	May be used in severe crisis to rapidly decrease thyroid hormone.
Prepare patient/family for surgery as indicated.	Subtotal or total thyroidectomy may be required once euthyroid state is attained.

Discharge or Maintenance Evaluation

- Patient will have stable vital signs and hemodynamic parameters will be within normal limits.

- Patient will have stable cardiac rhythm with no dysrhythmias.

- Patient will exhibit no signs/symptoms of cardiac failure.

- Patient will be able to tolerate activity without circulatory compromise.

- Patient will be able to accurately verbalize instructed information.

Risk for altered nutrition: less than body requirements
[See DKA]

Related to: hypermetabolic state, excessive thyroid hormone secretion, nausea, vomiting, elevated glucose levels

Defining characteristics: weakness, fatigue, weight loss, lack of inadequate food intake, increased glucose level

Risk for injury

Related to: cognitive impairment, altered protective mechanisms of body, hypermetabolic state

Defining characteristics: diminished attention span, agitation, restlessness, impaired judgment, weakness, impaired body functions

Outcome Criteria

Patient will be free of personal injury with all body systems functioning normally.

INTERVENTIONS	RATIONALES
Monitor patient for complaints of eye pain, photophobia, eye irritation, tearing, difficulty closing eyelids, and presence of periorbital edema.	May result from excessive catecholamine stimulation, and may require care until crisis is resolved.
Assess for decreasing visual acuity or blurring of vision.	May be a result of Graves' disease in which increased tissue behind the orbit causes exophthalmos and infiltration of extraocular muscles and weakness. Vision may worsen or improve without basis on medical therapy or disease progression.
Administer medications as indicated, especially eye lubricant drops and ointment.	Prevents eyes from drying and protects cornea when patient is unable to close eyelids completely because of edema.
Ensure interventions to prevent injury to patient are in place, such as bed in lowest position, side rails raised, restraints when necessary, etc.	Prevents injury due to physical risks in environment.
Assess for changes in mental status and ability; reorient patient as necessary.	Assists with identification of changes that may occur as a result of exhaustion, electrolyte or other chemical imbalance, or physiological problems and allows for prompt intervention.

Information, Instruction, Demonstration

INTERVENTIONS	RATIONALES
Discuss patient's feelings regarding alterations in appearance, methods to enhance self-image, and exercises for eyes.	Assists patient in verbalizing concerns regarding perceptions of unattractiveness and allows for discussion of methods to enhance appearance with makeup, shaded glasses, and exercises for extraocular muscles that can help maintain mobility of eyelids.

Discharge or Maintenance Evaluation

- Patient will be free of personal injury to any body system.

- Patient's eyes will remain moist, with decreased edema, and will have the ability to completely close the eyelids.

- Patient will be able to freely discuss concerns and problems and be able to utilize problem-solving skills.

Anxiety
[See Pheochromocytoma]

Related to: hypermetabolic state, increased catecholamine stimulation

Defining characteristics: apprehension, loss of control, panic, shakiness, distorted perception, restlessness, tremors, mental changes, lack of attention

Fatigue
[See DKA]

Related to: hypermetabolic state, increased thyroid hormone secretion, increased energy requirements, changes in body chemistry, central nervous system irritability, increased oxygen consumption and demand

Defining characteristics: lack of energy, inability to perform normal activities, inability to concentrate, lethargy, irritability, nervousness, tension, apathy, depression

Knowledge deficit

Related to: lack of information, unfamiliarity with resources, misinterpretation of information, lack of recall

Defining characteristics: requests for information, questions, misrepresentation of facts, inaccurate follow-through of instructions, development of preventable complications

Outcome Criteria

Patient will be able to accurately recall measures for managing hyperthyroidism and be able to decrease risk of complications.

INTERVENTIONS	RATIONALES
Discuss patient's perceptions and knowledge of disease.	Establishes knowledge base of patient and helps identify interventions and appropriate plan of care.
Ensure that family members are included in discussions and allowed to verbalize their concerns and questions.	Patient's physical condition may interfere with his ability to concentrate which can hinder the learning process. Instruction to the family can assist with reinstruction when needed.
Instruct in all medications, effects, side effects, complications, and symptoms to report to physician.	Provides knowledge and facilitates compliance with regimen. Antithyroid therapy will require long-term use in order to inhibit hormone production. Alternate drugs may be chosen if the patient develops symptoms of agranulocytosis from his therapy.
Instruct to notify physician for fever, sore throat, or rashes.	May be indicative of adverse reactions to thiourea therapy and facilitates prompt treatment.

INTERVENTIONS	RATIONALES
Instruct to avoid taking over-the-counter medications unless advised to do so by physician.	Antithyroid medicines can affect and/or be affected by several OTC drugs and may cause dangerous interactions.
Instruct in diet needs, avoidance of caffeine, artificial preservatives and dyes.	Hypermetabolic states require increased nutrients to maintain well-being and meet demand. Stimulants and additives may result in systemic problems.
Instruct in need/rationale for continued medical follow-up.	Compliance with monitoring medical regimen and identification of potential complications can be assessed for timely intervention.

Discharge or Maintenance Evaluation

- Patient/family members will be able to accurately recall all instructional information provided to them.

- Patient will be free of preventable complications.

- Patient will be able to correctly recall all medications and effects.

- Patient will be able to manage hyperthyroidism without crisis.

THYROTOXICOSIS (THYROID STORM)

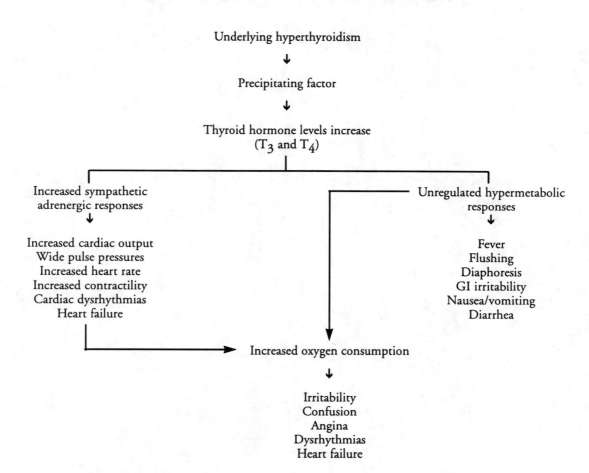

Underlying hyperthyroidism

↓

Precipitating factor

↓

Thyroid hormone levels increase
(T$_3$ and T$_4$)

Increased sympathetic
adrenergic responses

↓

Increased cardiac output
Wide pulse pressures
Increased heart rate
Increased contractility
Cardiac dysrhythmias
Heart failure

Unregulated hypermetabolic
responses

↓

Fever
Flushing
Diaphoresis
GI irritability
Nausea/vomiting
Diarrhea

Increased oxygen consumption

↓

Irritability
Confusion
Angina
Dysrhythmias
Heart failure

MUSCULOSKELETAL SYSTEM

Fractures

Amputation

Fat Embolism

Fractures

A fracture is a break in a bone that occurs when direct or indirect pressure is placed on the bone in a force sufficient to exceed the bone's normal elasticity and causes deformation. There are many types of fractures, but the major classifications include open or compound, closed or simple, complete, incomplete, and pathologic fractures.

In closed fractures, there is no contact of the bone with the environment. In open fractures, the skin surrounding the area of the break is open and the bone is exposed to the environment. The major goal in these types of fractures involves the prevention of infection in conjunction with achieving proper alignment. Many patients have severe bleeding associated with this type of fracture. A complete fracture is one that involves the complete cross-section of the bone and it is visibly misaligned. In an incomplete fracture, the actual break may only involve a part of the cross-section of the bone in which one side of the bone is broken and the other part is merely bent. Pathologic fractures occur without or with minimal trauma and are usually seen in diseases such as osteoporosis and cancer.

Fractures not only cause damage to the bone involved, but to the soft tissues, nerves, tendons, and vascular system as well. These structures are in close proximity to the bones and help to support skeletal weight and to facilitate joint movement. When the fracture occurs, this stability is lost, and in turn, results in pain, swelling and splinting. The surrounding muscles are usually flaccid initially after the injury, but within an hour or less, may commence to spasm and this may impair venous circulation and displace the fracture further.

Another complication that frequently occurs is called compartmental syndrome. After a fracture occurs to the arm or leg, the fascia surrounding the muscles form compartments with small openings for major arteries, nerves, and tendons. Edema can compress these structures and cause ischemia to muscle tissues. The initial ischemic changes result in a histamine release that causes dilation of the capillary bed and edema to the area. The edema further compresses the larger arteries, which in turn creates further ischemia, further histamine release, and a vicious cycle is formed. The nerves, veins, arteries, and muscles may receive irreversible damage within 6 hours, and contractures, paralysis, and paresthesia may occur within 24-48 hours without intervention.

Healing begins when the blood around the end of the bone forms a clot and is related to the revascularization process. An inflammatory response occurs with blood vessel dilatation, then the increased permeability of the capillaries allow protein and granulocytes to leak into the tissue. Fibrinogen converts to fibrin that collects proteins and other types of cells, and the granulation tissue allows for debris removal. When the pH of the fluid surrounding the bone fragments decreases, calcium goes into the solution and this begins the process that helps to form new bone. After a couple of weeks, the pH of the tissues rises, and calcium precipitates into the meshwork and a callus is formed as a bridge within the fragments of bone.

Frequently, if open fractures are present, fat particulate may embolize, and the patient must be monitored for this complication.
[See Fat Embolus]

MEDICAL CARE

X-rays: used to identify type, location, and severity of fractures or traumatic injuries and to evaluate healing process stage

Bone scans, CT scans, MRI scans: used to identify fractures and/or soft tissue damage

Arteriography: may be used to identify presence and severity of vascular damage associated with fracture

Laboratory: CBC may identify hemorrhage or hemoconcentration; WBC is usually increased due to the stress response after an injury but may indicate infection; coagulation profiles may be used to identify problems related to blood loss, liver injuries, or after blood transfusions

Surgery: may be required to repair and realign bone structure, nerve injury, soft tissue injury, or vascular injuries; may be required to stabilize skeletal integrity; may be required to relieve compartmental syndrome compression

Traction: used to realign fractured bones and to facilitate healing in proper alignment

NURSING CARE PLANS

Alteration in comfort

Related to: pain, muscle spasm, fracture, trauma, soft tissue injury, nerve injury, vascular injury, tendon injury, traction apparatus

Defining characteristics: communication of pain, moaning, facial grimacing, guarding of injured area, inability to be distracted, anxiety

Outcome Criteria

Patient will be free of pain or pain will be controlled to patient's satisfaction.

INTERVENTIONS	RATIONALES
Immobilize injured body part.	Reduces pain and prevents further skeletal displacement.
Support injured extremity gently and elevate using pillows as warranted.	Decreases edema, promotes venous return, and may help to decrease pain.

INTERVENTIONS	RATIONALES
Administer analgesics as warranted, and especially prior to painful activities.	Reduces pain, promotes muscle relaxation, and facilitates patient cooperation with medical treatment.
Provide backrubs, massage, position changes, and other comfort measures.	Helps to reduce pressure areas, enhances circulation, and may decrease pain.
Administer muscle relaxants as warranted.	Reduces muscle spasms which can decrease pain.

Information, Instruction, Demonstration

INTERVENTIONS	RATIONALES
Instruct on relaxation techniques, deep breathing exercises, visualization, guided imagery, therapeutic touch, etc.	Redirects attention from pain and provides patient with feelings of control; may assist patient in coping with discomfort.
Instruct patient in use of PCA as warranted.	Provides patient with control over his pain relief and has been shown to reduce the amount of narcotic analgesic the patient requires for pain control.
Instruct patient to notify nurse or MD of sudden different pain or pain that is unrelieved with analgesics.	May indicate infection, ischemia, or compartmental syndrome.

Discharge or Maintenance Evaluation

- Patient will have no complaints of pain.

- Patient will be able to control pain management by use of PCA with satisfaction.

- Patient will be able to recall information accurately and will notify medical personnel for signs/symptoms of complications.

- Patient will be able to demonstrate accurately and effectively the use of relaxation activity skills for use with controlling pain.

Impaired physical mobility

Related to: fractures, pain, immobilization, traction, neurovascular impairment

Defining characteristics: inability to move at will, limited range of motion, decreased muscle strength, decreased muscle control, reluctance to move injured body part

Outcome Criteria

Patient will achieve and maintain optimal mobility and function of injured area.

INTERVENTIONS	RATIONALES
Evaluate degree of immobility that has resulted from injury and patient's perception of his limitations.	After trauma, patient's perception of limitations may be out of proportion with their physical levels of activities and may require further information to dispel false concepts.
Maintain bedrest and move injured limbs gently, supporting areas above and below the fracture.	Decreases potential for further injury and impairment in alignment while stabilizing the injured area.
Reposition patient every 2 hours and prn.	Prevents formation of pressure areas and improves circulation.
Assist patient with range of motion exercises of all extremities as warranted.	Prevents muscle atrophy, increases blood flow, improves joint mobility, and helps prevent reabsorption of calcium due to disuse.
Encourage isometric exercises once bleeding and edema has resolved.	Helps to contract muscles without bending joints or moving extremities to facilitate maintenance of muscle strength. These exercises can exacerbate bleeding or edema if these problems are not resolved.
Ensure that adequate numbers of personnel are present for repositioning.	Casts and/or traction apparatus may be cumbersome and heavy and may require increased personnel to avoid injury to the patient or the nurses.

INTERVENTIONS	RATIONALES
Evaluate integrity of traction apparatus and set-up.	Traction provides for a pulling force on the long axis of a fractured bone to facilitate proper alignment and healing.
Maintain free hanging weights and unobstructed ropes when traction is utilized.	Ensures that the prescribed amount of weight is maintained on traction and reduces muscle spasms and pain.
Apply antiembolic hose and remove for 1 hour every 8 hours.	Prevents venous stasis and decreases potential for thrombophlebitis.
Observe for redness, tenderness, pain, or swelling to the calf; assess for positive Homan's or Pratt's signs.	May indicate thrombophlebitis.

Information, Instruction, Demonstration

INTERVENTIONS	RATIONALES
Instruct patient in use of spirometer and coughing and deep breathing exercises to be done every 2 hours.	Prevents atelectasis and facilitates lung expansion.
Do not routinely elevate the knees.	Elevation may place pressure on the lower extremities and decrease venous return and blood flow.

Discharge or Maintenance Evaluation

- Patient will achieve and maintain increased mobility and function of injured area.

- Patient will be free of complications that may occur as a result of immobility.

- Patient will be able to effectively demonstrate exercises to increase mobility.

- Patient will be able to recall accurately all information instructed.

Risk for peripheral neurovascular dysfunction

Related to: vascular injury, soft tissue injury, interruption of blood flow, edema, thrombus, hypovolemia

Defining characteristics: decreased or absent pulses, cyanosis, mottling, pallor, cold extremities, mental changes, abnormal vital signs, decreased urinary output

Outcome Criteria

Patient will be able to maintain adequate tissue perfusion.

INTERVENTIONS	RATIONALES
Monitor vital signs.	Systemic perfusion will be impaired if circulating blood volume is inadequate.
Palpate peripheral pulses and identify changes in equality or character of pulses distal to injury.	Decreased or absent pulse may indicate vascular injury that requires immediate intervention.
Monitor extremity involved for rapid capillary refill, skin color, warmth, and sensation.	Circulatory impairment may result in delayed refill times greater than 5 seconds. Arterial compromise may occur when skin is cool to cold and white, and venous compromise may occur with cyanosis. Sudden ischemic signs may be caused with joint dislocation due to injury to adjacent arterial structures.
Monitor for changes in neurovascular integrity every 1-2 hours as warranted. Notify MD for significant changes.	Paresthesias, numbness, tingling, or diffused pain may occur when nerves have been damaged or when circulation is impaired, and may require intervention.
Evaluate complaints of pain that are abnormal for the type of injury sustained, pain with passive muscle stretching, or	Hemorrhage and/or edema within the muscle fascia can impair blood flow and cause compartmental syndrome that

INTERVENTIONS	RATIONALES
decreases in muscle movement distal to the injury, and notify MD as warranted.	will require emergency intervention to restore circulation. Compartmental syndrome can result in permanent dysfunction and deformity within 24-48 hours and irreversible damage may occur after 6 hours without intervention.
Assist with monitoring of compartmental pressures as warranted.	Increases in pressure above 30 mmHg requires immediate intervention to prevent permanent damage.
Assess skin around cast edges for redness or pressure points, or for complaints of burning under the cast. Cover rough edges of cast with tape.	Rough edges of the cast may produce pressure and result in ischemia or tissue breakdown. Burning pain may indicate pressure areas that are inside cast and not visible.
Monitor cast for presence of flattened or dented areas.	May indicate that the cast is placing pressure to areas and may result in tissue necrosis.
Cut/bivalve cast as needed per hospital/MD protocol for circulatory impairment.	Relieves circulatory impairment that may occur from edema and swelling to injured area.
Apply ice packs to fracture site as warranted.	Reduces edema and hematoma formation.
Remove patient's jewelry from injured extremity.	May impair circulation when extremity swells.
Perform testing for tendon damage: Immobilize the two fingers on either side of the patient's middle finger and ask him to wiggle the middle finger; immobilize the proximal interphalangeal joint of a lacerated/injured finger and ask him to flex the finger.	May indicate superficial tendon damage if the patient cannot wiggle his finger, and deep tendon damage if the patient cannot flex the finger.

Information, Instruction, Demonstration

INTERVENTIONS	RATIONALES
Prepare patient for surgery as warranted.	Surgical intervention may be required to relieve compartmental pressure in order to avoid permanent dysfunction.

INTERVENTIONS	RATIONALES
Instruct patient in signs/symptoms to notify nurse/MD: increased pain, decreased sensation or movement, or changes in temperature or color of injured part.	Provides knowledge and allows for patient involvement in care. Provides method for prompt detection of potential complications to facilitate prompt intervention.

Discharge or Maintenance Evaluation

• Patient will have equally palpable pulses, warm and dry skin, and stable vital signs.

• Patient will have normal sensation to injured part.

• Patient will be able to recall information accurately and will be able to avoid potential complications.

Impaired skin integrity

Related to: compound fracture, traumatic injury, surgery, use of traction pins or other devices, use of fixation devices, immobilization

Defining characteristics: disruption of skin surface or other tissue layers, open wounds, pain, paresthesias

Outcome Criteria

Patient will achieve optimal wound healing and have no skin breakdown.

INTERVENTIONS	RATIONALES
Observe skin for open wounds, redness, discoloration, duskiness, cyanosis, mottling, or pallor.	Changes may indicate problems with circulation that may be caused by traction, casts, or splints, or by edema.
Apply eggcrate mattress, flotation mattress, air mattress, sheepskins, or use kinetic type bed.	Helps prevent formation of pressure areas caused by immobility.
Encourage patient to use trapeze bar and reposition frequently.	May minimize potential for abrasions to elbows from friction

INTERVENTIONS	RATIONALES
	during movement. Positioning helps to decrease pressure to skin areas.
Monitor integrity of traction set-up, pad areas that come in contact with patient's skin.	Improper set-up or positioning of apparatus may result in tissue injury or skin breakdown. Padding prevents pressure areas from forming on skin and enhances moisture evaporation to prevent skin excoriation.
Cover the ends of any traction pins or wires with cork or other protectors.	Prevents injury to other skin tissues.
Apply skin traction as ordered. Apply traction tape lengthwise on both sides of the injured limb after applying tincture of benzoin and extend the tape beyond the limb.	Benzoin provides a protective layer to prevent skin abrasion with removal of tapes. Traction tape that encircles a limb may impair circulation.
Mark a line on the tapes at the point when the tape extends beyond the limb.	Provides identification marker to assess whether traction tape has slipped.
Using elastic bandage, wrap the limb and tape (and padding, if needed) being careful to avoid wrapping too tight.	Allows prescribed traction without impairing circulation.
Remove skin traction at least daily and observe for any reddened or discolored areas. Provide skin care.	May provide evidence of any skin impairment and allows for cleansing of area to remove debris or drainage.
If cast is present, cleanse plaster off skin while still damp.	Dry plaster can flake and result in skin irritation.
Use padding, tape, and/or plastic to protect cast near perineal area.	Prevents skin breakdown and helps to prevent contaminants from adhering to cast.
Avoid use of lotions or oils around cast edges.	These agents can create a seal and prevent the cast from "breathing." Powder should be avoided because of the potential for accumulation inside the cast.

Information, Instruction, Demonstration

INTERVENTIONS	RATIONALES
Instruct the patient to avoid putting objects inside cast, such as fly swatters, coat hangers, etc.	Objects used for scratching may damage tissue.
Instruct patient in cast care.	Provides knowledge for future patient care and involves the patient in his medical treatment.

Discharge or Maintenance Evaluation

- Patient will have no further skin breakdown.

- Patient will have healed wounds without complications.

- Patient will be able to avoid complications of immobility.

- Patient will be able to accurately recall all instructive information.

Risk for infection

Related to: broken skin, disrupted tissues, exposed bone structure, traction devices, surgery, invasive procedures

Defining characteristics: temperature elevation, elevated white blood cell count, shift to the left, purulent drainage, redness, warmth, and tenderness

Outcome Criteria

Patient will be free of signs/symptoms of infection and wounds will heal without complications.

INTERVENTIONS	RATIONALES
Monitor vital signs. Observe for fever, chills, and lethargy.	Increased temperature and heart rate may indicate impending or present sepsis. Gas gangrene may result in hypotension and mental changes.

INTERVENTIONS	RATIONALES
Observe wounds for redness, drainage, dehiscence, failure to heal, etc.	May indicate presence of infection.
Perform wound care/pin care utilizing sterile technique.	Removes drainage and debris from wound which may prevent infection.
Obtain cultures as ordered.	Identifies causative organism and allows for specific antimicrobial therapy to eradicate the infection.
Observe prescribed isolation techniques.	Isolation may be required depending on type of infective organism. Precautions will prevent cross-contamination and spread of infection.
Observe wounds for presence of crepitus or fruity-smelling/frothy drainage.	May indicate the presence of gas gangrene infection.
Evaluate patient's complaints of sudden increase of pain or difficulty with movement in injured area.	May indicate development of compartmental syndrome or osteomyelitis.
Observe for hyperreflexia, muscle rigidity, spasticity in facial and jaw muscles, and decreases in ability to speak or swallow.	May indicate development of tetanus.

Information, Instruction, Demonstration

INTERVENTIONS	RATIONALES
Instruct patient to avoid touching wounds or pin sites.	Decreases potential for spread of infection.
Instruct patient/family in isolation procedures.	Provides knowledge and ensures compliance with procedures and decreases chance of cross-contamination.
Prepare patient for surgical procedures as warranted.	Surgical intervention may be required to remove necrotic bone or tissue to facilitate healing process and to prevent further infection.

Discharge or Maintenance Evaluation

- Patient will have appropriate wound healing with no signs/symptoms of infection.

- Patient will be able to accurately recall all instructions and avoid potential complications.

Knowledge deficit

Related to: lack of information, misunderstanding of information, inability to recall information

Defining characteristics: verbal requests for information, questions, inaccurate statements, lack of compliance with instructions, lack of follow-through, development of preventable complications

Outcome Criteria

Patient will be able to accurately verbalize understanding of disease process and treatment.

INTERVENTIONS	RATIONALES
Evaluate patient's understanding of disease process, injury, and treatment.	Provides baseline of patient's knowledge and helps identify need for instruction.
Instruct patient/family regarding mobility concerns.	Fractures usually require casts or splints during healing, and improper use may delay wound/bone healing.
Instruct patient in exercises to perform.	Prevents joint stiffness and muscle wasting.
Instruct in wound care/fixator pin care.	Enables patient to understand need for sterile/aseptic wound care to prevent further injury and infection.
Instruct patient to keep all follow-up appointments.	Provides for identification of complications and promotes patient compliance with medical regimen.

INTERVENTIONS	RATIONALES
Instruct in signs/symptoms to notify MD: pain, elevated temperature, chills, paresthesias, paralysis, color changes, edema, dislodged fixator, cracks in casts, etc.	Provides for prompt identification of problem to ensure prompt intervention.

Discharge or Maintenance Evaluation

- Patient will be able to accurately recall all instructional information.

- Patient will be free of preventable complications.

- Patient/family will be able to accurately perform demonstration of wound/pin care.

FRACTURES

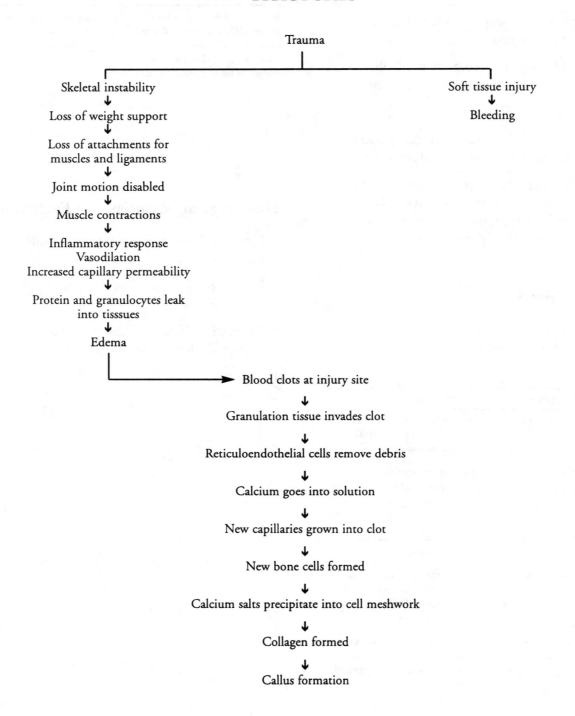

Trauma

Skeletal instability
↓
Loss of weight support
↓
Loss of attachments for
muscles and ligaments
↓
Joint motion disabled
↓
Muscle contractions
↓
Inflammatory response
Vasodilation
Increased capillary permeability
↓
Protein and granulocytes leak
into tisssues
↓
Edema

Soft tissue injury
↓
Bleeding

→ Blood clots at injury site
↓
Granulation tissue invades clot
↓
Reticuloendothelial cells remove debris
↓
Calcium goes into solution
↓
New capillaries grown into clot
↓
New bone cells formed
↓
Calcium salts precipitate into cell meshwork
↓
Collagen formed
↓
Callus formation

Amputation

Amputation may be caused by trauma, disease, or congenital problems. It may be required for uncontrolled infection, intractable pain, or gangrene due to inadequate tissue perfusion, and is usually performed as distally as possible to preserve viable tissue and bony structure for use with prosthetics.

A closed amputation utilizes a flap of skin for closure over the residual limb, and an open amputation requires future revisions and the wound heals by granulation. The open amputation is utilized in patients who are poor surgical candidates and with the presence of infection. Traumatic amputation is an accidental loss of a body part and is classified as complete when the part is totally severed, and partial when there is some connection with soft tissues.

Amputation may be considered as a last option when trying to salvage an extremity, and the surgeon may try revascularization, resection, or hyperbaric oxygenation in an attempt to save the limb. A lower extremity amputation is still considered a life-threatening procedure, especially when the patient is elderly or has peripheral vascular disease. With the advances in microsurgery, reimplantation of severed digits and limbs have become more successful.

MEDICAL CARE

Laboratory: culture and sensitivity of the wound may be done to identify the infection organism and the optimal antimicrobial agent required to eradicate the infection; sedimentation rate usually increased due to inflammatory response; CBC with differential used to identify elevated white blood cell count and presence of a shift to the left representing an infection process

Angiography, arteriography: used to assess blood flow and to identify the optimal amputation level

CT scans: used to identify neoplasms, osteomyelitis, or hematoma formation

Doppler ultrasound or flowmetry: used to assess blood flow to tissue areas

NURSING CARE PLANS

Alteration in comfort
[See Fractures]

Related to: injury, trauma, surgical procedure

Defining characteristics: complaints of pain, guarding of area, facial grimacing, moaning, discomfort

Alteration in tissue perfusion: peripheral

Related to: disease, surgical procedure, decreased blood flow, edema, hypovolemia

Defining characteristics: absent or diminished pulses, color changes, mottling, blanching, cyanosis, necrosis, gangrene, temperature changes, swelling

Outcome Criteria

Patient will have adequate peripheral perfusion with equal pulses, warm, pink skin, and optimal wound healing.

INTERVENTIONS	RATIONALES
Assess presence of peripheral pulses, strength, equality, and character. Notify MD for significant changes.	Changes in equality between limbs, diminished strength or absence indicates problems with perfusion.

INTERVENTIONS	RATIONALES
Perform neurovascular checks every 1-4 hours, noting changes in color, temperature, movement, or sensation.	Circulation may become impaired due to edema or tight dressings and may result in necrosis of tissues. Prompt detection of problems will allow for prompt intervention.
Evaluate non-operative leg for edema, inflammation, erythema, or positive Homan's or Pratt's signs.	Peripheral vascular disease may increase the incidence of post-operative thrombus formation.

Information, Instruction, Demonstration

INTERVENTIONS	RATIONALES
Instruct patient to report changes in sensation to operative site or any swelling.	Paresthesias may occur as a result of nerve damage or with impaired circulation. Swelling may result from fluid shifting or from continued bleeding which would require intervention.

Discharge or Maintenance Evaluation

- Patient will have strong, equal peripheral pulses, with no changes in sensation or temperature.
- Patient will be able to accurately recall signs/symptoms to report to nurse/MD.
- Patient will experience optimal wound healing.

Risk for infection

Related to: trauma, surgical incisions, open skin, invasive procedures, disease, decreased nutritional status

Defining characteristics: temperature elevation, elevated white blood cell count, shift to the left, sepsis, purulent drainage, reddened wound site, swelling, wound dehiscence

Outcome Criteria

Patient will be free of infection with no threat to wound healing.

INTERVENTIONS	RATIONALES
Monitor vital signs and notify MD for significant changes.	Sepsis may result in temperature elevation, tachycardia, and tachypnea.
Observe wound for signs of infection: redness, warmth, drainage changes, swelling, or dehiscence.	Prompt recognition of infection may result in prompt intervention and decrease the potential for further complications.
Culture wound drainage as warranted, and as per hospital protocol.	Identifies causative organism and allows for choice of optimal antimicrobial agent to eradicate infection.
Change dressing using aseptic or sterile technique as warranted.	Reduces spread of or introduction of bacteria to wound.
Ensure that drainage systems are functioning properly, and that measurement/emptying of drainage is being performed.	Drainage systems facilitate removal of drainage from wound which can decrease the chance of infection from stagnant body fluids. Measurement of drainage provides a trend to identify loss of fluid as well as potential healing or deterioration of wounds.
Administer antimicrobials as ordered.	Drug therapy may be given prophylactically using a broad-spectrum antibiotic until specific sensitivity reports are available to identify organism-specific antimicrobials.

Information, Instruction, Demonstration

INTERVENTIONS	RATIONALES
Instruct patient on signs/symptoms of infection to report.	Allows for prompt recognition of problems to facilitate prompt intervention.
Instruct on antimicrobial effects, side effects, and contraindications.	Provides knowledge and facilitates cooperation in the medical regimen.
Instruct patient/family on infection control procedures, isolation requirements, etc.	Provides knowledge and facilitates compliance with treatment; involves the family in patient care and reduces the potential for spread of infection.

Impaired skin integrity

Related to: amputation, surgical procedure, invasive procedures, broken skin

Defining characteristics: surgical wounds, puncture sites, abraded skin, disrupted skin or tissues

Outcome Criteria

Patient will have healed wounds with no skin or tissue disruption.

INTERVENTIONS	RATIONALES
Inspect wound daily to assess for healing, deterioration, color, character and amount of drainage, signs/symptoms of infection, etc.	Prompt detection of changes can facilitate prompt intervention for complications. Decreases in drainage amounts may indicate appropriate healing, whereas increasing amounts of drainage, or purulent/odiferous drainage may indicate the presence of fistulas, hemorrhage, or infective process.
If drainage amount is large, apply collection devices/bags over sites, recording amounts every 8 hours.	Helps reduce skin trauma by reducing surface area in contact with drainage, and facilitates more accurate measurement of drainage.
Cleanse wound per protocol at ordered frequency utilizing sterile or aseptic technique. (Many facilities use hydrogen peroxide followed by normal saline rinse.)	Helps reduce potential for infection; removes debris and caustic drainage from skin surface to preserve skin integrity and promote healing.
Utilize benzoin or other skin barrier products prior to the application of tape during dressing changes, or use Montgomery straps or stretch netting for dressings that may require more frequent changes.	Protects skin from abrasion with removal of tape. Use of netting or Montgomery straps prevent repeated removal of tape which can further disrupt skin integrity.

INTERVENTIONS	RATIONALES
Leave wound open to air, or cover with a light gauze dressing as soon as feasible.	Helps to facilitate healing; a light dressing may be required to prevent sutures or wound from becoming irritated by linens, clothes, etc.

Information, Instruction, Demonstration

INTERVENTIONS	RATIONALES
Instruct patient to avoid touching wound.	Prevents spread of infection or contamination of the wound.
Instruct patient in wound care as warranted.	Promotes knowledge and provides for patient involvement in his care.
Instruct in use of abdominal binder or supportive device as warranted.	Provides additional support for incisions at risk of dehiscence.

Discharge or Maintenance Evaluation

- Patient will have healed wounds with no impairment of skin integrity.

- Patient will be able to accurately perform wound care utilizing appropriate infection control techniques.

- Patient will be able to use supportive devices as needed to prevent wound dehiscence.

- Patient will be able to demonstrate appropriate behavior to prevent wound healing complications.

Risk for fluid volume deficit

Related to: nausea/vomiting, fever, excessive wound drainage, urine output, changes in vascular integrity, fluid shifts, oral fluid restriction

Defining characteristics: imbalance between intake and output, dehydration, poor skin turgor, tenting of skin

Outcome Criteria

Patient will achieve and maintain an adequate fluid balance, with stable vital signs and hemodynamic parameters, and palpable pulses.

INTERVENTIONS	RATIONALES
Monitor vital signs every 1-2 hours.	Fluid deficit symptoms may be manifested in low blood pressure, and increases in respiratory and heart rates. Changes in pulse quality or cool and clammy skin may indicate decreased perfusion and peripheral circulation and the need for replacement fluids.
Monitor intake and output q 1-2 hours, and notify MD of significant fluid imbalances or urine output less than 30 cc/hr for 2 hours.	Prompt recognition of imbalance and fluid loss provides for prompt intervention and replenishment of necessary fluids.
Evaluate for presence of nausea/vomiting; medicate as warranted.	Immediate postoperative nausea may result due to length of anesthesia and predisposition for nausea. Nausea/vomiting lasting longer than 3 days may result from adverse reactions to analgesics or other medications.
Observe wound sites for increases in drainage, swelling to area, or lack of drainage in drain tubes.	Sudden cessation of previously noted wound drainage may indicate an obstruction in the drainage system, with potential drainage then routed to tissues and other cavities. Edema to wound sites may indicate the formation of a hematoma or hemorrhage from the wound. Lack of swelling does not mean that hemorrhage is not occurring—retroperitoneal bleeding may not be visually noted until long after the patient has shown vital sign changes.
Administer IV fluids, blood and blood products as warranted.	Replaces necessary fluids and increases circulating volume.
Administer antiemetic drugs as warranted; may administer these in combination with analgesics.	Relieves nausea and vomiting which can result in the ability to ingest adequate fluid amounts.

INTERVENTIONS	RATIONALES
	Concurrent administration with analgesics may potentiate the analgesic in addition to controlling nausea and vomiting related to the pain medication.
Monitor lab values for hemoglobin and hematocrit, and notify MD for significant changes.	Hematocrit provides an indicator of fluid volume status and hydration. Blood losses that are not replaced may result in further fluid deficits.

Information, Instruction, Demonstration

INTERVENTIONS	RATIONALES
Instruct patient to report increases in wound drainage, leakage, or feelings of pressure sensation to wound areas.	Pressure sensation may result from retroperitoneal hemorrhage and should be evaluated immediately. Including the patient in his care provides for cooperation with medical regimen and provides for prompt recognition of potential problems that may lead to circulatory collapse from hypovolemia.

Discharge or Maintenance Evaluation

- Patient will be adequately hydrated, normotensive, with equal palpable pulses.

- Patient will have a balanced fluid intake with adequate urinary output.

- Patient will have normal skin turgor and moist mucous membranes.

- Patient will be able to accurately recall signs/symptoms to notify nurse/MD.

Body image disturbance

Related to: loss of body part, disease process, disfigurement, loss of function

Defining characteristics: negative feelings about body, preoccupation with missing part, avoidance of looking at missing part, perceptions of changes in lifestyle, preoccupation with previous function of missing part, feelings of helplessness

Outcome Criteria

Patient will be able to adapt and cope with changes in body image and demonstrate ability to accept self.

INTERVENTIONS	RATIONALES
Evaluate patient's ability to deal with amputation and his perception of need for amputation.	Provides input as to level of understanding of patient. Traumatic amputees most often have trouble in dealing with body image problems, as opposed to those who have reconciled that amputation may have been a life-saving procedure.
Observe for withdrawal, denial, or negativity regarding self.	Patients may not be able to deal with the trauma initially and may require time to come to terms with their new self. Recognition of stages of grief provides opportunity for interventions.
Provide time to discuss patient's concerns over the change in body structure and his perceptions of needs for a new/different lifestyle.	Provides opportunity to dispel false concerns and allows time for problem solving with realistic goals.
Encourage patient to help participate in his care and provide opportunities for patient to observe stump.	Promotes feelings of independence and allows time for patient to accept his body image. Positive reinforcement regarding the progress toward healing may further help his self-worth.
Discuss the availability of visits by another amputee.	Another person who has gone through the same experience may facilitate recovery and help the patient to recognize how he may attain a normal lifestyle.

INTERVENTIONS	RATIONALES
Encourage family members to assist with care and assess their ability to support patient.	Provides opportunity for family members to deal with the loss and to help in the rehabilitation phase.

Information, Instruction, Demonstration

INTERVENTIONS	RATIONALES
Instruct patient/family as to pre- and postoperative care, rehabilitation, and use of prosthetics.	Promotes knowledge and provides opportunity for patient to verbalize concerns and questions. May enhance postoperative recovery and facilitate compliance with medical treatment.
Obtain consultations as warranted with counselors or therapists.	May enhance patient's rehabilitation and ability to adapt to new body image.
Discuss concerns regarding sexuality as warranted.	Provides knowledge and helps with adjustment to body image, as well as provides opportunity to dispel any misconceptions.

Discharge or Maintenance Evaluation

- Patient will adapt and accept new situation and body image changes.

- Patient will be able to identify methods to adapt to changes and will be able to have positive self-esteem.

- Patient will be able to identify realistic goals and plans for rehabilitation and adapting to modification in body image.

Anticipatory grieving

Related to: actual loss of physical well-being

Defining characteristics: expressions of anger or

distress at loss, crying, sadness, guilt, alterations in sleep patterns, activity, eating or libido

Outcome Criteria

Patient will be able to express feelings appropriately and work through the stages of grief and grieving.

INTERVENTIONS	RATIONALES
Evaluate emotional status.	Anxiety, depression, and anger are normal reactions to loss of body parts. The patient may progress through the various stages of grief at their own rate and changes may be related to their physical condition as well.
Identify patient's stage in the grieving process.	Shock may be the initial response associated with the amputation, especially if it was traumatic. The patient may be so acutely ill that he is unable to express his feelings and concerns. Denial may initially be useful for patient's ability to cope with the injury, but continued denial may impair the patient's ability to effectively deal with the problem. Anger may be expressed either verbally, non-verbally, or physically, and the patient may displace his anger by placing blame. Depression may last from weeks to years and acceptance and support for these feelings will facilitate recovery.
Provide factual information to patient/family in regard to the diagnosis/prognosis. Do not give false reassurance.	Family may be where the initial instruction is directed if the patient's awareness is diminished due to his injury. The final outcome of a patient's injuries may not be initially known and so information should be kept simple.

INTERVENTIONS	RATIONALES
Assist patient to focus on needs he has now before changing focus to long-term goals. Encourage patient to take control in decisions regarding his care whenever possible.	Reduces frustration of facing an uncertain future, and allows the patient some control in dealing with current problems.
Provide acceptance of anger, hopelessness, and depression, but set limits on unacceptable behavior when warranted.	Acceptance of the patient's feelings acknowledges him as being worthwhile and a non-judgmental attitude is important in establishing trust and care. Limits may be needed to protect the patient and others from violent behavior while allowing the patient to express his negative feelings.
Provide consultation with therapists, social workers, or minister as warranted.	Physical and spiritual distress will be faced by the patient and his family and they will require long-term assistance and counseling in order to cope with the changes required by this injury.

Discharge or Maintenance Evaluation

- Patient will be able to progress through the various stages of grief and grieving effectively.

- Patient will be able to express his feelings and concerns appropriately without unacceptable violent behavior.

- Patient will be able to access community resources for long-term counseling and assistance to deal with his injury.

- Patient and family will be able to gain adequate support throughout the grieving process.

AMPUTATION

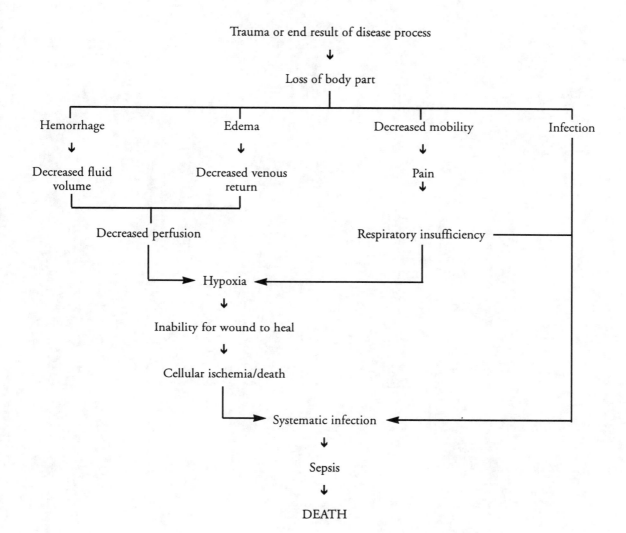

Trauma or end result of disease process

Loss of body part

Hemorrhage   Edema   Decreased mobility   Infection

Decreased fluid volume   Decreased venous return   Pain

Decreased perfusion   Respiratory insufficiency

Hypoxia

Inability for wound to heal

Cellular ischemia/death

Systematic infection

Sepsis

DEATH

Fat Embolism

A fat embolism usually occurs in patients with multiple fractures or fractures that involve the long bones or pelvis, when particles of bone marrow, tissue fat droplets, or combinations of platelets and free fatty acids are released and migrate to the lungs or brain. Embolization can occur within the first 24 hours up to 72 hours after injury.

The first signs/symptoms are usually changes in the mental status, with apprehension, confusion and restlessness noted. Petechiae to the chest, anterior axillae, shoulders, conjunctiva and buccal membranes occur due to capillary occlusion and are usually seen later. Respiratory distress with hypoxemia and hypoxia, pulmonary edema, and interstitial pneumonitis occur. The pulse rate increases, temperature elevates above 100 degrees and PaO_2 decreases.

MEDICAL CARE

Laboratory: serum lipase is elevated, sedimentation rate is increased; urine tests used to evaluate presence of free fat

Arterial blood gases: used to evaluate acid-base balance, presence of adequate oxygenation, and response to oxygen therapy

Electrocardiogram: used to evaluate changes in heart rate as well as cardiac changes, such as inversion of T waves and prominence of S wave in lead I showing myocardial and right ventricular failure

Corticosteroids: use is controversial, but may decrease inflammation and swelling

Heparin: use is controversial, but low dose heparin may be used to clear lipemic plasma and stimulate lipase activity

Dextran: low molecular weight dextran may be used to alter platelets and decrease intimal adhesions

X-rays: serial chest x-rays are used to evaluate pulmonary improvement or deterioration; x-rays of the bones involved in injury are used to evaluate healing process or alignment problems

NURSING CARE PLANS

Impaired gas exchange

Related to: altered blood flow due to embolism, shunting

Defining characteristics: abnormal acid-base balance, hypoxemia, hypoxia, tachypnea, tachycardia, air hunger, dyspnea, cyanosis, decreased oxygen saturation

Outcome Criteria

Patient will be able to achieve and maintain adequate respiratory function with arterial blood gases within normal ranges and with no evidence of respiratory distress.

INTERVENTIONS	RATIONALES
Monitor vital signs, especially respiratory status; assess for dyspnea, use of accessory muscles, retractions, nasal flaring, or stridor.	Dyspnea and tachypnea may be early signs of respiratory insufficiency. Other signs usually result from advanced respiratory distress, and all require prompt intervention.
Observe for changes in mental status, irritability, apprehension, or confusion.	Changes in mental status often are the very first signs in respiratory insufficiency. As hypoxemia and acidosis worsen, the level of consciousness may deteriorate to the point of lethargy or stupor.
Monitor pulse oximetry for oxygen saturation and notify MD for levels below 90%.	Oximetry may provide early warning of decreasing oxygenation and allow for prompt and timely intervention. In patients

INTERVENTIONS	RATIONALES
	who have decreased peripheral circulation however, the accuracy of pulse oximetry will be compromised and cannot be relied on totally.
Administer oxygen via nasal cannula or mask as warranted.	Provides supplemental oxygen and increases available supply of oxygen to ensure optimal tissue oxygenation.
Obtain ABGs as warranted.	Decreased PaO_2 and increased $PaCO_2$ indicate impending respiratory failure and impaired gas exchange.
Auscultate breath sounds for changes in equality and for presence of crackles (rales), rhonchi, wheezing, inspiratory stridor or crowing, or hyperresonant sounds.	Adventitious breath sounds may indicate progression of respiratory insufficiency. Inspiratory crowing may indicate upper airway edema frequently seen with fat emboli.
Observe for presence of blood in sputum.	May indicate hemoptysis that occurs with pulmonary embolism.
Observe for petechiae to chest, axillae, buccal mucosa, and conjunctiva.	Petechiae to these areas are frequently seen with fat emboli, and may occur 2-5 days after injury.
Encourage coughing, deep breathing exercises, and use of incentive spirometer.	Improves alveolar ventilation/ oxygenation and helps to minimize atelectasis.

Information, Instruction, Demonstration

INTERVENTIONS	RATIONALES
Prepare for placement on ventilator as warranted.	Deteriorating respiratory status may require mechanical ventilation to facilitate oxygenation. [See Mechanical Ventilation Care Plan.]
Use great care in repositioning patient especially during the first days post-injury.	Gentle handling of injured bones and tissues may prevent the development of a fat embolism.

INTERVENTIONS	RATIONALES
Monitor lab studies.	Patients with fat emboli frequently have anemia, elevated sedimentation rates, elevated lipase levels, fat in body fluids, hypocalcemia, and thrombocytopenia.
Administer corticosteroids as ordered.	Some physicians use steroids to prevent and treat fat emboli.

Discharge or Maintenance Evaluation

- Patient will have no respiratory dysfunction or distress.

- Patient will have arterial blood gases within his normal range.

FAT EMBOLISM

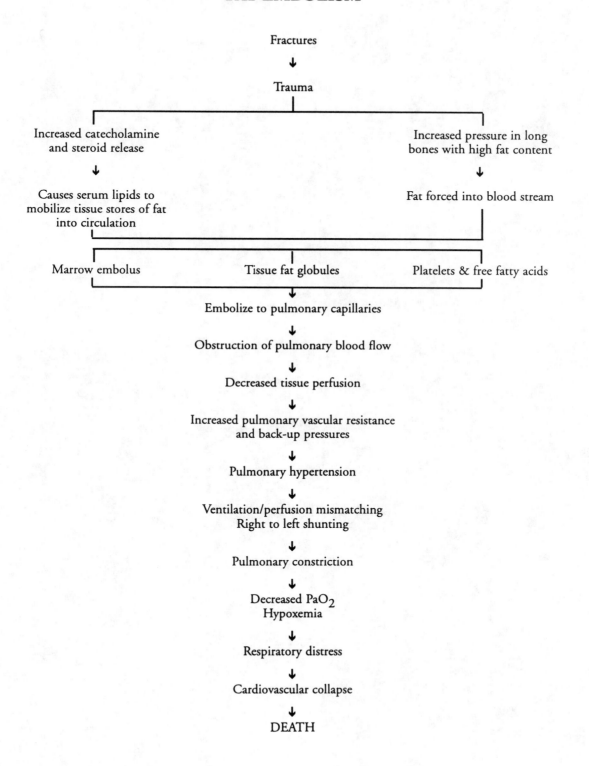

Fractures

↓

Trauma

Increased catecholamine
and steroid release

↓

Causes serum lipids to
mobilize tissue stores of fat
into circulation

Increased pressure in long
bones with high fat content

↓

Fat forced into blood stream

Marrow embolus   Tissue fat globules   Platelets & free fatty acids

Embolize to pulmonary capillaries

↓

Obstruction of pulmonary blood flow

↓

Decreased tissue perfusion

↓

Increased pulmonary vascular resistance
and back-up pressures

↓

Pulmonary hypertension

↓

Ventilation/perfusion mismatching
Right to left shunting

↓

Pulmonary constriction

↓

Decreased PaO$_2$
Hypoxemia

↓

Respiratory distress

↓

Cardiovascular collapse

↓

DEATH

INTEGUMENTARY SYSTEM

Frostbite/Hypothermia

Malignant Hyperthermia

Burns/Thermal Injuries

Frostbite/Hypothermia

Injuries from overexposure to cold, either air or water, occur in two types—localized injuries, such as frostbite, and systemic injuries, such as hypothermia. Untreated, both may be fatal.

Frostbite occurs after exposure to cold temperatures, usually below freezing. The severity of the injury is dependent on the amount of body heat lost, age and exacerbating factors such as wind chill, presence of wet clothing, and impairment of the circulatory status.

In frostbite, ice crystals form in the tissue fluids in and between the cells, causing injury to the red blood cells, which then develop sludging, and vascular damage. Blood is shunted to the heart and the brain. Skin is cold, hard, ashen white and numb, and with rewarming, becomes splotchy red or grayish in color, edematous, and very painful.

Frostbite can be either superficial, affecting skin and subcutaneous tissues, or deep, extending below subcutaneous tissues. With deep frostbite, the skin becomes white until thawed and then it becomes purplish-blue, with painful skin blisters, tissue necrosis, and development of gangrene when the tissue dies. At this point, amputation of the extremity may be required.

The most frequently seen sites that are involved with frostbite are the nose, ears, hands, and lower extremities. The goal of treatment is to restore body temperature to normal and prevent vascular damage to tissues. Supportive care is also important in restoring electrolyte imbalances and preventing hypovolemia.

Hypothermia occurs when the body's core temperature drops below 95° Farenheit and is noted by lethargy, mental dullness, decreasing level of consciousness, visual and auditory hallucinations, decreases in respirations and heart rate, and coma.

The core temperature may be as low as 80° Fahrenheit and below 90°, the body loses its self-warming mechanisms.

Hypothermia may also preclude successful resuscitation. Cardiac arrest is difficult to overcome if the core temperature is less than 85° Fahrenheit due to the increased ventricular fibrillation threshold.

Treatment is aimed at rewarming the body to increase the core temperature to adequate ranges, and to preserve organ and tissue viability.

MEDICAL CARE

Laboratory: CBC may indicate infection with shift to left; electrolytes will be required to restore balance from fluid shifts

IV fluids: used to restore circulating volume and prevent dehydration, and may be used to assist with rewarming

Dextran: low molecular weight dextran may be used to improve microcirculation to tissues

Reserpine: may be used to decrease sludging from injured cells and tissues

Antibiotics: may be necessary to treat infection if patient has open wounds or systemic infection

Analgesics: morphine and other drugs may be used to relieve severe pain from cold injuries; aspirin may be used to decrease platelet aggregation and sludging

Surgery: fasciotomy may be required to reduce tissue pressure caused from edema; amputation may be necessary for gangrenous injuries, or debridement may be required for necrotic tissues

Dialysis: peritoneal or hemodialysis may be used depending on severity of injury, in order to rewarm body

Rewarming techniques: warming blankets, warmed solutions for chest lavage or bladder irrigation, and warmed IV solutions may be utilized to increase temperature

NURSING CARE PLANS

Ineffective thermoregulation

Related to: exposure to cold, suppressed shivering response

Defining characteristics: temperature below 95° Fahrenheit, cold skin, mottling, cyanosis, pallor, poor judgment, apathy, decreased mental ability, level of consciousness changes, coma, lack of shivering, cardiopulmonary arrest, anuria, oliguria, decreased peripheral perfusion

Outcome Criteria

Patient will achieve and maintain an acceptable temperature with no complications.

INTERVENTIONS	RATIONALES
Obtain baseline temperature, and monitor every 15 minutes until stable.	Temperatures below 90 degrees result in suppression of normal body mechanisms to self-warming. Rewarming that is done too rapidly may cause peripheral vasodilation and may actually impede rewarming efforts.
Rewarm patient per hospital protocol. (Whole body or partial immersion into water that is 99-105 degrees, hypothermia blankets, gastric lavage with warmed solutions, peritoneal or hemodialysis, and IV infusions that are warmed are some methods currently used.)	Early rewarming decreases tissue damage from ice crystal formation, and helps to decrease cardiac instability and predisposition to ventricular fibrillation.

INTERVENTIONS	RATIONALES
Observe for mental changes and return of shivering response.	Shivering is suppressed at temperatures below 90 degrees F and is the body's normal response to facilitate self-warming. Patients have decreased mental abilities and levels of consciousness dependent on severity of hypothermia/injury, with hypoxia and hypoxemia occurring due to decreased perfusion.

Information, Instruction, Demonstration

INTERVENTIONS	RATIONALES
Instruct patient/family on appropriate procedures for rewarming.	Provides knowledge and reduces anxiety.

Discharge or Maintenance Evaluation

* Patient will be normothermic, with stable vital signs.

* Patient will be awake, alert, and oriented, with no alterations in abilities.

* Patient will be able to maintain thermoregulation.

* Patient will exhibit no complications from hypothermia.

Alteration in tissue perfusion: peripheral, cerebral, cardiopulmonary, renal, gastrointestinal

Related to: exposure to cold temperatures, frozen body parts, hypothermia, tissue necrosis, sludging of red blood cells, tissue ischemia

Defining characteristics: skin mottling, grayish skin color, purplish-blue color, cold skin, burning, tingling, numbness, pain, skin blisters, gangrene, diminished or absent pulses, decreased capillary refill, cardiac dysrhythmias, cardiac standstill, apnea, dyspnea, mental changes, unconsciousness, changes in consciousness level, coma, gangrene, oliguria, anuria, absent bowel sounds, ileus

Outcome Criteria

Patient will achieve and maintain normal body temperature with no lasting complications of decreased perfusion.

INTERVENTIONS	RATIONALES
Monitor EKG for rhythm changes, dysrhythmias, and cardiac standstill, and treat according to hospital policy.	Hypothermia affects heart rate and rhythm and may cause heart irregularities due to hypoxemia and conduction problems. Heart rhythm may be difficult to restore to sinus when body temperature is less than 85° F because of the increased ventricular fibrillation threshold. A 12-lead EKG may show an early J wave in the left ventricular leads.
Monitor vital signs every 15 minutes until stable, then every 1-2 hours.	During initial period after exposure, pulses and blood pressure may be too weak to be detectable. Rewarming too rapidly may result in heart irregularities.
Administer oxygen as ordered, with warmed humidification.	PaO_2 should be maintained above normal levels to treat hypoxia and hypoxemia that occurs with acidosis as a result of the injury and exposure.
Monitor pulse oximetry levels and notify MD if level drops below 90%. Monitor ABGs for changes.	Facilitates prompt identification of acid-base imbalances and changes in ventilation/oxygenation.
Monitor peripheral pulses for presence, character, quality, and changes.	Decreased or absent pulses may indicate impairment in circulation to extremities and may preclude tissue ischemia and necrosis.

INTERVENTIONS	RATIONALES
Move and handle patient and handle him gently when required.	Excessive movement may trigger lethal dysrhythmias or may cause tissue damage.
Administer warmed IV solutions as ordered.	Restores circulating volume, helps to maintain hydration and output, assists with rewarming efforts, and assists with treatment of hypotension.
Monitor hourly intake and output, and notify MD for significant changes or abnormalities.	Anuria or oliguria may indicate decreased perfusion to renal vessels or dehydration.
Evaluate patient's level of consciousness and mental status, and notify MD for significant changes.	Patients may have weakness, incoordination, apathy, drowsiness, and confusion with hypothermia. When body temperature is below 90 degrees F, stupor and coma are common.
Observe for muscle tremors, decreased reflexes, seizures, and Parkinson-like muscle tone.	Neurologic symptoms may occur due to hypothermic influences.
Remove constricting clothing and jewelry from patient.	Constriction especially in the presence of edema may impair circulation and perfusion.
Rewarm involved extremity in tepid water (37-40° Centigrade) until the tips of the injured part flush.	Prompt rewarming reverses ice crystal formation in tissues. Warmer water is not indicated due to the potential for burns. The appearance of skin flushing indicates that circulatory flow has been reestablished.
Avoid rubbing the injured extremity, and handle the area gently.	Helps to prevent further tissue damage.
Encourage patient to take warm liquids if possible.	Assists with rewarming.
Monitor vital signs; palpate for presence and character of pulses to extremities. Notify MD if pulse is absent after rewarming is accomplished.	When extremity has rewarmed, pulse should be able to be palpated. Absence of pulse may indicate decreased or absent circulation.

Information, Instruction, Demonstration

INTERVENTIONS	RATIONALES
Prepare patient for fasciotomy or amputation as warranted.	Edema may impair circulation requiring a fasciotomy to relieve pressure. If gangrene is present, amputation of the involved area will be necessary.
Instruct patient regarding long-term effects: increased sensitivity to cold, tingling, burning, increased sweating, etc.	Provides knowledge and identifies symptoms that patient may be faced with during his lifetime.
Instruct patient to avoid smoking.	Smoking causes vasoconstriction and may inhibit healing process.

Discharge or Maintenance Evaluation

- Patient will achieve optimal circulation and peripheral perfusion with equal palpable pulses.

- Patient will be able to recall and adhere to instructions and avoid preventable complications.

- Patient will be able to recall instructions accurately.

Alteration in comfort

Related to: tissue damage, surgical procedures, rewarming

Defining characteristics: communication of pain, facial grimacing, moaning, guarding, abnormal focus on pain, anxiety

Outcome Criteria

Patient will be free of pain, or pain will be controlled to patient's satisfaction.

INTERVENTIONS	RATIONALES
Evaluate pain level, and medicate with analgesics as ordered.	Rewarming process is extremely painful.
Elevate injured extremity on pillows as warranted.	Decreases edema which can result in pressure to tissues and pain.
Provide backrubs, repositioning, deep breathing exercises, visualization, guided imagery, etc.	Helps to refocus attention and enhances relaxation and ability to cope with pain.

Discharge or Maintenance Evaluation

- Patient will be pain free.

- Patient will be able to utilize comfort measures and techniques effectively to reduce or alleviate pain.

Risk for infection

Related to: frozen tissue, open wounds, decreased tissue perfusion, edema

Defining characteristics: elevated temperature, elevated white blood cell count, shift to left on differential, tachycardia, drainage, gangrene, edema

Outcome Criteria

Patient will be free of open wounds and infection process, and/or wounds will heal in a timely manner.

INTERVENTIONS	RATIONALES
When extremity has been rewarmed, apply a bulky sterile dressing to the area. Place gauze between toes or fingers.	Dressings between digits reduce moisture and help prevent tissue damage. Dressings help protect the area to reduce further injury.
If blisters are present, avoid rupturing them.	Reduces the risk of infection.

INTERVENTIONS	RATIONALES
Use sterile or strict aseptic technique for all dressing changes.	Frostbite makes the patient susceptible to infection.
Assist with whirlpool treatments for the injured extremity.	Treatments help to improve circulation, remove dead tissue, and help prevent infection.
Monitor vital signs and patient for presence of fever and chills.	Fever, tachycardia, and tachypnea may indicate presence of infection.
Administer antimicrobials as ordered.	Eradicates infective organism and may be given prophylactically.
Administer tetanus toxoid as ordered.	Concurrent trauma may necessitate administration to prevent onset of tetanus.

Discharge or Maintenance Evaluation

• Patient will be free of drainage from injury.

• Patient will be afebrile, with normal vital signs, and no symptoms of infection.

• Patient will have no systemic infection, or preventable complication.

FROSTBITE/HYPOTHERMIA

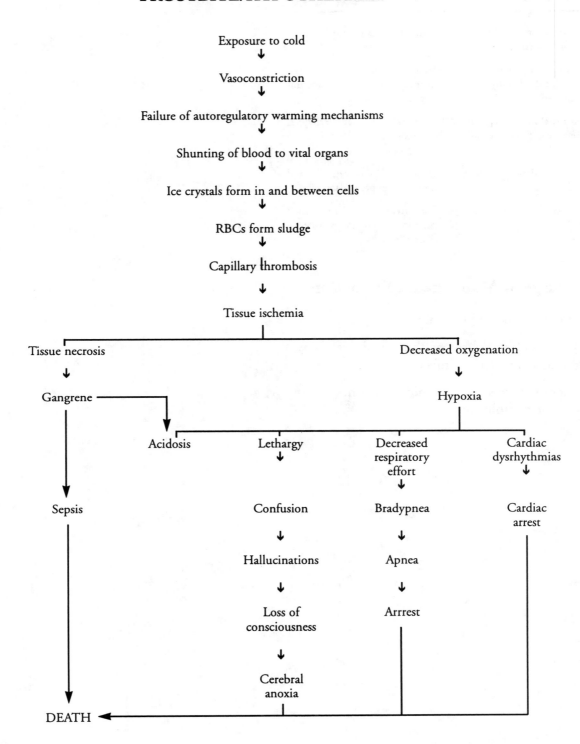

Malignant Hyperthermia

Malignant hyperthermia is a condition occurring from surgical procedures in which inhalation agents or muscle relaxants, such as succinylcholine, enflurane, fluroxene, ether, or halothane, are used. Although it occurs only about once in every 20,000 patients, the consequences may be lethal. Malignant hyperthermia results from excessive stores of calcium in the intracellular spaces that causes a hypermetabolic state with increased muscle contractions.

The inherited trait for this condition can be identified by increased creatine phosphokinase levels and/or muscle biopsy for histiochemistry and in vitro exposure to halothane. When this condition trait is identified in a patient who requires surgery, the preferred option is for local anesthesia.

The patient will notably have muscle rigidity, followed by tachycardia, dysrhythmias, rapidly increasing temperature, acidosis and shock. If left untreated, it has a mortality rate of 70%.

Treatment is aimed at recognition of the condition, with discontinuation of all anesthetic agents, and administration of dantrolene intravenously to slow down rate of metabolism. Supportive therapy to correct acidosis and fever should also be performed.

MEDICAL CARE

Electrocardiogram: used to identify conduction problems or dysrhythmias that may occur

Oxygen: used to supplement oxygen supply due to increased metabolic state

Dantrium: drug used to reverse effects of excessive calcium in intracellular areas; usually given until symptoms abate

Sodium bicarbonate: may be used to treat severe acidosis

Hypothermic treatment: cooling blankets, iced lavages and enemas, infusions of cooled IV solutions may be required to reduce temperature

NURSING CARE PLANS

Hyperthermia

Related to: reaction to anesthetic agents; hypermetabolic state

Defining characteristics: elevated temperature, tachycardia, tachypnea, muscle rigidity, tetany, cyanosis, presence of heart failure, acidosis, dysrhythmias, shock

Outcome Criteria

Patient will be free of fever, with stable vital signs, and will exhibit no evidence of muscle tetany.

INTERVENTIONS	RATIONALES
Monitor vital signs frequently; if able, continuously monitor temperature for changes.	Provides for prompt identification of worsening condition and allows for observation for effectiveness of therapy.
Monitor EKG for changes and treat dysrhythmias per hospital protocol.	Dysrhythmias may occur as a result of the marked hyperkalemia that may occur, or with electrolyte imbalances from fluid overload.
Administer dantrolene as ordered.	Normally given from 2-4 mg/kg IV rapidly through fast-running IV line; repeated every 15 minutes until a total of 10 mg/kg has been given, or symptoms subside. Dantrolene inhibits calcium release.
Monitor ABGs for changes.	May indicate metabolic or respiratory acidosis, and patients frequently have noted base excess -10 mmol.
Administer cooled IV solutions as ordered, utilize iced solutions	Methods may be required to decrease temperature to prevent

INTERVENTIONS	RATIONALES
for gastric lavage or enema, and/or place patient on cooling blanket.	further complication and body exhaustion.
Observe for shivering and administer Thorazine as ordered.	Shivering is a normal reaction to applications of cold, but is counterproductive because it increases metabolism to try to compensate for temperature changes. Thorazine is given to decrease shivering and reduce metabolic workload.

Information, Instruction, Demonstration

INTERVENTIONS	RATIONALES
Instruct patient/family in need of testing other members of the family for autorecessive trait.	May identify potential for anesthetic complications and avoid potentially life-threatening condition.
Instruct in utilization of hypothermic therapy methods.	Assists with understanding and facilitates compliance with discomfort.

Discharge or Maintenance Evaluation

• Patient will be normothermic with stable vital signs.

• Patient will have EKG with no rhythm aberrancies or conduction problems.

• Patient will exhibit no abnormal muscle contractions or tetany.

• Patient will be able to verbalize understanding of treatment and comply with regimen.

• Patient's family will comply and be tested for presence of trait that predisposes them to complications from anesthetic.

Risk for decreased cardiac output
[See Pheochromocytoma]

Related to: hypermetabolic state, fluid shifting

Defining characteristics: increased blood pressure and pulse, dyspnea, edema, confusion, restlessness, decreased urinary output, increased systemic vascular resistance, decreased cardiac output and cardiac index

Risk for altered nutrition: less than body requirements
[See Pheochromocytoma]

Related to: hypermetabolic state, anorexia

Defining characteristics: inadequate food intake, weight loss, muscle weakness, fatigue

Risk for impaired gas exchange
[See Pheochromocytoma]

Related to: increased respiratory workload, impaired oxygen to the heart, hypoventilation, altered oxygen supply, altered blood flow, change in vascular resistance

Defining characteristics: confusion, restlessness, hypercapnia, hypoxia, cyanosis, dyspnea, tachypnea, changes in ABG values, metabolic acidosis, respiratory acidosis, activity intolerance

MALIGNANT HYPERTHERMIA

Inherited autosomal dominant

PLUS

Muscle relaxants and/or general inhalation agents used for surgical procedures
↓
Excessive intracellular accumulations of calcium
↓

Increased metabolism rate   Hyperkalemia
↓   ↓
Increased muscle rigidity   Cardiac dysrhythmias
↓   ↓
Increased muscle contractions   Cardiac insufficiency
↓
Muscle tissue breakdown with
increased CPK and myoglobin
↓
Increased workload on renal system

Impaired oxygenation of tissues
↓
Metabolic acidosis
↓
Cardiovascular and renal compromise
↓
Organ failure
↓
DEATH

Burns/Thermal Injuries

Burns may be caused from thermal, chemical, electrical, or radioactive sources and may involve complex forms of trauma to multiple body systems. The depth of the injury is partially determined by the duration and intensity of exposure to the burning agent.

The initial treatment of a burn patient is to stop the burning process. This may be accomplished by cooling the skin, removal of contact with chemicals, removal from electrical current, or removal from radioactive environment. Often, inhalation injury also occurs because of inspiration of heated soot particles, chemicals and corrosives, or toxic fumes.

A severe burn, one in which the patient has 30% of his body involved, may take months to years to heal, and mortality is very high. Full-thickness, or third degree, burns involve all the layers of the skin and sometimes underlying tissues. Partial-thickness burns involve the epidermis and upper portions of the dermis. Fourth degree burns involve not only the epithelium, but fat, musculature, and bones, requiring extensive debridement and skin grafting.

There are several methods available for determination of the percentage of body burn involvement, but the "rule of nines" is frequently utilized. The body is sectioned off with each arm and head/neck area equaling 9%, front, back, and each leg equaling 18%, and the perineum equaling 1%. Extent of thickness, age, and other factors also play a significant role with treatment options. For acutely severe burns, transport to a burn center is recommended.

Shock may occur in adults who have burns covering greater than 15% of their body surface area, and with children when greater than 10% of their body surface area is involved. The burn injury causes dilation of the capillaries and small vessels which leads to increased capillary permeability and increased plasma loss. As edema increases, the destruction of the epidermis becomes a breeding ground for bacterial invasion and dead tissue sloughs off.

MEDICAL CARE

Laboratory: CBC will initially show elevated hematocrit due to hemoconcentration, and later decreased hematocrit may mean vascular damage to endothelium; white blood cell count may increase due to inflammatory response to the trauma and wound infection; electrolytes may show initially hyperkalemia due to injury, later changing to hypokalemia when diuretic phase begins; sodium initially decreased with fluid loss and later changes to hypernatremia when renal system attempts to conserve water; alkaline phosphatase elevated, glucose elevated due to stress reaction; albumin decreased; BUN and creatinine elevated due to renal dysfunction; carboxyhemoglobin may be done to identify carbon monoxide poisoning with inhalation injury

Radiography: chest-x-rays used to identify complications that may occur as a result of inhalation injury or with fluid shifting from rapid replacement

Arterial blood gases: used to identify hypoxia or acid-base imbalances; acidosis may be noted because of decreased renal perfusion; hypercapnia and hypoxia may occur with carbon monoxide poisoning

Lung scans: may be used to identify magnitude of lung damage from inhalation injury

Electrocardiogram: used to identify myocardial ischemia or dysrhythmias that may occur with burns or electrolyte imbalances

Analgesics: required to reduce pain associated with tissue damage and nerve injury

Tetanus toxoid: required to provide immunity against infective organism

Antimicrobials: may be required to treat infection

Surgery: may be required for skin grafting, fasciotomy, debridement, or repair of other injuries

IV fluids: massive amounts of IV fluids may be required for fluid resuscitation immediately post-burn, and will be required for maintenance of fluid balance as shifting occurs

NURSING CARE PLANS

Risk for fluid volume deficit

Related to: burn injury, loss of fluid through injured surfaces, hemorrhage, increased metabolic state, fluid shifts, third spacing, shock, increased cellular membrane permeability

Defining characteristics: tachycardia, hypotension, changes in mental status, restlessness, decreased urine output, prolonged capillary refill, pallor, mottling, diaphoresis, poor turgor

Outcome Criteria

Patient will achieve and maintain fluid balance with adequate urinary output.

INTERVENTIONS	RATIONALES
Monitor vital signs, and notify MD of significant changes or trends.	Hypotension may indicate that the circulating fluid volume is decreased. Changes in vital signs may indicate the amount of blood loss but may not change until loss is greater than 1000 cc. Hypovolemic shock may occur due to hemorrhage, third spacing, or coagulopathy.

INTERVENTIONS	RATIONALES
Measure hemodynamics if pulmonary artery catheter has been placed. Notify MD for abnormal parameters.	CVP, or right atrial pressure, gives estimate of fluid volume status. Dehydration may be reflected by CVP of less than 5, while overhydration may be reflected at levels over 18 cm H_2O. Hemodynamic values may help to evaluate the body's response to the circulating volumes.
Observe for restlessness, anxiety, mental changes, changes in level of consciousness, or weakness.	Changes may reflect the severity of fluid loss.
Observe for bleeding from all orifices and puncture sites, and for presence/development of ecchymoses, hematomas, or petechiae.	May indicate impaired coagulation, impending or present DIC, or inadequate replacement of clotting factors.
Monitor intake and output hourly and notify MD for significant imbalances.	May indicate fluid volume deficit, and establishes a guide for fluid and blood product replacement. Fluid replacement is titrated to ensure urinary output of at least 30-40 cc/hr. Myoglobin may discolor the urine red to black, and if present, urinary output should be at least 75-100 cc/hr to reduce potential for renal tubular necrosis.
Administer IV fluids as ordered. Two IV sites should be maintained.	Replaces fluid loss, allows for administration of vasoactive drugs, plasma extenders, and emergency medications, as well as the administration. Two sites are recommended to facilitate simultaneous fluid and blood resuscitation in critical settings. Crystalloids, such as Ringer's lactate, are used during the first 24 hours, then colloids are used because colloids help to mobilize extravascular fluids. Dextrose is usually not given during the first 24 hours after injury because dextrose does not remain in the vascular space where it is needed.

INTERVENTIONS	RATIONALES
Administer blood and/or blood products as ordered.	Whole blood may be required for acute bleeding episodes with shock due to the lack of clotting factors in packed red blood cells. Fresh frozen plasma and/or platelets may be required to replace clotting factors and to promote platelet function.

Information, Instruction, Demonstration

INTERVENTIONS	RATIONALES
Prepare patient for placement of pulmonary artery catheter.	Provides knowledge to the patient, and catheter is invaluable for identifying changes in fluid status and hemodynamic responses to those changes.

Discharge or Maintenance Evaluation

- Patient will have stable vital signs and urinary output.

- Patient will have balanced intake and output.

- Patient will have good turgor, moist membranes, and adequate capillary refill times.

- Patient will be free of hemorrhage or abnormal coagulation.

- Patient will have no transfusion reactions.

Risk for ineffective airway clearance

Related to: airway obstruction, edema, burns to the neck and chest, trauma to upper airway, pulmonary edema, decreased lung compliance

Defining characteristics: adventitious breath sounds, dyspnea, tachypnea, shallow respirations, apnea, cough with or without productivity, cyanosis, fever, anxiety, restlessness

Outcome Criteria

Patient will have clear breath sounds with stable respiratory status.

INTERVENTIONS	RATIONALES
Identify causative agent of burn.	May reflect type of exposure to toxic substances and potential for inhalation injury.
Monitor respiratory status for changes in rate, character, or depth; note tissue color changes with cyanosis, pallor, or cherry red color.	May indicate the presence or impending respiratory insufficiency and distress. Cherry red color may indicate carbon monoxide poisoning.
Auscultate lung fields for adventitious breath sounds.	Obstruction of airway and respiratory distress may happen quickly, but may be delayed up to 48 hours post injury. Identification of abnormal crackles, wheezing, or stridor may indicate impending airway compromise and require immediate intervention.
Observe for presence of cough, reflexes, drooling, or dysphagia.	Inhalation injury may result in patient's inability to handle salivary or pulmonary secretions as a result of pulmonary edema.
Elevate head of bed 30-45 degrees.	Promotes lung expansion and improves respiratory function.
Administer supplemental oxygen as warranted.	May be required to correct hypoxemia and acidosis; humidification of oxygen prevents drying out mucous membranes and keeps secretions less viscous.
Monitor ABGs and observe for trends or deterioration.	May facilitate timely identification of respiratory insufficiency and hypoxemia that requires intervention.
Monitor oximetry continuously.	Decreases in oxygen saturation may indicate impending hypoxemia or hypoxia.

INTERVENTIONS	RATIONALES
Monitor EKG continuously and treat dysrhythmias per protocol.	Cardiac dysrhythmias may occur as a result of hypoxia or electrolyte imbalances, and some conduction problems may occur in response to rapid fluid resuscitation.

Information, Instruction, Demonstration

INTERVENTIONS	RATIONALES
Instruct on coughing and deep breathing exercises.	Increases lung expansion and helps to mobilize secretions.
Prepare patient/family for potential placement on mechanical ventilation.	May be required for respiratory embarrassment and distress.

Discharge or Maintenance Evaluation

- Patient will be able to breathe spontaneously on his own with no adventitious breath sounds and adequate oxygen saturation.

- Patient will have arterial blood gases within normal limits.

- Patient will be able to comply with coughing and deep breathing exercises to help clear mucous secretions.

- Patient will not develop complications from injury.

Risk for impaired gas exchange
[See Mechanical Ventilation]

Related to: carbon monoxide poisoning, smoke inhalation, upper airway obstruction, burn

Defining characteristics: increased work of breathing, dyspnea, abnormal arterial blood gases, hypoxemia, hypoxia, decreased oxygen saturation, inability to effectively cough or clear secretions, viscous secretions, confusion, lethargy, restlessness, anxiety

Alteration in comfort
[See Snakebite]

Related to: burn injury, tissue destruction, wounds, debridement, surgery, invasive lines

Defining characteristics: communication of pain, moaning, crying, facial grimacing, inability to concentrate, tension, anxiety

Impaired skin integrity
[See Snakebite]

Related to: burn injury, surgical procedures, invasive lines

Defining characteristics: disruption of skin tissues, incisions, open wounds, drainage, edema

Fear/Anxiety
[See Snakebite]

Related to: burn injury, threat of death, fear of disfigurement or scarring, hospitalization, mechanical ventilation

Defining characteristics: expressions of apprehension, tension, restlessness, insomnia, expressions of concern, fear of unknown, tachypnea, tachycardia, inability to concentrate or focus

Alteration in nutrition: less than body requirements
[See Pheochromocytoma]

Related to: burn injury, increased metabolic rate, intubation

Defining characteristics: intake less than output, weight loss, abnormal electrolytes, weakness, lethargy, catabolic state

Impaired physical mobility
[See Fractures]

Related to: burn injury, dressings, imposed physical inactivity

Defining characteristics: inability to move at will, imposed inactivity, contractures, wounds, pain

Risk for infection
[See Frostbite]

Related to: burn injury, tissue destruction, open wounds, impaired skin integrity, ARDS

Defining characteristics: elevated white blood cell count, differential shift to the left, fever, tachycardia, tachypnea, wound drainage, necrosis, presence of systemic infection

BURNS/THERMAL INJURIES

(thermal, electrical, chemical)

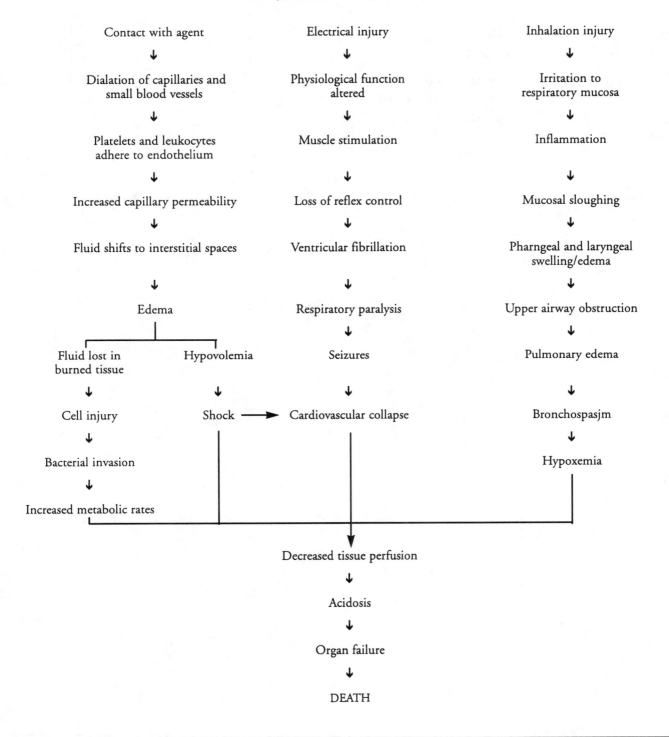

Contact with agent
↓
Dialation of capillaries and
small blood vessels
↓
Platelets and leukocytes
adhere to endothelium
↓
Increased capillary permeability
↓
Fluid shifts to interstitial spaces
↓
Edema

Fluid lost in   Hypovolemia
burned tissue
↓   ↓
Cell injury   Shock
↓
Bacterial invasion
↓
Increased metabolic rates

Electrical injury
↓
Physiological function
altered
↓
Muscle stimulation
↓
Loss of reflex control
↓
Ventricular fibrillation
↓
Respiratory paralysis
↓
Seizures
↓
Cardiovascular collapse

Inhalation injury
↓
Irritation to
respiratory mucosa
↓
Inflammation
↓
Mucosal sloughing
↓
Pharngeal and laryngeal
swelling/edema
↓
Upper airway obstruction
↓
Pulmonary edema
↓
Bronchospasjm
↓
Hypoxemia

Decreased tissue perfusion
↓
Acidosis
↓
Organ failure
↓
DEATH

OTHER

Multiple Organ Dysfunction Syndrome (MODS)

Sepsis denotes the presence of microorganisms or their by-products in the bloodstream that create a fulminating infection with resultant systemic involvement and shock. The hemodynamic changes that occur during septic shock may result in inadequate perfusion and the development of multiple organ dysfunction syndrome (MODS). Another syndrome which may lead to MODS is systemic inflammatory response syndrome (SIRS). Both sepsis and SIRS utilize the same inflammatory cascade with differing sources of infectious versus non-infectious causes, and can both potentially lead to MODS.

As the bacterial infection progresses, the immune system attempts to destroy the causative microorganism, and the endotoxins within the cell membrane are released into the vascular system. The endotoxins then trigger systemic inflammation, activation of the complement cascade, and histamine release. This results in vasodilation, increased capillary permeability, and leakage of the protein-rich plasma into the interstitial tissues.

As the plasma seeps into the alveoli, and platelets and white blood cells embolize in the microcirculation, resulting in release of more vasoactive materials, the lung's compliance decreases and ARDS develops. The liver is unable to detoxify the circulating endotoxins because of microembolization in the liver itself as well as sludge in the hepatic system. As fluid volume decreases, the heart rate increases and cardiac output is raised. As the abdominal organs are constricted from emboli in the microcirculation, myocardial toxic factor (MTF) is released and blocks the calcium ion action and contractility decreases. As more and more endotoxins are circulating, more and more body systems are affected with decreased perfusion, hypoxia, and anaerobic mechanisms that the body tries to use to maintain metabolic function.

The goal of treatment is to support cardiopulmonary function and to identify and eradicate the organisms responsible for the infection in the first place. With two organ systems involved, mortality is 50-60% despite treatment, with the percentage increasing to 90-100% mortality with four or more systems involved.

The most frequent precipitating factor is usually a temporary episode of a shock state that results in body cell ischemia. The typical pattern of MODS includes a hypotensive episode that is apparently successfully resuscitated, with elevation of heart rate and progressive respiratory failure. The patient is then intubated and appears to be doing better, but is in a hypermetabolic and hyperdynamic state that produces progressive changes in labwork. Inotropic support is required, then pseudomonas, yeast, or viral organisms progress, causing renal failure and involvement of all systems, with death ensuing approximately one month after the initial event.

MEDICAL CARE

Laboratory: CBC used to identify hemorrhage, platelet dysfunction, infection, shifts to the left on differential; electrolytes with sodium decreased; renal profiles used to evaluate renal dysfunction and therapeutic response to treatment; hepatic profiles to evaluate hepatic dysfunction; coagulation profiles to identify clotting dysfunction and DIC; fibrinogen elevated with DIC; cultures done to identify causative organism and determine appropriate antimicrobial therapy; glucose elevated due to metabolic state; lactate level increased with metabolic acidosis, shock, or hepatic dysfunction

Electrocardiogram: used to identify conduction disturbances or cardiac dysrhythmias; may have ST and T wave changes mimicking MI

Arterial blood gases: used to identify hypoxia, hypoxemia, acid-base imbalances and evaluate effectiveness of therapy; initially may have respiratory alkalosis and hypoxemia, and in later stages, metabolic and respiratory acidosis with compensatory mechanism failure

Radiography: chest x-rays used to identify pulmonary or cardiac changes in vasculature, edema, complications; abdominal x-rays used to identify potential sources of infection, i.e., free air in abdomen

Antibiotics: may be used to treat infectious cause of sepsis

Narcan: has been used to counteract some of the endotoxins that are circulating in system

Corticosteroids: have been used to decrease inflammatory response to toxins

NURSING CARE PLANS

Risk for infection
[See Renal Failure]

Related to: progression of sepsis to septic shock, secondary infections, compromised immune system, invasive lines, malnutrition, debilitation

Defining characteristics: increased white blood cell count, shift to the left, fever, chills, cough with or without sputum production, wound drainage, hypotension, tachycardia, impaired skin integrity, wounds, positive blood, urine or sputum cultures, cloudy concentrated urine

Hyperthermia
[See Pheochromocytoma]

Related to: circulating endotoxins, dehydration, hypermetabolic state

Defining characteristics: increased temperature, fever, flushed, warm skin, tachypnea, tachycardia

Risk for alteration in tissue perfusion: cerebral, gastrointestinal, cardiopulmonary, renal, and peripheral

Related to: vasoconstriction, microembolism, vascular occlusion, hypovolemia, increased oxygen consumption, inadequate oxygen delivery, alteration in utilization of oxygen by tissues

Defining characteristics: decreased peripheral pulses, prolonged capillary refill time, pallor, cyanosis, erythema, paresthesias, pain, tissue edema, lethargy, confusion, oliguria, anuria, abnormal ABGs

Outcome Criteria

Patient will have adequate perfusion to all body systems.

INTERVENTIONS	RATIONALES
Monitor vital signs, noting trends.	Hypotension occurs when microorganisms enter the bloodstream and activate chemical substances that result in vasodilation, decreased systemic vascular resistance, and hypovolemia. Tachypnea may be the first symptom of sepsis as the body responds to endotoxins and developing hypoxia.
Monitor hemodynamic pressures if available, at least every 1-2 hours and prn.	When shock progresses to cold stage, cardiac output decreases in response to decreased contractility and alterations in afterload and preload. Fluid shifting may cause third spacing and fluid overload, and monitoring hemodynamics can facilitate early identification of changes in trends.

INTERVENTIONS	RATIONALES
Monitor EKG for changes and treat according to hospital protocol.	Tachycardia occurs in response to hypovolemia and circulating endotoxins. Dysrhythmias may occur from hypoxia, acid-base imbalances, electrolyte imbalances, or shock.
Monitor mental status and level of consciousness for changes.	May indicate impending or present hypoxia or acidosis leading to decreased cerebral perfusion.
Auscultate lung fields for adventitious breath sounds.	May indicate fluid overload in response to fluid resuscitation or presence of congestive failure.
Observe for changes in peripheral skin color and temperature.	Vasodilation may occur in the early phase of shock with warm, pink, dry skin, but as shock progresses, vasoconstriction occurs and reduces peripheral blood flow resulting in mottling, or pale to dusky skin that is cold and clammy.
Monitor intake and output every hour.	As renal perfusion is compromised by vasoconstriction or microemboli, oliguria or anuria may develop.
Palpate abdomen and auscultate for bowel sounds.	Absence of bowel sounds may indicate decreased perfusion to the mesentery from vasoconstriction that may result in paralytic ileus.
Administer IV fluids as ordered.	Large volumes may be required to maintain circulating volume from hypovolemic state, but must be monitored to identify and treat fluid overloading.
Administer oxygen as ordered.	Provides supplemental oxygen necessary for cellular perfusion and to relieve hypoxia.
Administer vasoactive drugs as ordered.	May be required to maintain pressure and hemodynamics at adequate levels to maintain perfusion to body systems.

Information, Instruction, Demonstration

INTERVENTIONS	RATIONALES
Observe for oozing at puncture sites, petechiae, ecchymoses, or bleeding from any area.	May indicate presence or impending DIC or coagulation problem.
Monitor for drug toxicity signs and symptoms.	Decreased perfusion may increase half-life and decrease metabolism of therapeutic drugs and cause toxic reactions.

Discharge or Maintenance Evaluation

- Patient will have stable vital signs and hemodynamic parameters.

- Patient will have warm skin, with palpable peripheral pulses that are equal bilaterally.

- Patient will be neurologically stable, and have adequate perfusion to all body systems.

Risk for impaired gas exchange
[See Mechanical Ventilation]

Related to: endotoxins in circulation, hyperventilation, hypoventilation, respiratory alkalosis, increased capillary permeability, alterations in blood flow due to microembolism, capillary damage

Defining characteristics: dyspnea, tachypnea, hypoxia, hypoxemia, hypercapnia, confusion, restlessness, cyanosis, inability to move secretions, tachycardia, dysrhythmias, abnormal ABGs, decreased oxygen saturation

Risk for fluid volume deficit
[See GI Bleeding]

Related to: vasodilation, third spacing, fluid shifting, increased capillary permeability

Defining characteristics: weight loss, output greater than intake, hypotension, tachycardia, decreased central venous pressure, decreased hemodynamic pressures, increased temperature, dilute urine with low specific gravity, oliguria with high specific gravity, weakness, stupor, lethargy

MULTIPLE ORGAN DYSFUNCTION SYNDROME (MODS)

Acute Poisoning/Drug Overdose

Attempts to end one's life by use of excessive amounts of medication may be executed for many reasons. Active self-destructive behavior usually results from the patient's perception of an overwhelming catastrophic event in his life, in conjunction with the lack of appropriate coping strategies, and is visualized as a means of escape from the sensed threat to himself.

Suicidal patients are frequently ambivalent about wanting to die, and may have visions of last-minute rescue. The suicidal person may feel despair, guilt, shame, hopelessness, boredom, depression, weariness, or dependency, and when the point is reached when the person perceives that life no longer has meaning and despair is overwhelming, the patient acts on those emotions. Suicide may be considered the last logical step when the person perceives that others do not want them around or that the problem can never be reconciled.

Usually, an attempt at causing death is the culmination of a process in which the person had ideations about killing himself, verbal or nonverbal threats of his intention, and gestures in which attempts of causing self-injury without actual intentions to cause death.

Suicide is the eighth leading cause of death in this country today, and the second leading cause of death in young people. Drug ingestion is the most frequent method utilized with suicide attempts, partially because of the availability of medications, and partially to avoid more violent means of death, such as with weapons or by hanging.

MEDICAL CARE

Laboratory: drug screens may be used to identify agent used for suicide attempt; alcohol level to assess concurrent use or toxicity; electrolytes may be abnormal due to trauma or interaction with medication; hematocrit may be decreased with hypovolemia; drug levels, such as phenobarbital or acetaminophen, may be elevated due to toxicity; renal profile may show renal insufficiency; liver profile may show hepatic dysfunction, especially with acetaminophen overdose; coagulation profiles may be abnormal; urinalysis may show low specific gravity, increased protein, hematuria, oxalate crystals, or metabolic by-products from drug overdose

Radiography: chest x-rays may show aspiration pneumonia or pulmonary edema complications

Electrocardiogram: used to identify conduction problems or dysrhythmias that may occur from drug overdosage, electrolyte disturbances, or with congestive failure

Dialysis: hemodialysis or hemoperfusion may be performed to remove some drugs when levels are severely elevated

Diuretics: may be required to force osmotic diuresis with agents such as mannitol, to manage certain forms of overdose

Acetylcysteine: Mucomyst is treatment of choice with acetaminophen overdose

Charcoal: used to bind poisons, toxins, or other irritants, increases absorption in the GI tract, and helps to inactivate toxins until excreted

NURSING CARE PLANS

Risk for ineffective breathing pattern
[See Mechanical Ventilation]

Related to: respiratory depression from drug, obstruction, pulmonary edema, pneumonia

Defining characteristics: apnea, dyspnea, lethargy, stupor, coma, abnormal arterial blood gases, decreased oxygen saturation, shallow respirations, tachypnea, stridor, adventitious breath sounds

Risk for injury

Related to: toxic effects of ingested drugs

Defining characteristics: respiratory arrest, pulmonary edema, shock, cardiac dysrhythmias, conduction changes, encephalopathy, amblyopia, edema, bronchoconstriction, blindness, blurring of vision, hypotension, hypothermia, seizures, hypertension, rhabdomyolysis, oliguria, anuria, heart failure

Outcome Criteria

Patient will achieve and maintain function of all organ and body systems and be able to eliminate ingested drug.

INTERVENTIONS	RATIONALES
Monitor vital signs every 1-2 hours and prn.	Facilitates early identification of changes and prompt interventions. Drug overdose may cause CNS depression with hypothermia, cardiac dysfunction from toxic drug levels, and pressure changes with volume imbalances.
Monitor EKG for changes in rhythm, dysrhythmias, or conduction problems, and treat according to hospital protocol.	Overdoses of tricyclic antidepressants may cause prolongation of PR, QT, and QRS complex; ST segment and T wave abnormalities, intraventricular conduction defects, bundle branch blocks, and dysrhythmias that may lead to cardiac arrest.
Maintain airway and provide supplemental oxygen as warranted.	Patients with overdoses may be unable to protect their own airway and have bronchocon-

INTERVENTIONS	RATIONALES
	striction or obstruction leading to respiratory arrest and death. Supplemental oxygen may be required to offset acid-base imbalances that result from overdosage.
Auscultate lung fields for breath sounds and presence of adventitious sounds.	Pulmonary edema may result from overdoses of barbiturates, sedatives, hypnotics, and tranquilizers. Changes in breath sounds may identify impending edema or heart failure.
Auscultate heart for tones and presence of abnormal sounds.	Gallops, murmurs, and rubs may indicate the presence or impending presence of complications such as pulmonary edema or heart failure.
Administer IV fluids as ordered.	Crystalloid solutions are normally used to treat hypovolemia which may occur due to compromised circulatory status.
Administer naloxone as ordered.	Reverses effects of narcotic agents and may be required to manage CNS depression or respiratory depression.
Monitor intake and output every 2 hours; compare 24-hour totals, and observe for changes in urine character and color.	Assists with estimation of fluid balance within body. Myoglobin may be present if rhabdomyolysis occurs as a result of overdose.
Insert nasogastric tube, aspirate fluid for analysis, lavage stomach, and administer activated charcoal as ordered.	Lavage is done to remove any drugs that may be left in stomach to prevent further absorption of the drug. Aspirate may be sent to lab for analysis of drugs ingested to provide identification for appropriate treatment. Charcoal is given to absorb drugs from gastric contents to prevent systemic absorption.
Administer osmotic diuretics as ordered.	May be required to manage overdoses of ethanol, methanol, ethylene glycol, and isoniazid, but must be done using caution to avoid fluid overload and electrolyte imbalances.

INTERVENTIONS	RATIONALES
Administer sodium bicarbonate as ordered.	May be required for management of salicylate poisoning to alkalinize urine.
Administer ascorbic acid or ammonium chloride as ordered.	May be required for management of amphetamine or PCP overdoses to acidify urine.
Administer Mucomyst as ordered.	May be required for management of acetaminophen overdose to decrease absorption and limit hepatic dysfunction.
Administer physostigmine as ordered.	May be required for management of tricyclic antidepressant overdoses to reverse the anticholinergic effects, but should be given cautiously to prevent cholinergic toxicity.

Information, Instruction, Demonstration

INTERVENTIONS	RATIONALES
Prepare patient/family for dialysis procedures.	Hemodialysis or hemoperfusion may be required for removal of drugs from system in severe intoxication when levels are potentially lethal or the toxin may be metabolized to a more lethal substance.
Ensure suicide precautions are exercised—removal of all potentially dangerous items from room and reach, close observation at all times, keeping exiting windows and doors impenetrable, providing all medications in liquid form, accompanying the patient to other ancillary areas, and avoidance of secret pacts with patient.	Maintenance of precautions facilitate a safe environment and allows for identification of potential problems. A patient who has made one attempt at suicide may attempt to complete the job and may be quite resourceful with items to perform the deed. Medications should be given in liquid form to ensure that the patient has swallowed the medication rather than saving it to use as suicide attempt later.
Provide padded side rails, with rails elevated at all times.	Provides safe environment and reduces risk of injury, especially if patient has a seizure.

Discharge or Maintenance Evaluation

- Patient will have stable vital signs and neurological status.
- Patient will have stable function of all body systems.
- Patient will have absorption of drugs minimized and maximal elimination of absorbed drugs.
- Patient will remain free of other injury.

Risk for violence directed at self

Related to: drug overdose, psychological status

Defining characteristics: feelings of loneliness, hopelessness, helplessness, perceived or real loss of significant person, job, health status, or control, unpredictable behavior, threats, low self-esteem, dependence on drugs or alcohol, withdrawal from substances, communication of suicidal ideations, depression, hostility

Outcome Criteria

Patient will achieve and maintain psychologic stability and seek assistance with mental health providers.

INTERVENTIONS	RATIONALES
Ensure environment is calming, darkened, with enough light for observation of patient.	Facilitates decreased fear and anxiety which may result with violent behavior.
Approach patient in a nonjudgmental, nonthreatening manner.	May have a calming effect on patient.
Listen to patient and what he has to say about his current situation without reacting emotionally.	Allows patient to verbalize problems. Emotional responses from caregivers may exacerbate hostile reactions from patient.
Confirm understanding of patient's problem, but do not reinforce denial.	Fosters communication and facilitates realistic feelings and methods for coping.

INTERVENTIONS	RATIONALES
Assist patient to verbalize emotions, anger, and other stressors, and to develop a plan for dealing with them.	Provides safe outlets for patient to express feelings and helps to work out realistic solutions for solving problems.

Information, Instruction, Demonstration

INTERVENTIONS	RATIONALES
Instruct patient/family on community resources, hot lines, crisis centers, ministerial counselors, etc.	Provides knowledge and assistance of resources available once patient is discharged.
Consult mental health provider/professional as warranted.	Allows for effective therapeutic psychological treatment to discern appropriate methods of coping with crisis.
Encourage family members to discuss their feelings and methods of coping.	Validates their feelings and responses and may assist them in finding more appropriate methods to cope with crisis.
Discuss actions to take if patient expresses suicidal ideations or attempts.	Patient may be more likely to try suicidal attempt again if situations or coping strategies are not changed. Understanding that if the patient has a definite plan for suicide, the more likely it is that he will be successful at ending his life, and that immediate intervention will be required.

Discharge or Maintenance Evaluation

- Patient will achieve psychological equilibrium and have no further suicidal attempts/gestures.

- Patient will be able to cope with crises in an appropriate manner, and will be able to effectively search out community resources for assistance.

- Patient and family will be able to verbalize feelings and effectively achieve therapeutic communication.

- Patient and family will be able to access available resources.

Risk for ineffective individual coping
[See Mechanical Ventilation]

Related to: crisis, drug overdose, loss of control, depression

Defining characteristics: verbal manipulation, inability to meet basic needs, inability to effectively deal with crisis, ineffective defense mechanisms, irritability, hostility

ACUTE POISONING/DRUG OVERDOSE

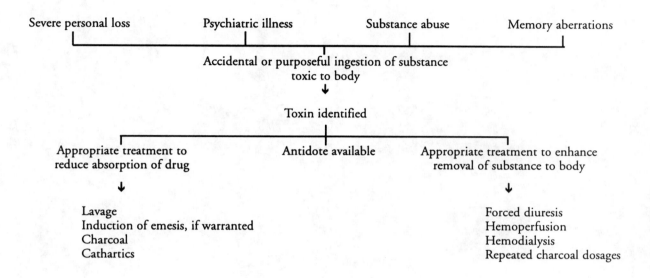

Severe personal loss   Psychiatric illness   Substance abuse   Memory aberrations

Accidental or purposeful ingestion of substance
toxic to body
↓
Toxin identified

Appropriate treatment to   Antidote available   Appropriate treatment to enhance
reduce absorption of drug   removal of substance to body
↓   ↓

Lavage   Forced diuresis
Induction of emesis, if warranted   Hemoperfusion
Charcoal   Hemodialysis
Cathartics   Repeated charcoal dosages

SYMPTOMS WILL BE DIFFERENT BASED ON ACTUAL SUBSTANCE INGESTED

System involved

CNS   Cardiac   Resp   Kidney   Liver

Decreased perfusion
Increased demand on tissues

Cerebral edema   Dysrhythmias   Metabolic acidosis   Coagulation
Seizures   Ischemia   Respiratory failure   problems
↓   Cardiac failure   Kidney failure   ↓

Coma   Hemorrhage

DEATH

Snakebite

In the United States, there are actually two types of poisonous snakes—coral snakes and pit vipers, which include rattlesnakes, water moccasins, and copperheads. Coral snakes are usually nocturnal creatures and less active than pit vipers, but tend to bite with a chewing motion and cause significant tissue damage.

Snakebites may occur on any portion of the body, but usually are noted on the extremities. Pit viper bites with envenomation result in immediate pain and edema within 10-20 minutes. Other symptoms include fever, ecchymoses, blisters, and local necrosis, as well as nausea, vomiting, diarrhea, metallic or rubbery taste, tachycardia, hypotension, and shock. Neurotoxins may cause numbness, tingling, fasciculations, twitching, convulsions, dysphasia, occasional paralysis, respiratory distress, coma, and death. Pit viper bites may also impair coagulation and cause internal bleeding.

Coral snake bites usually have a delayed reaction up to several hours, and may result in very little or no tissue pain, edema, or necrosis. The neurotoxic venom produces paresthesias, weakness, nausea, vomiting, dysphagia, excessive salivation, blurred vision, respiratory distress and failure, loss of muscle coordination, paralysis, abnormal reflexes, shock, cardiovascular collapse, and death. Coral snake bites may also result in coagulopathy problems.

The snake venom is a mixture of several proteins, enzymes, and polypeptides, and may produce several toxic reactions in patients who have been bitten. Correct diagnosis is imperative to treat the specific envenomation accurately and in a timely manner. Snakebites are critical emergencies and require precise identification of the snake as well as presence of envenomation. Designation of severity of the bite is commonly rated as minor, moderate, or severe, and depends on the presence of symptoms, depth of envenomation, and laboratory findings.

Treatment of snakebite involves administration of antivenin after a test dose for horse serum sensitivity is performed. If this sensitivity is present, diphenhydramine may be given prior to the antivenin. Swelling may necessitate surgical intervention to relieve the pressure and to prevent further vascular damage, and ensuing complications are usually related to secondary infection, renal failure, disseminated intravascular coagulation, or gangrene.

MEDICAL CARE

Laboratory: CBC used to identify blood loss and hemoconcentration; fibrinogen level, platelets, PT, PTT, and APTT to evaluate clotting; blood type and cross-matching to provide blood products as warranted; renal and liver studies to identify dysfunction, elevated BUN, creatinine, bilirubin, or creatine kinase

Electrocardiogram: used to establish a baseline for identification of problems that may occur with hemodynamic changes and to identify dysrhythmias and conduction problems

Surgery: fasciotomy may be required to relieve pressure caused from swelling or compartmental syndrome; amputation may be required for gangrene or necrosis

Analgesics: used to alleviate and/or control the pain related to envenomation and swelling; morphine is usually not given due to its vasodilator action

Antivenin: required as the antidote for snakebite; amount of antivenin is dependent on the severity of the reaction rather than patient weight, and ranges from 3 to 15 or more vials; children usually require more antivenin because of the ratio of venom to body size

Sedation: may be required to alleviate anxiety and to facilitate compliance with treatments

Tetanus toxoid: given to prevent complication that may be induced with infection from snakebite

Corticosteroids: usually are not recommended in the initial phase after snakebite because of the enhancement of the venom action and blocking of antivenin; may be warranted to treat shock or allergic reactions

Diphenhydramine: used when the patient has a reaction to the horse serum used for antivenin, or for other anaphylactic reactions

NURSING CARE PLANS

Risk for fluid volume deficit

Related to: hemorrhage, third spacing, altered coagulation, increased cellular membrane permeability, shock

Defining characteristics: tachycardia, hypotension, changes in mental status, restlessness, decreased urine output, prolonged capillary refill, pallor, mottling, diaphoresis, poor turgor

Outcome Criteria

Patient will achieve and maintain fluid balance with adequate urinary output.

INTERVENTIONS	RATIONALES
Monitor vital signs, and notify MD of significant changes or trends.	Hypotension may indicate that the circulating fluid volume is decreased. Changes in vital signs may indicate the amount of blood loss but may not change
	until loss is greater than 1000 cc. Hypovolemic shock may occur due to hemorrhage, third spacing, as well as the release of vasoactive substances and coagulopathy from the snakebite.
Measure hemodynamics if pulmonary artery catheter has been placed. Notify MD for abnormal parameters.	CVP, or right atrial pressure, gives estimate of fluid volume status. Dehydration may be reflected by CVP of less than 5, while overhydration may be reflected at levels over 18 cm H_2O. Hemodynamic values may help to evaluate the body's response to the circulating volume and bleeding status.
Observe for restlessness, anxiety, mental changes, changes in level of consciousness, or weakness.	Changes may reflect the severity of fluid loss.
Observe for bleeding from all orifices and puncture sites, and for presence/development of ecchymoses, hematomas, or petechiae.	May indicate impaired coagulation, impending or present DIC, or inadequate replacement of clotting factors.
Monitor intake and output hourly and notify MD for significant imbalances or urinary output less than 30 cc/hr for two hours.	May indicate fluid volume deficit, and establishes a guide for fluid and blood product replacement.
Administer IV fluids as ordered. Two IV sites should be maintained.	Replaces fluid loss, allows for administration of vasoactive drugs, plasma extenders, and emergency medications, as well as the administration of antivenin. Two sites are recommended to facilitate simultaneous fluid and blood resuscitation in critical settings. Crystalloids do not work as well as colloids because of the increased capillary permeability.
Administer blood and/or blood products as ordered.	Whole blood may be required for acute bleeding episodes with shock due to the lack of clotting factors in packed red blood cells. Fresh frozen plasma and/or platelets may be required to replace clotting factors and to promote platelet function.

Information, Instruction, Demonstration

INTERVENTIONS	RATIONALES
Instruct on use of antivenin, effects, side effects. Test dose for horse serum.	Provides knowledge and decreases anxiety. Skin test is required to identify hypersensitivities to the antivenin and frequently is repeated to ensure that the results are not false. If a reaction is noted, the antivenin is still given but is preceded by diphenhydramine.
Prepare patient for placement of pulmonary artery catheter.	Provides knowledge to the patient, and catheter is invaluable for identifying changes in fluid status and hemodynamic responses to those changes.

Discharge or Maintenance Evaluation

- Patient will have stable vital signs and urinary output.

- Patient will have balanced intake and output.

- Patient will have good turgor, moist membranes, and adequate capillary refill times.

- Patient will be free of hemorrhage or abnormal coagulation.

- Patient will have no transfusion reactions.

Risk for alteration in tissue perfusion: peripheral, cardiopulmonary, renal, cerebral

Related to: envenomation, edema, compartmental syndrome, coagulopathy, hemorrhage, hypovolemia, neurotoxins

Defining characteristics: hypotension, tachycardia, edema, decreased or absent pulses, inflammation, reddened or cyanotic skin, necrosis, gangrene, mental changes, restlessness, anxiety, abnormal hemodynamic parameters, abnormal arterial blood gases

Outcome Criteria

Patient will have adequate tissue perfusion to all organ systems.

INTERVENTIONS	RATIONALES
Observe puncture wound for bleeding, color, temperature, and note changes from baseline.	Skin normally changes after a snakebite from inflamed to a dark, cyanotic color. Changes in the wound and local tissues may reflect the action of the venom and potential complications.
Measure the circumference of the extremity involved initially and then every 2-4 hours.	Monitors for swelling and inflammation, and helps to identify the need for fasciotomy.
Palpate, or use doppler, to discern peripheral pulses distal to the snakebite, and notify MD for absence or decrease.	Edema may result in compartmental syndrome and obstruct circulation to the extremity causing ischemia, necrosis, and gangrene.
Assist with fasciotomy or insertion of catheter into the tissues of the edematous extremity.	Reduces tissue pressure and prevents tissue dehiscence and other complications.
Administer oxygen as warranted.	Provides supplemental oxygen which may be decreased due to hemorrhage or oxygen-carrying capability.
Evaluate extremity and site of snakebite for pain, ecchymoses, blisters, or blebs.	Venom effects may jeopardize tissue perfusion. Swelling and discoloration usually begin to dissipate after 48 hours, and continued problems may indicate the presence of other complications.
Apply ice packs over dressings as warranted. DO NOT apply ice directly over snakebite and surrounding tissues.	May reduce swelling. Ice packs may increase damage to skin tissues and cause necrosis.
Monitor for complaints of paresthesias, weakness, muscle incoordination, or fasciculations.	May indicate advancement of neurotoxic venom.
Observe for increases in salivation, dysphasia, dysphagia, or lethargy.	May indicate advancement of venom and further complications that will require life-saving treatment.

INTERVENTIONS	RATIONALES
Observe for changes in respirations, increased work of breathing, nasal flaring, retractions, dyspnea.	May indicate impending respiratory distress and may lead to cardiovascular failure and death.

Information, Instruction, Demonstration

INTERVENTIONS	RATIONALES
Prepare patient for fasciotomy.	Provides knowledge and reduces anxiety. Incision may be required to prevent skin dehiscence from edema.
Instruct patient in signs to notify MD or nurse: swelling, paresthesias, color changes, temperature changes, etc.	Provides for prompt identification of problem and prompt intervention to prevent further complications.
Prepare patient for amputation.	Provides knowledge and facilitates understanding of need for procedure, risks, and benefits, and allows the patient to make an informed choice. Amputation may be required for gangrene/necrosis.

Discharge or Maintenance Evaluation

* Patient will achieve and maintain adequate perfusion to all body systems.

* Patient will have palpable, equal peripheral pulses, with no paresthesias or evidence of ischemia.

* Patient will have adequate urine output and balanced intake/output.

* Patient will have adequate cerebral perfusion with no mental status changes.

* Patient will be able to accurately recall all information.

* Patient will be able to make an informed consent for procedures and will comply with treatment modalities.

* Patient will not exhibit any preventable complications.

Alteration in comfort
[See Fractures]

Related to: snakebite, swelling, edema, surgical procedures, decreased tissue perfusion, anxiety, envenomation

Defining characteristics: communication of pain, moaning, crying, facial grimacing, inability to concentrate

Impaired skin integrity

Related to: snakebite, envenomation, surgical procedures, invasive lines, necrosis, gangrene

Defining characteristics: disruption of skin tissues, incisions, open wounds, drainage, edema

Outcome Criteria

Patient will have wound healing occurring in a timely manner.

INTERVENTIONS	RATIONALES
Assess wound and surrounding tissues for appearance, drainage, swelling, healing, deterioration, etc.	Provides baseline for comparison and for identification of deterioration.
Cleanse wound with soap and water, or other agents per hospital protocol, as warranted.	Removes debris and drainage from skin surfaces and helps to prevent infection.
Apply gauze dressing as warranted and change every day utilizing sterile technique.	Dressing may help to control bleeding, absorbs drainage, and provides barrier for wound. Using proper technique for wound care prevents potential complications.
Elevate extremity as warranted.	Reduces swelling and pain, and helps to keep skin tissues free of pressure that might cause ischemia or necrosis.
Monitor extremity and wound for changes.	Swelling and discoloration should begin to subside by 48 hours. If swelling increases, or tissue perfusion is impaired, surgical intervention may be required.

Information, Instruction, Demonstration

INTERVENTIONS	RATIONALES
Prepare patient for fasciotomy or amputation, as warranted.	Provides knowledge to patient to facilitate an informed choice, and reduces anxiety.

Discharge or Maintenance Evaluation

- Patient will have healed wounds with no circulatory impairment.

- Patient will be able to circumvent preventable complications.

Impaired gas exchange

Related to: envenomation, ARDS, neurotoxins, cardiotoxins, hematotoxins, lactic acidosis, edema, snakebite, anaphylactic reactions, bronchospasm

Defining characteristics: dyspnea, tachypnea, air hunger, abnormal arterial blood gases, altered acid-base balances, cyanosis, inadequate oxygen saturation levels

Outcome Criteria

Patient will maintain own airway and have optimal ventilation and perfusion.

INTERVENTIONS	RATIONALES
Monitor respiratory status for changes: dyspnea, tachypnea, decreased oxygen saturation levels, cyanosis, decreases in mentation, restlessness, etc.	May indicate hypoxemia and hypoxia.
Administer oxygen as ordered.	Provides supplemental oxygen to increase availability, and to saturate red blood cells with oxygen.
Observe for laryngeal spasm, bronchospasm, or excessive salivation.	May indicate worsening respiratory status which may require mechanical ventilation.

INTERVENTIONS	RATIONALES
Obtain ABGs as warranted for signs of respiratory distress.	Will identify acid-base imbalances as well as hypoxemia, hypercarbia, and other ventilatory problems.
Prepare for intubation and mechanical ventilation, as warranted.	Hypoxemia that is not able to be corrected will require mechanical ventilation to facilitate adequate oxygenation

Discharge or Maintenance Evaluation

- Patient will be free of respiratory distress and able to maintain own airway and oxygenation on room air.

- Patient will have no respiratory complications.

Fear/Anxiety

[See Mechanical Ventilation]

Related to: snakebite, threat of death, fear of disfigurement or scarring, hospitalization, mechanical ventilation, envenomation

Defining characteristics: expressions of apprehension, tension, restlessness, insomnia, expressions of concern, fear of unknown, tachypnea, tachycardia, inability to concentrate or focus

SNAKEBITE

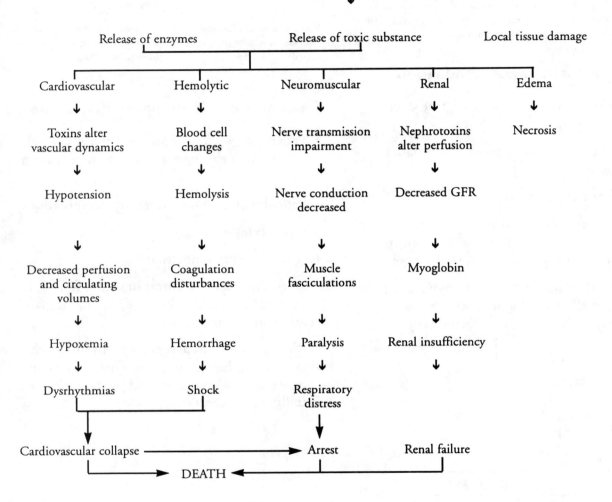

Envenomation
↓

Release of enzymes   Release of toxic substance   Local tissue damage

Cardiovascular   Hemolytic   Neuromuscular   Renal   Edema
↓   ↓   ↓   ↓   ↓

Toxins alter   Blood cell   Nerve transmission   Nephrotoxins   Necrosis
vascular dynamics   changes   impairment   alter perfusion
↓   ↓   ↓   ↓

Hypotension   Hemolysis   Nerve conduction   Decreased GFR
                             decreased

↓   ↓   ↓   ↓

Decreased perfusion Coagulation   Muscle   Myoglobin
and circulating   disturbances   fasciculations
volumes
↓   ↓   ↓   ↓

Hypoxemia   Hemorrhage   Paralysis   Renal insufficiency
↓   ↓   ↓   ↓

Dysrhythmias   Shock   Respiratory
                         distress
                           ↓

Cardiovascular collapse ⟶ Arrest   Renal failure
         ⟶ DEATH ⟵

Transplants

Transplantation of living tissues, cells, or organs from one individual to another is one method of treatment for several end-stage organ diseases. Often, transplantation is the last resort for a variety of disorders after conventional medical or surgical therapies have failed to provide adequate functioning. Recent advances in technique and treatment have improved the rate of success, and transplantation has improved the quality of life for many patients who otherwise would either die or be resigned to lives of dialysis or suffering.

Transplants are categorized by the relationship between the donor and the recipient. An autograft relates to the transplantation of tissue from one location to another in the same person. An isograft is a graft between identical twins, and an allograft, or homograft, is a graft between members of the same species. A xenograft, or heterograft, is a graft between members of different species.

Bone marrow transplants are performed in order to restore immunologic and hematologic function to patients who have aplastic anemia, leukemia, or severe combined immunodeficiency disorder. Multiple aspirations of bone marrow are obtained and then infused intravenously with red blood cells.

Heart transplants are performed to attempt to restore function in end-stage cardiac failure that has been unresponsive to other medical therapeutics, and usually involve patients who have cardiomyopathy, rheumatic heart disease, congenital heart disease, or coronary artery disease. After the patient is placed on cardiopulmonary bypass and the diseased heart is removed, the donor allograft heart is implanted. Frequently, a combined heart-lung transplant is performed due to the increased success rate as a result of fewer vascular anastomoses being required.

Renal transplants are performed to restore kidney function in end-stage renal disease. Allografts are usually obtained from living relatives or cadavers. The kidney is usually implanted in a retroperitoneal position against the psoas muscle in the iliac fossa. When cadaver kidneys are used approximately half of the recipients may require dialysis because of the presence of acute tubular necrosis.

Liver transplants are performed to restore function in patients with chronic active hepatitis, hepatitis B antigen-negative postnecrotic cirrhosis, primary hepatocellular tumor, or congenital anomalies of the bile duct or inborn errors of metabolism in children. The liver is implanted into the right upper abdominal quadrant and the vasculature is anastomosed. Biliary drainage anastomosis problems often result in bacteremia.

Pancreas transplants are performed on patients with insulin-dependent diabetes mellitus to provide insulin-producing tissue. The pancreas, either total with a small amount of duodenum, or partial segment of the distal pancreas, is transplanted. This type of transplant is performed as a life-enhancing procedure and is most successful prior to the development of severe secondary diabetic complications.

The goal in transplantation is to maintain optimal functioning of the organ and to prevent rejection. This goal is facilitated by antigen matching, tissue typing for histocompatibility, tests for prior sensitization, transfusions of whole blood, and immunosuppressive therapy.

Despite a small increase in the available donor

organs, the number of candidates for transplant far exceeds the organs available, and many patients die prior to undergoing transplantation. Complications of infection, rejection, and immunosuppressive drugs are a very real part of the process.

Transplantation of almost any tissue is feasible but rejection is the most frequent complication when the body tries to destroy the graft tissue. Rejection occurs when the immune system recognizes the graft as being foreign to the body and begins a responsive action to the antigens of the graft. Thus begins a cell-mediated immune response in the lymph tissues. Antibody-mediated immune responses, inflammatory responses, and complement activation also play a significant role in the rejection process.

Rejection may occur immediately after transplantation or up to years later, and most transplant patients experience at least one rejection episode during their lives. Signs/symptoms of rejection vary depending on the type of graft. Corneal transplant rejection is evidenced by corneal clouding, corneal edema, or conjunctival hyperemia. Cardiac transplant rejection is evidenced by decreased QRS, right axis shift, atrial dysrhythmias, conduction defects, S_3 gallop, jugular vein distention, decreased exercise tolerance, low grade fever, malaise, weight gain, dyspnea, right ventricular failure, and peripheral edema. Liver transplant rejection may be manifested with changes in urine or stool color, jaundice, hepatomegaly, ascites, pain in the center of the back, right flank, or right upper quadrant of the abdomen, low grade fever, malaise, or anorexia. Renal transplant rejection may involve low grade fever, decreased urine output, pain, swelling and/or tenderness in the kidney, increased blood pressure, malaise, weight gain, or peripheral edema. Pancreas transplant rejection may show

symptoms of increased glucose levels, polyuria, polydipsia, polyphagia, weight loss, low grade fever, and tender or enlarged pancreas. Bone marrow transplantation rejection is usually evidenced by severe diarrhea, jaundice and skin changes.

Rejection can be classified as being acute, hyperacute, or chronic depending on the mechanisms of rejection and the duration of time prior to the appearance of symptoms. Acute reactions may occur anywhere from 7 days to several weeks after transplant. A cell-mediated acute reaction occurs when the graft develops interstitial edema, ischemia, and necrosis, but high dose steroid therapy may reverse the reaction. Antibody-mediated acute reactions occur when fibrin, platelets, and polymorphonuclear cells adhere to the graft cells, resulting from recipient antibody-donor antigen responses. This aggregation produces ischemia and eventually necrosis. Hyperacute reactions develop immediately after the transplant up to a few days after. Immediate hyperacute reactions happen when the recipient has preformed antibodies against the donor antigens and is usually caused by previous blood transfusions, previous transplants, or from pregnancy. An accelerated hyperacute reaction happens when the recipient lymphocytes and neutrophils infiltrate the graft and may be prevented with the use of antisera to T lymphocytes. Chronic reactions occur over many months and eventually leads to loss of graft function. This occurs when the vascular endothelium becomes inflamed, and the arterial lumen decreases. Fibrin and platelets aggregate and over time, result in decreased blood flow to the organ and ischemia and dysfunction prevail.

The principal mechanism of rejection is GVH (graft versus host) disease. This occurs when an immunocompetent donor graft is transplanted into an immune-impaired recipient. If the donor and the recipient are not histocompatible, foreign cells will initiate an attack against the host cells, which are then unable to reject them. This usually occurs with bone marrow or liver transplants.

MEDICAL CARE

Laboratory: renal profiles used to assess kidney function; hepatic profiles used to assess liver function; CBC used to evaluate anemia, infection, and blood loss; glucose levels used to monitor pancreatic function; ABO blood grouping; Lewis antigens used to evaluate compatibility for kidney transplants; microtoxicity assays for evaluation of bone marrow; tissue typing for histocompatibility; lymphocyte antibody screen to evaluate preformed antibodies; lymphocyte cross-matching used after a suitable donor is found; serology, HIV, hepatitis screens to evaluate suitability for transplantation

Surgery: required for transplantation of tissues/organs

Biopsy: tissue biopsies used as the most accurate diagnostic tool to determine the extent of lymphocyte infiltration and potential tissue damage; serial biopsies can be used to monitor course of treatment

Immunosuppressive drugs: used to decrease or eliminate the body's ability to reject new transplanted tissues; can increase the risk for opportunistic organisms; usually a combination of drugs are used rather than just one

Blood transfusions: used to improve graft survival of certain organisms

Radiation therapy: used in some instances for pretransplantation immunosuppression

Thoracic duct drainage: used in some instances for pretransplantation immunosuppression

NURSING CARE PLANS

Risk for infection

Related to: immunosuppression, effects of transplantation, invasive procedures, invasive lines/catheters, trauma, surgery

Defining characteristics: increased immature white blood cells, differential with a shift to the left, fever, chills, cough, hypotension, tachycardia, presence of wounds, positive blood, urine, or sputum cultures, cloudy urine, purulent drainage

Outcome Criteria

Patient will have no signs/symptoms of infection after transplant surgery.

INTERVENTIONS	RATIONALES
Patient should be in private room, with appropriate isolation techniques in use. Visitors with illness must be restricted from visiting.	Decreases potential of infection when patient is already immunocompromised.
Observe for signs/symptoms of infection to all body systems.	Provides for prompt identification of complication and facilitates timely intervention.
Provide diet with appropriate nutrients and fluids. Restrict fresh fruits and vegetables.	Proper nutrition facilitates antibody formation and prevents dehydration. Fresh fruits/vegetables may harbor parasitic spores or bacteria that may result in an infection.
Monitor CBC, especially WBC count for abrupt changes in neutrophils.	Sudden decreases in mature WBCs may result from chemotherapy and further compromise the immune response.
Use sterile/aseptic technique with dressing changes, IV site changes, or other invasive care.	Immunosuppressive drugs or effects of the patient's disease process may slow wound healing. Drainage is a potential medium for bacterial growth.
Observe mouth and oral cavity for presence of lesions or thrush. Use nystatin as warranted.	Steroid and antibiotic administration may result in an overgrowth of fungal colonization resulting in candidiasis.

Discharge or Maintenance Evaluation

- Patient will exhibit no signs of infection post-transplant.

- Patient will have stable vital signs and hemodynamics.

- Patient will not develop any complication.

Risk for injury

Related to: rejection of transplanted organ, tissue, or bone marrow, allergic reaction to transplant

Defining characteristics: fever, chills, diaphoresis, peripheral edema, weight gain, decreased urine output, hypertension, urticaria, enlargement of the graft, oliguria, anuria, hypotension, right-sided heart failure, right flank pain, light-colored stools, anorexia

Outcome Criteria

Patient will not have rejection of new transplant.

INTERVENTIONS	RATIONALES
Monitor patient for fever, chills, hypotension, flushing, inflammation, thrush, cough, urinary changes.	May indicate impending rejection of transplant, or adverse reaction to immunosuppressants. Acute rejection is common and usually occurs during the first weeks or months following the transplant.
Monitor for increased bilirubin levels, hepatomegaly, encephalopathy, or heart failure.	May indicate complication as a result of bone marrow transplant and is usually seen in 25% of patients.
Observe for rash or skin ulcerations.	May indicate presence of graft-versus-host (GVH) disease and may occur up to 2 weeks post-transplant.
Administer immunosuppressive therapy as ordered.	Drugs interfere with some step in the body's response against the graft to decrease the immune

INTERVENTIONS	RATIONALES
	response. Imuran suppresses DNA and RNA synthesis; cyclosporine blocks the release of interleukin-1 and gamma-interferons and blocks activated T lymphocytes; prednisone and other corticosteroids inhibit T-cell proliferation, decreases production of interleukin-2 and gamma-interferons, and decreases IgG synthesis; muromonab blocks T cells that foster renal rejection.
Administer blood products as warranted.	Anemia and blood dyscrasias may be present after bone marrow transplants and require supplementation of blood products until transplantation is successful and may occur up to 2 weeks after infusion. Granulocyte infusion may be deemed necessary if antibiotic therapy is not effective to treat bacterial infections.
Monitor lab studies for significant changes.	Provides data that may be indicative of impending or present rejection.

Information, Instruction, Demonstration

INTERVENTIONS	RATIONALES
Prepare patient for biopsies as warranted.	Cardiac transplants require periodic endomyocardial biopsies to identify cellular rejection.
Instruct patient/family on signs/symptoms of rejection of particular transplanted organ/tissue.	Promotes knowledge, facilitates compliance, and allows for prompt notification to decrease severity of complications or rejection episode.
Prepare patient for surgery as warranted.	If excessive immunosuppression is required or if rejection is inevitable, kidney transplants may require removal and patient will need placement back of dialysis.

INTERVENTIONS	RATIONALES
Instruct patient on all medications taken, side effects, adverse effects, contraindications, and potential drug interactions.	Decreases risk of self-medication, and provides for prompt notification of adverse reactions that may require further intervention.

Discharge or Maintenance Evaluation

- Patient will have minimal rejection of transplanted organ/tissue.

- Patient will be able to comply with drug regimen to prevent rejection.

- Patient will be able to verbalize understanding of signs/symptoms to report to physician, and will be able to seek prompt medical care.

- Patient will be cognizant of all medications being taken, purposes, and potential side effects, and will have no adverse reactions.

- Patient will avoid further surgery.

Alteration in tissue perfusion: cardiopulmonary, cerebral, renal, gastrointestinal, peripheral
[See Renal Failure]

Related to: transplant rejection, allergic reactions, infection, pulmonary edema, DIC

Defining characteristics: oliguria, anuria, polyuria, fever, chills, increased white blood cell count, differential shift to the left, bleeding, ecchymoses, hematuria, guaiac positive stools, DIC, blood dyscrasias, decreased platelet count, headache, mental status changes, adventitious breath sounds, gallops, abnormal heart tones, dysrhythmias, rashes, ulcerations, nausea, vomiting

Social isolation

Related to: changes in health status, changes in physical status, imposed physical isolation, inadequate support system

Defining characteristics: feelings of loneliness, feelings of rejection, absence of family members/friends, sad, dull affect, inappropriate behaviors

Outcome Criteria

Patient will be able to participate in activities as tolerated and be able to have effective interaction with people within confines of medical disease process.

INTERVENTIONS	RATIONALES
Determine patient's comprehension of medical situation and rationales.	Identifies potential misconceptions and allows for realistic input to facilitate understanding.
Utilize appropriate isolation techniques based on patient's condition, and when possible, limit use of protective equipment.	Facilitates providing safe environment for patient yet providing social interaction to decrease feelings of social isolation. Appropriate use of gowns, masks, and gloves may be required due to patient's suppressed immune system.
Encourage visitation of family as much as possible. Provide a telephone so that patient may contact family and friends.	Transplantation costs are high and done in major hospital settings, so that family members may not be able to travel great distances for the length of time the patient may be hospitalized. Methods of communication are important to promote feelings of inclusion in family matters.
Identify significant family members or friends who are important to patient and involve them in care.	Support systems decrease sense of isolation and loneliness and helps to reestablish communication.
Assist patient to develop strategies for coping with isolation.	Promotes feelings of self-control while developing goals for achievement.
Contact social services, counselors, organizations, ministers, or other resources.	May be helpful to continue care once patient is discharged, and may be able to facilitate supportive encounters.

Discharge or Maintenance Evaluation

- Patient will be able to verbalize understanding of necessity for isolation procedures and will comply.

- Patient will have fewer feelings of loneliness and isolation.

- Patient will be able to meet sensory demands by family and friends.

- Patient will be able to effectively access community resources for referrals.

Alteration in comfort
[See Cardiac Surgery]

Related to: transplant operation, invasive lines and catheters, immobility

Defining characteristics: communication of pain, facial grimacing, increased blood pressure, increased heart rate, diaphoresis, moaning, splinting

Alteration in skin integrity
[See Cardiac Surgery]

Related to: transplant operation, invasive lines and catheters, biopsies, wounds

Defining characteristics: surgical incisions, disruption of skin surfaces, abrasions, redness, warmth, drainage

Knowledge deficit
[See Renal Failure]

Related to: transplant operation, changes in health status, anxiety

Defining characteristics: lack of knowledge, presence of preventable complications, verbalized questions

TRANSPLANTS

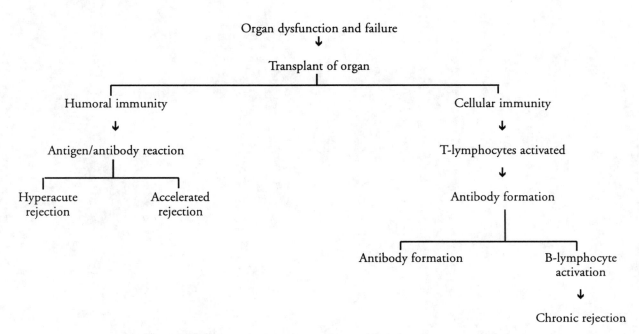

Signs of rejection will vary depending on particular organ that is transplanted.

Cardiogenic Shock

Cardiogenic shock is a severe form of pump failure that occurs when damage to the heart muscle is sufficient enough to impair contractility and reduce stroke volume and cardiac output. Usually the patient must necrotize 40% or more of the left ventricular myocardium to result in shock. In this type of shock, blood volume is adequate and fluid challenges will not improve cardiac output because the problem is that the heart fails to pump effectively. This decreases the stroke volume, and eventually tissue ischemia and hypoxia occurs. Cardiac output is decreased and hypotension ensures. Because of inadequate tissue perfusion, anaerobic metabolism produces lactic acid, leading to an acidotic state in the body. Despite treatment, 80% of patients who suffer this shock state will die.

Cardiogenic shock may result from mechanical interference with ventricular filling, from interference with ventricular emptying, from disturbances in heart rate or rhythm, or from inadequate myocardial contraction. Other causes that may predispose the patient to cardiogenic shock include acute dysrhythmias, severe congestive heart failure, cardiac tamponade, papillary muscle rupture, rupture of the interventricular septum or wall of the ventricle, ventricular aneurysm, mural thrombi, cardiomyopathy, pulmonary embolism, tension pneumothorax, or damage to the myocardial valves.

Patients with cardiogenic shock usually have increased CVP with jugular vein distention, cardiac index less than 2.0 L/min/m^2, systolic blood pressure less than 80 mmHg, mean arterial pressure less than 60 mmHg, PCWP greater than 18 mmHg, increased systemic vascular resistance, oliguria less than 20 cc/hr, peripheral edema, and pulmonary congestion. In the early stages of this shock, the initial decrease in cardiac output and blood pressure may be masked by the nervous system and compensatory mechanisms from the baroreceptors, which attempt to compensate for the increases in the body's cardiac workload and myocardial oxygen demand. Unless the cycle is interrupted, the scenario is always death.

MEDICAL CARE

Oxygen: to increase available oxygen supply

Alpha-adrenergic agonists: phenylephrine (Neo-Synephrine) used to improve blood pressure through vasoconstriction without inotropic effect

Beta-adrenergic agonists: isoproterenol (Isuprel) and dobutamine (Dobutrex) used to act directly on the myocardium to improve contractility, and to lower preload and afterload

Alpha-beta adrenergic agonists: norepinephrine (Levophed), epinephrine (Adrenalin), and dopamine (Intropin) used to improve contractility through vasoconstriction and direct action on myocardium

Vasodilators: nitroglycerin (Tridil) and nitroprusside (Nipride) used to reduce venous return to the heart by promoting peripheral pooling of blood, reduces preload, afterload, and myocardial oxygen consumption

Diuretics: furosemide (Lasix) used to reduce cardiac congestion and pulmonary edema

Enzyme inhibitors: amrinone (Inocor) used to inhibit the enzyme phosphodiesterase, increase available calcium, and increases cyclic adenosine monophosphate, or cAMP, levels to strengthen contractions

Cardiac catheterization: used to assess pathophysiology of the patient's cardiovascular disorder, to provide left ventricular function information, to allow for measurement of heart pressures and cardiac output, and to measure mixed venous blood gas content

Intra-aortic balloon pump: used to decrease workload on the heart by decreasing preload and afterload, and to improve coronary artery perfusion

Ventricular assist devices: used when other measures have failed; VADs allow blood to bypass the ventricle(s) which allows the heart to rest and lowers myocardial oxygen demands

Arterial blood gases: used to evaluate hypoxia and hypoxemia, metabolic acidosis, and other imbalances

NURSING CARE PLANS

Decreased cardiac output

Related to: circulatory failure, bradycardia, tachycardia, congestive failure

Defining characteristics: SBP < 80 mmHg, oliguria, cold clammy skin, weak thready pulses, dyspnea, tachypnea, cyanosis, confusion, restlessness, mental lethargy, dysrhythmias, chest pain

Outcome Criteria

Patient will have adequate cardiac output to maintain perfusion to all body systems.

INTERVENTIONS	RATIONALES
Monitor EKG for dysrhythmias and changes in heart rhythm.	Decreased cardiac output will decrease perfusion to the heart and dysrhythmias may occur.
Monitor vital signs every 15 minutes, or every 5 minutes during active titration of vasoac-	Bradycardia may result in decreased cardiac output, which leads to lowering of blood pres-

INTERVENTIONS	RATIONALES
tive drugs. Maintain MAP at >60 mmHg.	sure, increased respiratory rate, and can increase heart rate. Compensatory mechanisms in the body can easily fail within a short time. MAP < 60 is inadequate to perfuse coronary or cerebral vessels.
Monitor hemodynamic pressures and calculate CI, SVR, TPR, left and right stroke work and stroke work index. Measure CO.	Evaluates effectiveness of treatment and allows for efficient titration of vasoactive drugs. Determines actual cardiac output by measurement. In cardiogenic shock, CVP will be elevated >10 mmHg, CO will be <2.2 L/min, SVR will be increased, PVR and TPR will be increased, and stroke volume will be decreased. A good predictor of mortality is the LVSWI, with 95% death rate if <25 gm m/m^2.
Administer oxygen as ordered. Monitor oxygenation by use of pulse oximetry or ABGs.	Provides supplemental oxygen to increase available oxygen to tissues and reduce hypoxia.
Monitor for mental changes and changes in level of consciousness.	Decreased cardiac output may decrease perfusion to cerebral tissues.
Monitor urine output every hour and notify MD if <30 cc/hr.	Decreased cardiac output results in decreased renal perfusion and may lead to oliguria or renal failure.
Monitor for weak/thready pulses, capillary refill >5 seconds, cool clammy skin, pallor or cyanosis.	Decreased cardiac output results in decreased peripheral perfusion and tissue compromise.
Auscultate lungs for crackles (rales) or wheezes, and heart tones for S$_3$ gallop.	May indicate increasing fluid to lungs and impending congestive heart failure.
Observe for cough and pink frothy sputum.	May indicate pulmonary edema.
Auscultate heart tones for systolic murmur.	May indicate ventricular septal rupture or mitral insufficiency which may cause cardiogenic shock.

INTERVENTIONS	RATIONALES
Observe for abnormal precordial movement at 3-5 intercostal space.	May indicate cardiogenic shock.
Place head of bed no higher than 30 degrees if blood pressure is within acceptable parameters. Avoid trendelenburg position.	Elevation of the head of the bed may promote lung expansion and facilitate easier breathing. Blood pressure may be too low to have HOB elevated and patient should be supine to maintain blood pressure and perfusion to vital organs. Placement in trendelenburg position may increase preload, increase the workload on the heart, inhibit lung expansion, and prevent baroreceptors from sensing decreases in cardiac output.
Administer vasoactive drugs and titrate to maintain vital signs and hemodynamic pressures within MD ordered parameters.	Through a variety of actions, these drugs allow alteration of hemodynamic status to achieve and maintain optimal perfusion.
Administer morphine IV as ordered.	Relieves pain and helps to improve blood pressure and cardiac output by decreasing preload.
Administer atropine as ordered.	May be used to reverse bradycardia and help prevent some of the vagal effects from morphine.
Avoid using isoproterenol with MI patients except for temporary use prior to transvenous pacing, and only if shock is associated with severe bradycardia.	Isuprel increases myocardial oxygen consumption and workload of the heart while it increases heart rate.
Prepare patient for placement on IABP or for VAD usage.	Provides knowledge and decreases fear.

Information, Instruction, Demonstration

INTERVENTIONS	RATIONALES
Instruct on equipment, procedures, medications.	Provides knowledge and decreases fear.

Discharge or Maintenance Evaluation

- Patient will have cardiac output/cardiac index and hemodynamic pressures within normal limits.

- Urine output will be adequate.

- Vital signs will be normal and without overt signs of impaired perfusion to any body system.

- Lung fields will be clear with adequate oxygenation.

- Patient will be alert and oriented, with no mental changes.

Anxiety
[See MI]

Related to: change in health status, fear of death, threat to body image, threat to role functioning, pain

Defining characteristics: restlessness, insomnia, anorexia, increased respirations, increased heart rate, increased blood pressure, difficulty concentrating, dry mouth, poor eye contact, decreased energy, irritability, crying, feelings of helplessness

Knowledge deficit
[See MI]

Related to: lack of understanding, lack of understanding of medical condition, lack of recall

Defining characteristics: questions regarding problems, inadequate follow-up on instructions given, misconceptions, lack of improvement of previous regimen, development of preventable complications

CARDIOGENIC SHOCK

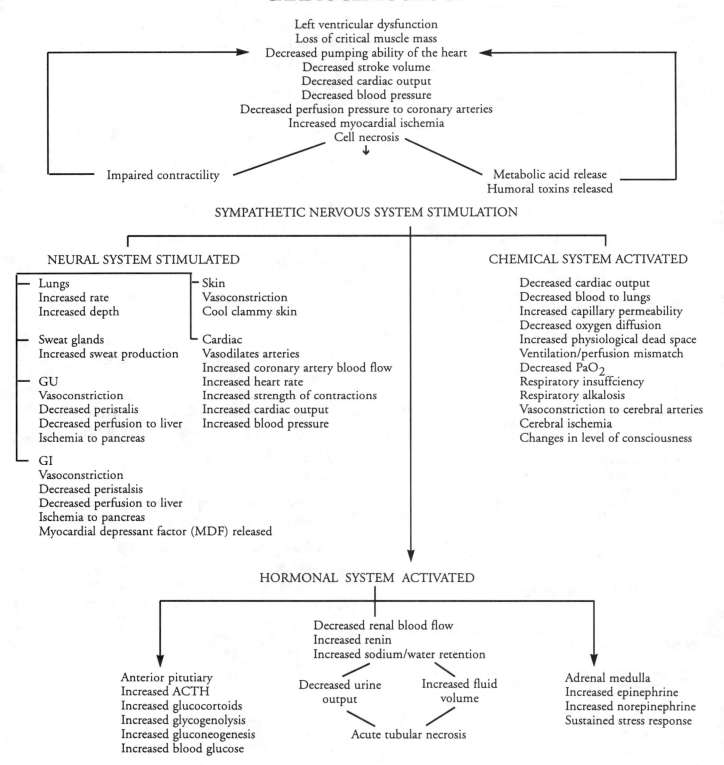

Left ventricular dysfunction
Loss of critical muscle mass
Decreased pumping ability of the heart
Decreased stroke volume
Decreased cardiac output
Decreased blood pressure
Decreased perfusion pressure to coronary arteries
Increased myocardial ischemia
Cell necrosis

Impaired contractility

Metabolic acid release
Humoral toxins released

SYMPATHETIC NERVOUS SYSTEM STIMULATION

NEURAL SYSTEM STIMULATED

Lungs
Increased rate
Increased depth

Skin
Vasoconstriction
Cool clammy skin

Sweat glands
Increased sweat production

Cardiac
Vasodilates arteries
Increased coronary artery blood flow
Increased heart rate
Increased strength of contractions
Increased cardiac output
Increased blood pressure

GU
Vasoconstriction
Decreased peristalis
Decreased perfusion to liver
Ischemia to pancreas

GI
Vasoconstriction
Decreased peristalsis
Decreased perfusion to liver
Ischemia to pancreas
Myocardial depressant factor (MDF) released

CHEMICAL SYSTEM ACTIVATED

Decreased cardiac output
Decreased blood to lungs
Increased capillary permeability
Decreased oxygen diffusion
Increased physiological dead space
Ventilation/perfusion mismatch
Decreased PaO_2
Respiratory insufficiency
Respiratory alkalosis
Vasoconstriction to cerebral arteries
Cerebral ischemia
Changes in level of consciousness

HORMONAL SYSTEM ACTIVATED

Decreased renal blood flow
Increased renin
Increased sodium/water retention

Anterior pitutiary
Increased ACTH
Increased glucocortoids
Increased glycogenolysis
Increased gluconeogenesis
Increased blood glucose

Decreased urine
output

Increased fluid
volume

Adrenal medulla
Increased epinephrine
Increased norepinephrine
Sustained stress response

Acute tubular necrosis

INDEX OF NURSING DIAGNOSES

Index

REFERENCES

References

Books

Berkow, Robert, Editor. <u>The Merck Manual</u>, 16th Ed., Merck, Sharp, & Dohme Inc., Rahway, NJ, 1993.

Guyton, Arthur. <u>Human Physiology and Mechanisms of Disease</u>, 6th Ed., W. B. Saunders Co., Philadelphia, PA, 1997.

Guyton, Arthur. <u>Textbook of Medical Physiology</u>, 9th Ed., W. B. Saunders Co., Philadelphia, PA, 1995.

Minssen, Beth. <u>Critical Care Core Curriculum</u>, 6th Ed., Panhandle Education For Nurses, Lubbock, TX, 1995.

Minssen, Beth. <u>Multiple Organ Failure Syndrome</u>, 2nd ed., Panhandle Education For Nurses, Lubbock, TX, 1995.

Skidmore-Roth, Linda. <u>Mosby's 1997 Nursing Drug Reference,</u> Mosby Year-Book Inc., St. Louis, MO, 1997.

Suddarth, Doris Smith. <u>The Lippincott Manual of Nursing Practice</u>, 6th Ed., J. B. Lippincott, Philadelphia, PA, 1996.

Swearington, Pamela and Keen, Janet. <u>Manual of Critical Care</u>, 3rd Ed., Mosby, St. Louis, MO, 1995.

Tierney, Lawrence M., et al., <u>Current Medical Diagnosis and Treatment</u>, 35th ed., Appleton and Lange, Stamford, CT, 1996.

Periodicals

Ahrens, Susan G. "Managing Heart Failure: A Blueprint for Success," Nursing 95, 25 (12): 26-31, 1995.

Blanford, Nickie. "Renal Transplantation: A Case Study of the Ideal," Critical Care Nurse, 13 (1): 46-55, 1993.

Bright, Linda D. "Deep Vein Thrombosis," American Journal of Nursing, 95 (6): 48-49, 1995.

Huston, C. J. and Boelman, R. "Autonomic Dysreflexia," American Journal of Nursing, 95 (6): 55, 1995.

Mee, Cheryl L. "Ventilator Alarms—How to Respond with Confidence," Nursing 95, 25 (7): 61-64, 1995.

Meissner, Judith E. "Caring for Patients with Meningitis," Nursing 95, 25 (7): 50-51, 1995.

Merkley, Kathleen. "Assessing Chest Pain," RN, 57 (6): 58-62, 1994.

Teplitz, Linda. "Hypertensive Crisis: Review and Update," Critical Care Nurse, 13 (6): 20-35, 1993.

Weinman, Steven A. "Emergency Management of Drug Overdose," Critical Care Nurse, 13 (6): 45-51, 1993.

SKIDMORE-ROTH PUBLISHING, INC.

400 Inverness Drive South, Suite 260, Englewood, CO 80112
Ph. 1-800-825-3150

title	code	isbn #	price	qty
INSTANT INSTRUCTOR SERIES				
AIDS HIV, Bradley-Springer 1995	ADIN01	1-57930-010-0	$9.95	
C.C.U., Randall 1995	CCINC1	1-56930-022-4	$9.95	
Geriatric, Jaffe 1992	GRN01	0-944132-68-5	$9.95	
Hemodialysis, Fowlds 1994	DLN01	1-56930-020-8	$9.95	
I.C.U., Randall 1995	ICUI01	1-56930-021-6	$9.95	
IV	IVI01	1-56930-043-7	$9.95	
Obstetric, Jaffe 1992	OBIN01	0-944132-67-7	$9.95	
Oncology, Gale 1994	ONIN01	1-56930-023-2	$9.95	
Pediatric, Keller 1992	PDIN01	0-944132-66-9	$9.95	
Psychiatric, Yard 1992	PSYI01	0-944132-69-3	$9.95	
NURSING CARE PLANS SERIES				
Critical Care, Comer 1998	CNCP01	1-56930-035-6	$38.95	
Geriatric (2nd ed.), Jaffe 1996	GNCP02	1-56933-052-6	$38.95	
HIV/AIDS (2nd ed.), Bradley-Springer 1998	ADSC02	1-56930-097-6	$38.95	
Oncology, Gale 1996	ONCP01	1-56930-004-6	$38.95	
Pediatric (2nd ed.), Jaffe 1998	PNOP02	1-56930-057-7	$38.95	
SURVIVAL SERIES				
Geriatric Survival Handbook (3rd ed.), Acello 1997	G8G001	1-56930-061-5	$26.95	
Nurse's Survival Handbook (3rd ed.), Acello 1998	NSGD03	1-56930-040-2	$39.95	
Obstetric Survival Handbook (2nd ed.), Masten 1998	OBSG01	1-56930-083-6	$35.95	
Pediatric Nurse's Survival Guide, Rebeschi 1996	PNGD01	1-56930-018-6	$29.95	
NURSING/OTHER				
Body in Brief (3rd ed.), Rayman 1997	BBRF03	1-56930-055-0	$35.95	
Diagnostic and Lab Cards (3rd ed.), Skidmore-Roth, 1998	DLC03	1-56930-065-8	$28.95	
Drug Comparison Handbook (2nd ed.), Reilly 1995	DRUG02	1-56930-16-x	$35.95	
Essential Laboratory Mathematics, Johnson & Timmons, 1997	ELM01	1-56930-056-9	$29.95	
Geriatric Long-Term Procedures & Treatments (2nd ed.), Jaffe 1994	GLTP02	1-56930-045-3	$34.95	
Geriatric Nutrition and Diet (3rd ed.), Jaffe 1998	NUT03	1-56930-096-8	$25.95	
Handbook of Long-Term Care (2nd ed.), Vitale 1997	HLTC02	1-56930-068-6	$28.95	
Handbook for Nurse Assistants (2nd ed), Nurse Asst. Consort. 1997	HNA02	1-56930-059-3	$23.95	
I.C.U. Quick Reference (2nd ed.), Comer 1998	ICQU02	1-56930-071-2	$35.95	
Infection Control, Palmer 1996	INFO01	1-56930-061-8	$94.95	
Nursing Diagnosis Cards (2nd ed.), Weber 1997	NDC02	1-56930-060-7	$29.95	

title	code	isbn #	price	qty
Nurse's Trivia Calendar, Rayman	NTC98	1-56930-073-9	$11.95	
OBRA (3rd ed.), Jaffe 1998	OBRA03	1-56930-047-X	$119.95	
OSHA Book (2nd ed.), Goodner 1997	OSHA	1-56930-069-0	$119.95	
Procedure Cards (3rd ed.), Jaffe 1996	PCCU03	1-56930-054-2	$24.95	
Pharmacy Tech, Reilly 1994	PHAR01	1-56930-005-4	$25.95	
Spanish for Medical Personnel, Meizel 1993	SPAN01	1-56930-001-1	$21.95	
Staff Development for the Psych Nurse, Finkelman 1992	STDEV0	0-944132-78-2	$59.95	
OUTLINE SERIES				
Diabetes Outline, Barnwell 1995	DBOL01	1-56930-031-3	$23.95	
Fundamentals of Nursing Outline, Chin 1995	FUND01	1-56930-029-1	$23.95	
Geriatric Outline, Morice 1995	GER01	1-56930-050-x	$23.95	
Hemodynamic Monitoring Outline, Schactman 1995	HDMO01	1-56930-034-8	$23.95	
High Acuity Outline, Reynolds 1995	HAT001	1-56930-028-3	$23.95	
Med-Surgical Nursing Outline (2nd ed.), Reynolds 1998	MSN02	1-56930-068-2	$23.95	
Obstetric Nursing Outline (2nd ed.), Masten 1997	OBS02	1-56930-070-4	$23.95	
Pediatric Nursing Outline, Froese-Fretz et al 1998	PN02	1-56930-067-4	$23.95	
RN NCLEX REVIEW SERIES				
PN/VN Review Cards (3rd ed.), Goodner 1998	PNRC03	1-56930-093-3	$32.95	
RN Review Cards (3rd ed.), Goodner 1998	RNRC03	1-56930-092-5	$32.95	

Name_____

Address_____

City_____ State_____ Zip_____

Phone (_____)_____

❑ VISA   ❑ MasterCard   ❑ American Express   ❑ Check/Money Order

Card #_____ Exp. Date_____

Signature (required)_____

Prices subject to change. Please add $6.95 each for postage and handling. Include your local sales tax.

MAIL OR FAX ORDER TO:
   SKIDMORE-ROTH PUBLISHING, INC.
   400 Inverness Drive South, Suite 260
   Englewood, Colorado 80112
   1-800-825-3150

Visit our website at: http://www.skidmore-roth.com